Alzheimer's Disease:
A Complete Guide for Nurses

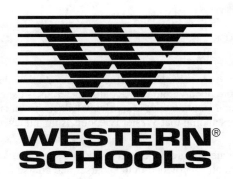

WESTERN® SCHOOLS

By
Patricia N. Allen, MSN, RN, APRN

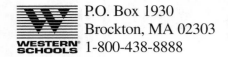

P.O. Box 1930
Brockton, MA 02303
1-800-438-8888

ABOUT THE AUTHOR

Patricia N. Allen, MSN, RN, APRN, has been teaching undergraduate nursing courses in the Adult Health Department at Indiana University School of Nursing at Bloomington since 1999. She is the current coordinator of gerontology content for all nursing courses on the Bloomington campus and represents the campus in The John A. Hartford Center of Geriatric Nursing Excellence group for Indiana University School of Nursing. She is also a gerontology content writer for several grants and projects, including a recent Fund for the Improvement of Postsecondary Education (FIPSE) awarded to the Indiana University Center on the Aged and Aging. She has codeveloped continuing education courses for care of older adults and a web-based course for multidisciplinary care of older adults through Indiana University at Bloomington.

> **Patricia N. Allen** has disclosed that she has no significant financial or other conflicts of interest pertaining to this course book.

THIS BOOK WAS EXPANDED FROM *ALZHEIMER'S: THINGS A NURSE NEEDS TO KNOW* WRITTEN BY

Joan Cagley-Knight, MSN, ARNP, is a registered nurse consultant/supervisor in field operations with Managed Care & Health Quality, Agency for Health Care Administration, Area 8, Fort Myers, FL. She holds a Master of Science in Nursing from the University of South Florida, Tampa, and a Master of Arts in Counseling from the University of Northern Iowa in Cedar Falls, IA. For 10 years, Ms. Cagley-Knight was a nursing instructor at Hawkeye Community College in Waterloo, IA. She is a certified federal and state surveyor for long-term care facilities and is the former director of educational services at a national educational video company, where she wrote and/or produced 50 educational videotapes for long-term-care and home-care staff use.

ABOUT THE SUBJECT MATTER REVIEWER

Joan Garity, EdD, RN, is an associate professor at the College of Nursing and Health Sciences, University of Massachusetts, in Boston. She teaches courses in ethics, law, and health policy issues at the undergraduate and graduate levels and teaches nursing research at the undergraduate level. The focus of her nursing research is Alzheimer family caregivers, particularly their needs in coping, resilience, learning style, and postplacement. Dr. Garity is certified in end-of-life issues by the national End-of-Life Nursing Education Consortium (ELNEC).

> **Joan Garity** has disclosed that she has no significant financial or other conflicts of interest pertaining to this course book.

Nurse Planner: Amy Bernard, RN, BSN, MS

Copy Editor: Jaime Stockslager Buss

Indexer: Sylvia Coates

Western Schools' courses are designed to provide nursing professionals with the educational information they need to enhance their career development. The information provided within these course materials is the result of research and consultation with prominent nursing and medical authorities and is, to the best of our knowledge, current and accurate. However, the courses and course materials are provided with the understanding that Western Schools is not engaged in offering legal, nursing, medical, or other professional advice.

Western Schools' courses and course materials are not meant to act as a substitute for seeking out professional advice or conducting individual research. When the information provided in the courses and course materials is applied to individual circumstances, all recommendations must be considered in light of the uniqueness pertaining to each situation.

Western Schools' course materials are intended solely for your use and not for the benefit of providing advice or recommendations to third parties. Western Schools devoids itself of any responsibility for adverse consequences resulting from the failure to seek nursing, medical, or other professional advice. Western Schools further devoids itself of any responsibility for updating or revising any programs or publications presented, published, distributed, or sponsored by Western Schools unless otherwise agreed to as part of an individual purchase contract.

Products (including brand names) mentioned or pictured in Western School's courses are not endorsed by Western Schools, the American Nurses Credentialing Center (ANCC) or any state board.

ISBN: 1-57801-122-1

IMPORTANT: Read these instructions *BEFORE* proceeding!

Enclosed with your course book, you will find the FasTrax® answer sheet. Use this form to answer all the final exam questions that appear in this course book. If you are completing more than one course, be sure to write your answers on the appropriate answer sheet. Full instructions and complete grading details are printed on the FasTrax instruction sheet, also enclosed with your order. Please review them before starting. *If you are mailing your answer sheet(s) to Western Schools, we recommend you make a copy as a backup.*

ABOUT THIS COURSE

A Pretest is provided with each course to test your current knowledge base regarding the subject matter contained within this course. Your Final Exam is a multiple choice examination. **You will find the exam questions at the end of each chapter.**

In the event the course has less than 100 questions, leave the remaining answer boxes on the FasTrax answer sheet blank. **Use a black pen to fill in your answer sheet.**

A PASSING SCORE

You must score 70% or better in order to pass this course and receive your Certificate of Completion. Should you fail to achieve the required score, we will send you an additional FasTrax answer sheet so that you may make a second attempt to pass the course. Western Schools will allow you three chances to pass the same course…*at no extra charge!* After three failed attempts to pass the same course, your file will be closed.

RECORDING YOUR HOURS

Please monitor the time it takes to complete this course using the handy log sheet on the other side of this page. See below for transferring study hours to the course evaluation.

COURSE EVALUATIONS

In this course book, you will find a short evaluation about the course you are soon to complete. This information is vital to providing Western Schools with feedback on this course. The course evaluation answer section is in the lower right hand corner of the FasTrax answer sheet marked "Evaluation," with answers marked 1–17. Your answers are important to us; please take a few minutes to complete the evaluation.

On the back of the FasTrax instruction sheet, there is additional space to make any comments about the course, the school, and suggested new curriculum. Please mail the FasTrax instruction sheet, with your comments, back to Western Schools in the envelope provided with your course order.

TRANSFERRING STUDY TIME

Upon completion of the course, transfer the total study time from your log sheet to question 17 in the course evaluation. The answers will be in ranges; please choose the proper hour range that best represents your study time. You **MUST** log your study time under question 17 on the course evaluation.

EXTENSIONS

You have two (2) years from the date of enrollment to complete this course. A six (6) month extension may be purchased. If after 30 months from the original enrollment date you do not complete the course, *your file will be closed and no certificate can be issued.*

CHANGE OF ADDRESS?

In the event you have moved during the completion of this course, please call our student services department at 1-800-618-1670, and we will update your file.

A GUARANTEE TO WHICH YOU'LL GIVE HIGH HONORS

If any continuing education course fails to meet your expectations or if you are not satisfied in any manner, for any reason, you may return it for an exchange or a refund (less shipping and handling) within 30 days. Software, video, and audio courses must be returned unopened.

Thank you for enrolling at Western Schools!

WESTERN SCHOOLS
P.O. Box 1930
Brockton, MA 02303
(800) 438-8888
www.westernschools.com

Alzheimer's Disease:
A Complete Guide for Nurses

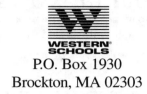

WESTERN SCHOOLS
P.O. Box 1930
Brockton, MA 02303

Please use this log to total the number of hours you spend reading the text and taking the final examination (use 50-min hours).

Date	Hours Spent
7/2/06	6
7/3	3
7/4	1
7/5	4
7/6	5
7/7	2
7/8	3

TOTAL | 24 |

Please log your study hours with submission of your final exam. To log your study time, fill in the appropriate circle under question 17 of the FasTrax® answer sheet under the "Evaluation" section.

Alzheimer's Disease:
A Complete Guide for Nurses

WESTERN SCHOOLS
CONTINUING EDUCATION EVALUATION

Instructions: Mark your answers to the following questions with a black pen on the "Evaluation" section of your FasTrax® answer sheet provided with this course. You should not return this sheet.

Please use the scale below to rate how well the course content met the educational objectives.

A	**Agree Strongly**	**C**	**Disagree Somewhat**
B	**Agree Somewhat**	**D**	**Disagree Strongly**

After completing this course, I am able to

1. Define and discuss Alzheimer's disease (AD) and how it impacts older adults today.

2. Discuss the pathology (etiology) of AD and its implications for diagnosis and treatment.

3. Discuss the nursing process, including best-practice interventions, for treating communication disabilities of patients with AD.

4. Discuss the nursing process for incontinence and nutritional concerns in patients with AD.

5. Discuss falls and identify the need for safety interventions.

6. Outline the prevalence of, assessment of, interventions for, and outcomes for pain in patients with AD, and discuss pharmacological treatment of pain in these individuals; identify reasons for hospitalization of people with AD and the care they should receive while hospitalized.

7. Recognize the need to incorporate holistic care into nursing practice, discuss the concepts of spirituality and religion as they relate to persons with AD, and acknowledge and provide for the special end-of-life needs of people with dementia.

8. Recognize common therapeutic approaches for managing the behavior of patients with AD and incorporate these approaches into nursing practice.

9. Identify and implement the pharmacological principles that guide the care of older adults with AD.

10. Identify issues faced by caregivers of persons with AD, as well as interventions designed to improve their quality of life and recognize the affect of stress, depression, and other demands on the risk of abuse or neglect of the AD patient and measures that may be necessary to protect the person with AD.

11. The content of this course was relevant to the objectives.

12. This offering met my professional education needs.

13. The objectives met the overall purpose/goal of the course.

14. The course was generally well written, and the subject matter explained thoroughly. (If no, please explain on the back of the FasTrax instruction sheet.)

15. The content of this course was appropriate for home study.

16. The final examination was well written and at an appropriate level for the content of the course.

17. **PLEASE LOG YOUR STUDY HOURS WITH SUBMISSION OF YOUR FINAL EXAM.**
    Please choose the response that best represents the total study hours it took to complete this 25-hour course.

    A. Less than 21 hours   C. 24-27 hours
    B. 21-23 hours   D. Greater than 27 hours

CONTENTS

FIGURES AND TABLES

Chapter 7

Chapter 8

Chapter 9

Chapter 10

PRETEST

1. Begin this course by taking the pretest. Circle the answers to the questions on this page, or write the answers on a separate sheet of paper. Do not log answers to the pretest questions on the FasTrax test sheet included with the course.

2. Compare your answers to the PRETEST KEY located in the back of the book. The pretest answer key indicates the course chapter where the content of that question is discussed. Make note of the questions you missed, so that you can focus on those areas as you complete the course.

3. Complete the course by reading each chapter and completing the exam questions at the end of the chapter. Answers to these exam questions should be logged on the FasTrax test sheet included with the course.

1. The only method that can be used to definitively diagnose Alzheimer's disease (AD) is

    a. complete blood count and electroencephalography.

    b. brain scan.

    c. magnetic resonance imaging.

    d. autopsy.

2. Three types of illness that affect the mental health of elderly people are

    a. pneumonia, renal impairment, and delirium.

    b. dementia, delirium, and depression.

    c. dementia, depression, and drug withdrawal.

    d. Creutzfeldt-Jakob disease, Ménière's disease, and depression.

3. One promising diagnostic method for AD is

    a. biochemical markers, such as cerebral spinal fluid.

    b. surgical analysis of brain lesions.

    c. magnetic imaging of the brain.

    d. positive electron imaging of the brain.

4. Creutzfeldt-Jakob disease is a form of dementia characterized by

    a. a long incubation period.

    b. a rapid onset.

    c. a lack of methods to control the spread of the disease.

    d. visual hallucinations of cows.

5. Lingering characteristics of people with AD that can enhance communication include

    a. inability to speak.

    b. decision-making capability.

    c. repetitious questioning.

    d. value and use of humor and hope.

6. One significant barrier to adequate nutrition in a long-term care nursing facility is

    a. lack of laboratory test results for albumin, etc.

    b. lack of accurate weight measurements.

    c. too much assistance for residents.

    d. lack of time for nursing assistants to observe residents eating, chewing, and swallowing.

7. Malnutrition in older adults can be caused by such personal issues as

   a. wandering and poorly cooked food.

   b. inability to sit at a table to eat, wandering, and delirium.

   c. personal loss, dependency, loneliness, and chronic illness.

   d. the process of aging and medication use.

8. An effective intervention for incontinence is

   a. diaper use.

   b. behavior modification.

   c. fluid restriction.

   d. medication administration.

9. When staff members are busy or a nursing home or hospital is operating without a full staff, the first duty likely to be overlooked is

   a. feeding residents.

   b. dressing residents.

   c. allowing visitors.

   d. toileting residents.

10. Common causes of falls in older adults include

    a. reclining-type chairs, low sofas, and wheel chairs.

    b. alcohol abuse, medications, and pets.

    c. linoleum floors, wall-to-wall carpeting, and no-skid stair runners.

    d. tennis shoes, no-skid socks, and handrails.

11. The Centers for Medicare and Medicaid Services (CMS) and the Joint Commission on Accreditation of Healthcare Organizations (JCAHO) physical restraint requirements require

    a. use of restraints only in critical care settings.

    b. assessment by the patient's clinician within 48 hours of restraint application.

    c. education of staff on safe and proper application and use of restraints.

    d. use of restraints to ensure patient safety when staff members are out of the room.

12. Assessing pain in an individual with cognitive impairment is a difficult task. The best practice for managing pain in people with AD is to

    a. expect every old person to complain of pain.

    b. assume that older adults expect to experience pain and that they consider it a normal and inevitable part of the aging process.

    c. assess pain in a systematic way to successfully detect it.

    d. simply ask questions of the person with AD, such as "How long have you had this pain?" or "When did your pain start?"

13. *Spirituality* is a broad term that

    a. encompasses religious preferences, affiliations, rites, and rituals.

    b. refers to a system of beliefs and formal practices that take place individually or in a community group to provide focus and meaning to life, to explain death, and maintain hope for the future.

    c. encompasses the formal beliefs and rituals a person uses to search for the meaning of life.

    d. refers to individual beliefs about relationships, love and intimacy, forgiveness, hopes for the future, and methods of making peace with the past.

14. A family caregiver for a frail older adult in an African American home is most likely to

    a. continue working the same number of hours outside the home.

    b. be someone other than the spouse.

    c. be the person's spouse.

    d. experience feelings of shame about signs of dementia.

15. The therapeutic approach that is typically only helpful during the early stages of dementia or AD is

    a. validation therapy.

    b. reality orientation.

    c. the Need-Driven Dementia-Compromised Behavior Model.

    d. humor.

16. The philosophy of an organization

    a. sets the priorities and guides the actions of the practitioners.

    b. outlines what will happen in an organization without management intervention.

    c. is the gradual unhampered evolution of an organization's principles.

    d. represents the format for the procedures of a facility.

17. When a person with AD exhibits a behavior problem, you should first

    a. identify and examine the behavior.

    b. try to convince the person to change his or her behavior.

    c. allow yourself to express your anger because the person needs to know that you are upset.

    d. teach the person not to demonstrate the behavior.

18. Common ways to handle fatigue in a person with memory loss include

    a. taking frequent naps.

    b. exercising strenuously three times per day.

    c. using the most alert time to see friends, go to the doctor, and perform other activities.

    d. changing the environment and engaging in many different forms of stimulation.

19. An 80-year-old woman is taking haloperidol, an antipsychotic drug, three times per day. A common side effect this woman may experience while taking this type of drug is

    a. lip smacking.

    b. high blood pressure.

    c. confusion.

    d. low-grade fever.

20. Frequent tardiness or absence by a staff member in a long-term care facility may be a sign of

    a. fatigue.

    b. overworking.

    c. caregiver burnout.

    d. too many family obligations.

INTRODUCTION

In the latter part of the 20th century, we saw a focus on sound theory and research about adults and age-appropriate care. We also saw explosive growth in the older adult population, partially due to the number of aging baby boomers. As a result of these trends, now in the start of the 21st century, gerontologic-geriatric nursing is becoming an area for graduate study, research, and care. There is currently a greater emphasis in the undergraduate curriculum as well.

With this increased focus on gerontologic care, we must also focus on the disease processes that are specific to this population, including dementia. As a nurse, it is important to understand advances in research on dementia, new medications, and the suspected causes of dementia. This study course is designed to be an up-to-date and thorough review of the major issues, leading to understanding of the clinical and social concerns for individuals with one form of dementia — Alzheimer's disease (AD). AD is the most common form of dementia and probably the most feared condition that is associated with aging.

Although the portion of the older adult population acquiring some form of dementia is low, lapses of memory can commonly occur with aging. These lapses are often misinterpreted as signs that a person is suffering from dementia. Health practitioners must understand the differences between expected aging processes and the pathophysiology of AD. This course focuses on identification of underlying conditions and the nurse's participation in the course of these situations. The new knowledge available to nurses is derived from advances made in understanding the physiology, psychology, and sociology of aging. Not only does this research demystify the aging process but it also gives direction to nursing practice. This knowledge is also extremely important for the teaching that nurses must accomplish with family members and other staff.

Much research has been directed at finding ways to alleviate the cognitive decline associated with AD and the behavioral problems that are characteristic of the disease. Understanding why people with AD do and say the things they do can and has led to the development of frameworks of therapeutic approaches that help caregivers. For example, reality orientation, reminiscing, validation, and the Need-Driven Dementia-Compromised Behavior Model are presented in this course as potential contexts for comprehending bizarre or mysterious behaviors.

Furthermore, new medications for AD are being developed at a rapid pace. These newly developed drugs are based on the biochemical understanding of dementia and AD. Before administering one of these medications, the nurse should read and understand as much of the available information as possible in order to avoid costly mistakes, such as dosage and administration errors. For a review of pharmacology principles, including pharmacokinetics and pharmacodynamics, see the appendix on pharmacology at the end of this study course.

Nurses, family members, and professional caregivers may all provide care for a patient with AD. The role of caregiver has been widely studied. The focus of much of this research has been identification of the burdens and stressors associated with caregiving. However, some attention is now being directed toward recognition of the benefits of caregiving as well. Individuals with AD may live at home or in a health care facility. This course helps nurses and nursing students examine the overall experience of caregiving as either a professional caregiver or a family caregiver. It also introduces the reader to ways of looking at what happens in the daily lives of caregivers. Considerations of caregiving and suggested interventions are also presented. Care of a person with AD can be expensive. However, the financial and legal implications of care can be managed by planning ahead.

The term "best practices" is used to acknowledge interventions that work well in a practice setting. For people with dementia, best practices are the actions that can be taken to address a variety of holistic needs. Obstacles to communication, bowel and bladder incontinence, and barriers to meeting nutritional needs are presented along with strategies for dealing with them. Unfortunately, pain and hospitalization are two issues a caregiver will likely address when caring for patients with dementia; most individuals with AD suffer from pain and are hospitalized at some point. The nurse must also be sure to address the less obvious needs of these individuals, including spiritual, religious, and activity needs.

Sometimes people with AD can be dangerous to themselves or the person providing care. Many individuals are quick to use, or suggest the use of, restraints in management of problem behaviors. This is generally not a positive resolution to the problem behavior. Nurses interact with others in the management of these complex or difficult behaviors and should model the desired interactions with patients who are demonstrating these behaviors. Simply through their positive management of behaviors, nurses can help others to understand that restraint use is not necessary to manage difficult behaviors. The use of physical and chemical restraints for elderly persons with dementia means a loss of personal freedom of movement and can cause numerous problems. Research on the benefits and harms of restraints has led to changes in the use of restraints in long-term care facilities; these changes are now being implemented in acute care settings with conflicting results. Federal regulations and many states now mandate the limited use of restraints with rigorous assessment and time limits as well as the banishment of restraint protocols. Alternatives to restraint use are available and documented in the literature. This course offers strategies that nursing staff and families can use to manage difficult behaviors. Understanding contributing factors to the behaviors of all patients with AD and factors specifically related to a particular patient's behavior makes implementation of effective interventions more likely.

CHAPTER 1

DEFINING ALZHEIMER'S DISEASE

CHAPTER OBJECTIVE

After completing this chapter the reader will be able to define and discuss Alzheimer's disease (AD) and how it impacts older adults today.

LEARNING OBJECTIVES

After studying this chapter, the reader will be able to

1. differentiate indications of dementia, depression, and delirium.

2. recognize the impact of AD on the American family and financial system.

3. identify clinical manifestations of depression in older adults.

4. discuss depression demographics in older adults and how depression affects the diagnosis of AD and quality of life of older adults.

5. identify progressive degenerative dementia and the resulting depression in older adults.

6. describe the stages of AD and their relationship to the overall progression of the disease.

7. review the financial burden of AD and its implications for diagnosis and treatment.

INTRODUCTION

How will we age? Each of us wonders about this question. Probably the best way to judge the answer is to examine how we are handling our "middle age." We tend to become "more of ourselves" as we grow older. Someone who has always been outspoken and opinioned or fun loving and sociable most likely will act the same way when he or she is older. It is important to recognize that confusion, memory loss, and behavioral problems should not be an expected part of aging.

Consider the poem "I Can't Remember."

Just a line to say I'm living,
that I'm not among the dead,
though I'm getting more forgetful
and mixed up in my head.
　　I got used to my arthritis,
　　　to my dentures I'm resigned.
　　I can manage my bifocals,
　　　but, God, I miss my mind.
For sometimes I can't remember
when I stand at the foot of the stairs,
if I must go up for something
or have just come down from there.
　　And, before the fridge so often,
　　　my poor mind is filled with doubt,
　　have I just put food away,
　　　or have I come to take some out?
And, there are times when it is dark,
with my nightcap on my head,
I don't know if I'm retiring
or just getting out of bed.
　　So if it's my turn to write you,
　　　there's no need for getting sore

1

I may think I've written
and don't want to be a bore!
So remember that I love you
and wish that you were near,
but now it's nearly mail time,
so I must say "Good-bye, Dear."
    P.S. Here I stand beside the mailbox
    with a face so very red,
    Instead of mailing you my letter,
    I have opened it instead!

—Anonymous

What is AD?

As defined by Clark and Karlawish (2003), AD "is a complex neurodegenerative dementing illness [that] has become a major public health problem because of its increasing prevalence, long duration, high cost of care, and lack of disease-modifying therapy."

Although AD is not a normal part of aging, patients, caregivers, and physicians frequently mistake its physiologic effects as normal aging changes. Diseases of the brain can include several features, such as memory impairment; a disturbance of thinking function, which usually displays itself as amnesia; difficulty learning; and trouble recalling new information. AD is also a progressive language disorder that usually begins with anomia and develops to fluent aphasia. The disease progresses until a physical loss of function occurs. The AD patient may experience focal abnormalities, alterations in gait, and seizures. This physical loss usually does not occur until the final years of the disease.

AD is not a new phenomenon. However, before the last two decades, little was known about it. The ancient Greeks and Romans described signs and symptoms similar to those associated with AD. Even in the 16th century, Shakespeare noted that in extreme old age, the signs of second childishness or mere oblivion were known and recognized.

In the early 1900s, during an autopsy of a former patient, Dr. Alois Alzheimer detected signs of the brain disease that is now named after him. When the patient was alive, Dr. Alzheimer thought she was experiencing a mental illness. During the autopsy, however, he found dense deposits outside and around the nerve cells in her brain. These deposits are now called neuritic plaques. Inside the cells, he found neurofibrillary tangles, or twisted threads of nerve fibers. Today, detection of plaques and tangles during autopsy remain the best way to diagnose AD.

TYPES OF COGNITIVE IMPAIRMENT

Three types of illness affect the mental health of the elderly: dementia, delirium, and depression (see Table 1-1). Note that the onset and progression of these illnesses differ. For example, the onset of delirium is abrupt compared with depression (slow, uneven) and dementia (slow, even). Also, the mood state varies for each: depression being constant, withdrawn, or sad; delirium, anxious and restless; and dementia fluctuating from apathy to outgoing or catastrophic. The significance of nursing observations and assessment is apparent given these characteristic differences.

The clinical criteria for mental disorders is defined by the American Psychiatric Association's *Diagnostic and Statistical Manual of Mental Disorders,* 4th Edition (*DSM-IV*). As stated in the *DSM-IV*, there must be a cognitive impairment sufficient to interfere with usual functioning in order to meet the diagnostic criteria.

Dementia

Dementia is an organic mental disorder characterized by a loss of or impairment in mental functioning or cognition. The loss of the ability to think and reason manifests as changes in behavior and intellectual functioning. These changes affect memory, verbal skills, math skills, and spatial-visual perceptions. The term "dementia" is accepted by the medical community and families as being less judg-

TABLE 1-1: COMPARISON OF THE CLINICAL FEATURES OF DELIRIUM, DEMENTIA, AND DEPRESSION

Clinical feature	Delirium	Dementia	Depression
Onset	Acute or subacute, depending on cause; often at twilight or in darkness	Chronic, generally insidious, depending on cause	Coincides with major life changes, often abrupt
Course	Short, diurnal fluctuations in symptoms, worsens at night, in darkness, and on awakening	Long, no diurnal effects, symptoms progressive yet relatively stable over time	Diurnal effects, typically worse in the morning; situational fluctuations but less than with delirium
Progression	Abrupt	Slow but even	Variable, rapid or slow but uneven
Duration	Hours to less than 1 month; seldom longer	Months to years	At least 6 weeks, can be several months to years
Awareness	Reduced	Clear	Clear
Alertness	Fluctuates, lethargic or hyper-vigilant	Generally normal	Normal
Attention	Impaired, fluctuates	Generally normal	Minimal impairment, easily distracted
Orientation	Generally impaired, severity varies	Generally normal	Selective disorientation
Memory	Recent and immediate impaired	Recent and remote impaired	Selective or "patchy" impairment, "islands" of intact memory
Thinking	Disorganized, distorted, fragmented, incoherent speech, either slow or accelerated	Difficulty with abstraction, thoughts impoverished, judgment impaired, words difficult to find	Intact but with themes of hopelessness, helplessness, or self-depreciation
Perception	Distorted: illusions, delusions, and hallucinations; difficulty distinguishing between reality and misperceptions	Misperceptions usually absent	Intact, delusions and hallucinations absent except in severe cases
Psychomotor behavior	Variable (hypokinetic, hyperkinetic, and mixed)	Normal, may have apraxia	Variable (psychomotor retardation or agitation)
Sleep-wake cycle	Disturbed, cycle reversed	Fragmented	Disturbed, usually early-morning awakening
Associated features	Variable affective changes, symptoms of autonomic hyperarousal, exaggeration of personality type, associated with acute physical illness	Superficial, inappropriate, and labile affect; attempts to conceal deficits in intellect; personality changes; aphasia; possible agnosia; lacks insight	Affect depressed, dysphoric mood, exaggerated and detailed complaints, preoccupied with personal thoughts, insight present, verbal elaboration
Assessment	Distracted from task, numerous errors	Failings highlighted by family, frequent "near miss" answers, struggles with test, great effort to find an appropriate reply, frequent requests for feedback on performance	Failings highlighted by individual, frequently answers "don't know," little effort, frequently gives up, indifferent toward test, does not care or attempt to find answer

Note. Reprinted from "Assessing Cognitive Function" by M.D. Foreman, K. Fletcher, L.C. Mion, & L. Simon, 1996, *Geriatric Nursing, 17*(5), 228–33, with permission from Elsevier.

mental than other, outdated terms, such as "organic brain disease" and "senile dementia."

Delirium

Acute and reversible dementias with a number of known causes are referred to as delirium. The causes of delirium appear to lie outside the central nervous system (CNS). Unfortunately, transient delirium is common among elderly patients, especially those who are hospitalized, recovering from surgery, or restricted to bed rest or other forms of immobility. Recognition of delirium superimposed on dementia is an overlooked and unreported phenomenon leading to early discharge from the hospital with untreated and unrecognized medical conditions. In other words, a person can have dementia but, if delirium is also present, delirium may be believed to be the result of the dementia and not another cause. Studies indicate that patients with delirium superimposed on dementia are also much more likely to be restrained, with subsequent functional declines. Nurses need to acknowledge the significance of this condition, perform careful assessments of mental state, stabilize the environment during hospitalization, and aggressively seek treatment of any physiological causes of delirium.

Dementia and delirium are not chronic and are potentially reversible. Delirium is often precipitated by a physical illness and manifests as psychiatric complications. Extreme sleepiness, lethargy, partial consciousness, hallucinations, delusions, and excitability can be indications of acute states of delirium. In some instances, patients have a mixture of these features.

Depression

Depression is a brain disorder of biological origin that is one of the most treatable, yet possibly the most undertreated, diseases of the elderly. Depression commonly goes undiagnosed and therefore goes untreated (Teresi, Abrams, Holmes, Ramirez & Eimicke, 2001).

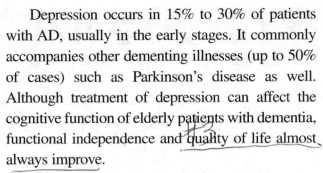

Depression occurs in 15% to 30% of patients with AD, usually in the early stages. It commonly accompanies other dementing illnesses (up to 50% of cases) such as Parkinson's disease as well. Although treatment of depression can affect the cognitive function of elderly patients with dementia, functional independence and quality of life almost always improve.

Depression has been associated with cognitive impairment in older persons, and depressive symptoms are common among AD patients. Because of this commonality of depressive symptoms, nurses can benefit from knowing the risk factors for depression in all elderly people. Depression frequently occurs in elderly patients who suffer from vascular disorders. However, many cases go undiagnosed and untreated. Clinicians, caregivers, family members, and patients may incorrectly attribute depressive symptoms to the aging process. Depression is, however, a clinical syndrome — not a normal part of aging.

Many people assume that a depressed mood is the hallmark sign of depression. In fact, other depressive symptoms are more likely to be apparent. These symptoms can include loss of interest in activities of daily living (ADLs), sleeplessness, and loss of appetite. The signs and symptoms of depression can also overlap those of neurological diseases. These symptoms can include fatigue, sleeplessness, agitation, and motor retardation. AD patients' cognitive symptoms may be exacerbated when depression is superimposed. This fact negatively impacts early diagnosis of AD.

Some intriguing preliminary studies in Sweden and the Netherlands indicate that depressed mood and lack of interest with loss of energy and depressive symptoms may be components of preclinical AD, a correlation that was found among a group of educated people (Berger, Fratiglioni, & Forsell, 2000; Geerlings, Schmand, Braam, et al., 2000; Wilson et al., 2002).

Facts About Depression

The following facts are helpful to gain insight into the magnitude of depression in the older adult population:

- Clinical depression ranges from 8% to 15% among community-dwelling older persons and up to 30% among institutionalized older adults.

- Older white men have the highest rate of completed suicide of any age-group, gender, or ethnic group. The risk of suicide is 50% higher among older adults than the risk among younger people.

- Between 35% and 40% of Parkinson's patients have depressive symptoms.

- Up to 20% of AD patients experience depression.

- Chronic depression in older adults occurs in 7% to 30% of cases of depression, with one-third of those who recover relapsing in the first year.

- In the next 20-30 years, as younger people with a high prevalence of depression age, they will contribute to the increasing incidence of depression as they age.

- Depression rates are significantly higher in people with coexisting medical conditions.

- The numerous functional losses that most older adults experience may partially explain the onset of depression.

- Fewer than 5% to 7% of older adults in care facilities receive mental health care.

RISK FACTORS FOR AD

Stroke and AD are the third most common causes of death in the United States. The elderly population is very familiar with this statistic and it induces fear and anxiety in many people. Here are some risk factors for AD:

- Increasing age (primary risk factor) — Both the incidence and prevalence of AD increase with age. When mild cases of AD are included, the prevalence approaches 10.5% of noninstitutionalized white people older than age 65. Research estimates for Hispanic and black populations are even higher.

- Sex — AD occurs in the female population more frequently than in the male population, at a ratio of 2:1. This may be because women live longer, in general, than do men.

- Heredity — may influence the development of AD

- Previous head injury

- Low serum levels of folate and vitamin B_{12}

- Education — individuals with fewer years of formal education are more likely to suffer from AD

- Lower income

- Lower occupational status.

Factors associated with lower risk of AD include:

- higher levels of education

- moderate levels of daily wine consumption

- higher levels of dietary fish consumption.

Nun Study

In the Nun study, researchers examined the medical and personal histories of 678 nuns for more than 10 years. The researchers also tested the nuns' cognitive function and, at death, dissected their brains. From this intensive evaluation of a part of the population, researchers concluded that a college education and an active intellectual lifestyle may protect a person from some effects of AD. Nuns who had lower linguistic capabilities early in their lives were more susceptible to reduced cognitive function and, eventually, AD (Kemper, Greiner, Marquis, Prenovost, & Mitzner, 2001; Danner, Snowdon, & Friesen 2001).

DEMOGRAPHICS OF AD

Here are some facts and demographics associated with AD:

- The number of Americans with AD is approximately 4.5 million.

- The rate of AD increases as the population ages.

- The percentage of people over age 65 with AD is approximately 10%.

- The percentage of people over age 85 with AD is approximately 50%.

- Between 100,000 and 120,000 new cases of AD in people over age 85 are diagnosed each year.

- By 2050, an estimated 11.3 to 16 million (10% prevalence) noninstitutionalized white people older than age 65 will have AD. This number could be even higher for black and Hispanic people.

- The monetary cost of AD in the United States is $100 billion per year.

- The average life span after onset of dementia is approximately 8 to 10 years.

- Nearly 50% of nursing home residents have AD or another cognitive disorder.

- The average annual cost of nursing home care per capita is $42,000.

- The total number of nursing home beds in 1986 was 1.7 million; in 1995, 1.75 million; in 2000, 1.8 million; and in 2001, 1.78 million.

- Nursing home care expenditures are expected to increase by 70% between 1998 and 2007.

(Alzheimer's Organization, 2004; Mariano, 1999)

STAGES OF DEMENTIA

The course of Alzheimer's dementia involves a gradual deterioration. Generally, the younger a person is when AD occurs, the more severe the disease becomes. (For a summary of these changes, known as the Global Deterioration Scale, see Table 1-2.)

Signs and symptoms in the first stage of AD, which may last as long as 15 years, are often vague and inconclusive. The onset of the disease is insidious and usually occurs between ages 50 and 80. Patients experience forgetfulness and personality changes, such as social withdrawal, apathy, and occasional outbursts of irritability. Usually, the person is well-groomed and socially appropriate.

During the confusional stages, more severe cognitive impairments become apparent. The beginning, or initial, confusional stage may persist for 7 years and is characterized by the earliest recognizable deficits. Manifestations of these deficits include loss of direction when driving a car, poor performance at work that is noticeable to coworkers, inability to come up with a word or name, and decreased accomplishment in demanding business and social situations.

In the late confusional stage, which lasts an average of 2 years, the person exhibits decreasing knowledge of current events and personal history, an inability to handle money, and a flattening of affect (withdrawal). Denial of any cognitive problems is the affected person's major defense mechanism.

Moderate cognitive decline occurs during the early dementia phase. During this clinical phase, which lasts an average of 18 months, the person cannot survive without assistance. Both the ability to judge the safety of a situation and fine motor coordination are impaired. Some disorientation to time and place occurs, and the person may need help with choosing clothes but not with eating or toileting. The person may know his or her name but may not remember telephone numbers or grandchildren's names.

Over a period of approximately 2 years, the manifestations of the middle phase of dementia appear. The person becomes totally dependent on the caregiver for survival and needs progressive assistance with all ADLs. Urinary and fecal incontinence begin, and emotional and personality changes

TABLE 1-2: CHARACTERISTIC PROGRESSION OF ALZHEIMER'S DISEASE: GLOBAL DETERIORATION SCALE

Stage	Characteristics	Diagnosis	Duration (avg)	Mood change*
1 Normality	No subjective or objective complaints	Normal adult	50–75 yr	None
2 Forgetfulness	Subjective deficits in word finding and locating objects	Normal aged adult	15 yr	Concern
3 Early confusional	Difficulty handling complex occupational tasks	Compatible with incipient Alzheimer's disease	7 yr	Anxiety
4 Late confusional	Needs assistance with complex tasks, such as handling finances and planning holiday meals	Mild Alzheimer's disease	2 yr	Flattening of affect, denial, emotional withdrawal, and sometimes tearfulness
5 Early dementia	Can no longer function independently; needs assistance choosing proper attire	Moderate Alzheimer's disease	18 mo	Increase in flattening of affect; sometimes displays anger or tearfulness at loss of independence
6 Middle dementia Substage A	Needs assistance dressing	Moderately severe Alzheimer's disease	5 mo	Agitation and psychotic symptoms
Substage B	Needs assistance bathing and adjusting water temperature		5 mo	
Substage C	Needs assistance in mechanics of toileting and brushing teeth		5 mo	
Substage D	Urinary incontinence		4 mo	
Substage E	Fecal incontinence		10 mo	
7 Late dementia Substage A	Speech ability limited to a half-dozen intelligible words	Severe Alzheimer's disease	1 yr	Pathologic passivity
Substage B	Intelligible vocabulary limited to one word		18 mo	
Substage C	Ability to walk is lost		1 yr	
Substage D	Ability to sit up is lost		1 yr	
Substage E	Ability to smile is lost		18 mo	
Substage F	Ability to hold up head is lost		Survival from this point is variable	

*The patient's change in mood is less consistent in the evolution of the disease.

Note. From "The Global Deterioration Scale for assessment of primary degenerative dementia" by B. Reisberg, S.H. Ferris, M.J. deLeon, & T. Crook, 1982, *American Journal of Psychiatry, 139*(9), 1136–39. Copyright © 1983 by Barry Reisberg, MD. Reprinted with permission.

increase. In many cases, the person no longer remembers the name of his or her spouse.

Finally, in the late phase of dementia, the person becomes aphasic and inattentive. The person cannot walk, sit up, or hold up his or her head. Generalized signs of CNS involvement include quadriparesis and seizures.

THE FINANCIAL BURDEN OF AD

The steady growth in the population of people living to be 90- to 100-years-old comes with implicit financial burdens to the public health system. AD imposes substantial burdens both physically and financially on the people with the disease as well. If the disease is slowed, higher costs of care are delayed and decreased.

Survival rate estimates and associated costs are impacted by the decrease in cognitive and functional ability and age at the time of diagnosis. These variables are also associated with lower probabilities of surviving 10 years after diagnosis. Shorter than 10-year survival rates are associated with more years spent in institutions. Fifty to fifty-nine percent of AD patients live 5 years after diagnosis, and thirty percent live 10 years after diagnosis.

Because women are affected with AD two times as much as men, women incur higher costs related to the disease. These costs include higher institutional costs for women. Researchers claim that women receive 15% more total hours of care per day than men and incur 70% higher total costs (Kinosian, Stallard, Lee, et al., 2000).

Costs Associated with AD

Previously, Medicare beneficiaries who had AD were denied reimbursement for the costs of mental health services, hospice care, and home care. Why? Some people rationalized that AD patients were incapable of medical improvement. However, AD is now diagnosable in early stages, when patients are most likely to achieve significant benefits from treatment. As a result, in April 2002, Medicare changed its coverage for patients with AD by no longer denying reimbursement for such services as medications and speech, occupational, and physical therapy (Humphrey, 2002; Centers for Medicare and Medicaid Services, 2002c). Approximately 70% of people with AD remain at home, and families pay most of the associated costs of care out of their own pockets — approximately 75% of total costs. Only an average of $12,500 is paid annually for the care of each person with AD. The average lifetime cost for an individual with AD is approximately $174,000 (Koppel, 2002).

The Alzheimer's Association estimates that by 2010, Medicare costs will increase by more than 50%, from approximately $32 billion in 2000 to approximately $50 billion. It also estimates that residential care of people with dementia will increase by 80% (Koppel, 2002).

According to the Alzheimer's Association (Koppel, 2002), AD costs American businesses $61 billion a year. This $61 billion is expended in two areas: $24.6 billion is spent on the direct care of AD patients, and $36.5 billion is paid in some form to caregivers of AD patients. This expenditure can be equated to the net profits of the top ten Fortune 500 companies. In 1998, this total cost equaled $33 billion.

A multitude of research studies have demonstrated that behavioral symptoms are significant independent predictors of direct costs of care in patients with AD. Significant increases in costs are also associated with increases in severity of dementia. These costs are associated with greater caregiver distress and increased risk of institutionalization.

Computation and prediction of the costs of AD must include all costs associated with care of AD patients, including formal and informal costs. Direct formal costs are payments made for such services as physicians, medications, hospital care, paid home care, and long-term care services. Direct informal costs are the economic values placed on unpaid caregiving, including the care for AD patients that is provided by family members and volunteers. Unfortunately, for many individuals who develop AD, access to nonpaid care is not available (Murman, Chen, Powell, et al., 2002; Koppel, 2002).

Until recently, economic evaluations of pharmacological therapies were unnecessary because these therapies had insufficient benefits for patients with AD. However, new medications can improve cognitive function and may delay functional deterioration. Many of these new medications are expensive, and their effectiveness varies among patients. Although these medications do not save lives, they improve the quality of life for AD patients by reducing associated disability.

Drugs that treat symptoms of memory loss and other cognitive loss in patients with AD have demonstrated that their clinical effectiveness does justify their costs. One such medication is donepezil (Aricept). Studies have demonstrated the cost-effectiveness of donepezil in treatment of mild or moderate AD. When drugs are effective, cognitive function improves and therefore costs of medical and supportive care decrease. This improvement delays admittance to in-patient care settings, which are also associated with high costs (Feldman, Gauthier, Hecker, et al., 2001; Jones, 2003; Neumann, 1999; Rogers & Friedhoff, 1996; Rogers, Doody, Mohs, & Friedhoff, 1998; Tariot, et al., 2001).

Another study evaluated the economics of the drug galantamine (Reminyl). It reviewed the estimated need for full-time care and its associated costs. The results suggest that galantamine use in patients with AD in the United States could reduce the use of costly resources, such as formal home care and nursing home care, leading to cost savings over time. Specifically, the need for full-time care was reduced by 6 to 7 months, with a dollar savings of $9,000 to $11,500 per patient (Migliaccio-Walle, Getsios, Caro, et al., 2003).

SUMMARY

The reason one person ages so differently than another and at such a different rate is still a great mystery. Nurses can benefit from learning how to recognize both the normal physiological manifestations of aging and the mental changes that affect aging people. AD is characterized by a gradual mental and physical decline; however, it is not a part of the expected mental changes that can occur as one ages.

The mental health concern occurring with the most frequency and consequence among aging people is depression. Depression is a common early finding in people with AD. However, diagnosing depression in people with AD is commonly difficult because they may exhibit nonspecific somatic complaints rather than classic symptoms. It is essential to assess patients for concurrent illnesses that can mimic AD or dementia. Due to the relatively long period of illness, increasing age of the general population, and the need for various levels of care for people with AD, the financial burden on people with AD, their families, and society can be significant. New treatments and earlier recognition and intervention for AD may be able to significantly reduce the costs associated with this disease.

EXAM QUESTIONS

CHAPTER 1
Questions 1-10

1. Dementia in AD is characterized by

   a. sleep patterns interrupted by early morning awakenings.

   b. reduction in the person's awareness of surroundings.

   c. attitudes of giving up or answering "I don't know" to questions.

   d. difficulty with abstractions, judgment, and finding the right words.

2. Acute states of confusion accompanied by lethargy, partial consciousness, or hallucinations are best categorized as

   a. delirium.

   b. dementia.

   c. depression.

   d. deficiency of vitamin B or E.

3. Depression in older adults

   a. when treated, almost always enhances quality of life.

   b. commonly occurs in the late stages of AD.

   c. occurs in as much as 60% of patients with AD.

   d. rarely impacts cognitive symptoms and thus the diagnosis of AD.

4. The best means of diagnosing AD is through

   a. family reports.

   b. an autopsy.

   c. behavior observation.

   d. blood tests.

5. Depression in people with AD can be problematic because

   a. it occurs in all patients with AD.

   b. many cases go undiagnosed and untreated.

   c. clinicians, caregivers, family members, and patients may correctly attribute depressive symptoms to the aging process.

   d. families and nurses are unable to identify depression in older adults.

6. The best indicators of depresson in older adults are

   a. a depressed mood and increased appetite.

   b. a decreased appetite and sleeplessness.

   c. sleeplessness and an increased appetite.

   d. a hyperactive mood and sleeplessness.

7. The primary risk factors for AD include

   a. male sex and increasing age.

   b. head injury and male sex.

   c. increasing age and female sex.

   d. genetic factors and male sex.

8. A true statement regarding AD is

   a. adults older than age 65 represent 50% of people with AD.

   b. the annual cost of AD in the United States is approximately $150 billion.

   c. the average annual cost of nursing home care is approximately $42,000.

   d. the average life span after onset of dementia is approximately 18 to 20 years.

9. During the early stages of Alzheimer's dementia

   a. urinary incontinence is a major problem.

   b. the patient may not know the names of his or her spouse and grandchildren.

   c. social withdrawal and occasional irritability are common.

   d. the person cannot survive without assistance.

On answer sheet — choice was C →

10. The middle dementia stage of AD is characterized by

    a. a duration time frame of 15 years.

    b. urinary and fecal incontinence.

    c. aphasia and inability to walk or sit up.

    d. denial as the affected person's major defense mechanism.

CHAPTER 2

PATHOLOGY AND DIAGNOSIS OF ALZHEIMER'S DISEASE

CHAPTER OBJECTIVE

After completing this chapter the reader will be able to discuss the pathology (etiology) of Alzheimer's disease (AD) and its implications for diagnosis and treatment.

LEARNING OBJECTIVES

After studying this chapter, the reader will be able to

1. examine the pathology (etiology) of AD and its implications for diagnosis and treatment.

2. identify the neurological losses patients with AD experience.

3. differentiate among dementia, depression, and delirium.

4. identify the four A's that indicate areas of loss in cognitive impairment.

5. discuss the array and most effective tools used to diagnose AD.

6. recognize the importance of early diagnosis of AD and its influence on patient outcomes.

7. discuss the stages, features, and ten warning signs of AD.

8. analyze mild cognitive impairment (MCI) and its role in AD.

INTRODUCTION

This chapter reviews the components of the clinical diagnosis of AD, including the pathophysiology of dementia, the most common symptoms of AD, and the relationship of the pathology of the disease to the potential for developing a cure and better diagnostic tools.

PATHOLOGY

The myth that old age is invariably linked to serious intellectual and physical declines has been debunked. However, aging is associated with normal biological declines in every body system, beginning with visual changes in the midtwenties. These cumulative age-related changes influence the lives of aging people (Cavanaugh & Blanchard-Fields, 2002). They may manifest as an inability to cope with acute or chronic illnesses as a person grows older. It is helpful to recognize both the normal physiological manifestations of aging and the mental changes that affect aging persons.

In general, aging occurs at the cellular level. One theory states that each cell has a genetically determined life span, during which it can replicate itself a limited number of times. Structural cell changes occur with age, including changes in the structures of deoxyribonucleic acid (DNA) and ribonucleic acid (RNA). Possible causes include genotypical programming, X-rays, noxious chemicals, and certain food products. In the central nervous system (CNS), neurons show age-related signs of degeneration. As circulation to the brain decreases, cell loss speeds up, especially in the brain. On average, brain weight decreases by 17% in both men and women by the time they are 80-years-old.

The Brain and AD

Changes in memory and learning ability also occur with normal biological aging. These changes reflect not declining intelligence or ability to learn, but rather decreased speed of learning. Simple recall ability declines, but verbal ability and learning skills continue.

All areas of the body are affected by aging, and no single cause of aging has been proven. Genetic factors are implicated in some disorders that commonly occur with age, such as hypertension, coronary artery disease, and malignant neoplasms of the breast and stomach.

Pathology of the Brain

Understanding the pathology of AD has led to clinical advances in its diagnosis and treatment. Remember that several forms of dementia exist, but AD dementia is the most frequently occurring type of dementia in older adults. AD pathology typically begins in or near the hippocampus and later spreads to the frontal, temporal, and parietal lobes. This progression and sequence of events in the brain help to explain the consistent appearance of memory loss before other cognitive deficits in AD and the clinical features of its later stages (Royall, 2003).

Structural lesions of the cerebral hemispheres and diencephalons are associated with dementia. The exact origin and cause of these lesions remains a mystery. The relentless neuronal cell damage and death that occur as a result of these lesions may be diffuse and frequently involve the temporal and frontal lobes. Cell death is responsible for the brain atrophy that marks the progression of AD, as indicated by impaired cognition and ultimately brain failure and, therefore, death.

Autopsy has been touted as the only means of confirming AD. Because the brain naturally degenerates as a person ages, the validity of the diagnosis of AD can be questionable in people who are approximately age 80 and older. It is hard to absolutely differentiate the brain of a person with AD from one in the later years of older adulthood. In cases in which autopsy has been conducted on people older than age 79, the cause of death has been cited as "probable AD" in only 20% to 25% of cases.

The damage that occurs in the brains of people with AD involves changes in three nerve cell mechanisms: communication, metabolism, and repair. During normal metabolism, amyloid precursor protein (APP), which is found partially inside the cell and partially outside the cell, is sliced apart (cleaved) by enzymes. When there is a problem with the sequence of metabolism events, APP is sliced at the wrong place and beta amyloid is produced. Beta-amyloid eventually moves into and around nerve cells. How it does this is not fully understood, but it finally joins up with other beta-amyloid filaments or fragments and creates plaques (deposits) that cause nerve cells to die.

Beta-amyloid plaques can be one of two types: diffuse or neuritic. Neuritic plaques are associated with more mature forms of plaque and are closely associated with the clinical signs and symptoms of AD. There has been much discussion, without conclusion, about whether these plaques are the cause of AD or form as a result of it.

Neurofibrillary tangles of tau (neural thread protein) are a main component of the pathology of AD. In fact, they are the second major histopathological feature of AD. Tau proteins normally bind and provide stabilization of microtubules (a cell's skeleton). In AD, they become abnormally paired helical filaments known as neurofibrillary tangles — bundles that get twisted up inside the cell. Because the tau proteins no longer provide support to the cell skeleton, the brain tissue atrophies (Copstead & Banasik, 2000).

Although a relationship exists between the amyloid plaques and neurofibrillary tangles, neither are unique to AD; they are also found in diseases such as Creutzfeldt-Jakob disease as well as in the brains of people without AD. These amyloid plaques must be present in order to diagnosis AD; however, by themselves, they are insufficient to account for the extent of cognitive impairment seen in AD patients. It is known that the greater the number of plaques, the greater the degree of AD. In addition, the neurofibrillary tangle seems to be the lesion that closely correlates with the degree of dementia.

Other Causes of AD

Other suggested pathological causes of AD include the presence of a slow-growing virus (with an incubation period of 2 to 30 years). It is hypothesized that trauma occurs, causing a disruption in the tissues that provides a means for the virus to enter. Infection and environmental exposure are two additional suggested risk factors for AD.

Determination of neurochemical deficits in AD has focused on the neurotransmitters of the cholinergic system. Neurotransmitters are the chemical substances that, along with electrical impulses, relay messages or impulses from neuron to neuron in the brain and peripheral tissues. Recall from your early physiology course work that acetylcholine is a neurotransmitter that acts as the brain's chemical messenger. Deficits in the neurotransmitter acetylcholine were the first ones discovered in AD. Later, deficits in norepinephrine, dopamine, and serotonin were also discovered, either in their production or in the availability of receptor sites, where the neurotransmitter action occurs. Since the recognition of deficits in neurotransmitters in patients with AD, many pharmacological treatments that add to (potentiate), or antagonize the effects of neurotransmitters have been developed (Copstead & Banasik, 2000).

Acetylcholine plays a major role in the formation of memories. It is found in abundance in the hippocampus and cerebral cortex, two of the regions devastated by AD. A dysfunction of acetylcholine production is known as a cholinergic abnormality. In AD, a significant decline in acetylcholine also occurs. Dysregulation of cholinergic, dopaminergic, and g-aminobutyric acid transmitter is found in cases of dementia. Significant cholinergic distribution deficiencies can occur in different brain regions of AD patients. This helps explain why AD and other forms of dementia seem so similar. This knowledge also helps clinicians diagnose other causes of dementia associated with anticholinergic medications. It can also help explain why certain medications impact AD patients (see chapter 9). This knowledge also helps increase understanding of the memory and behavioral abnormalities of AD.

Psychopathological Features of AD

Psychopathological features, such as hallucinations or delusions, are integral elements of AD, and present numerous problems for family members and care givers of demented patients. Wandering, agitation, physical aggression, hallucinations, and delusions are some of the most common behavioral signs of decreased cognitive losses. The psychopathological features correlate with the progression of the stages of AD (see Table 2-1). The prevalence and persistence of wandering and agitation increase as a function of time and decreased cognitive status. Physical aggression is less prevalent and increases as a function of cognitive decline but persists only in severely impaired patients. Delusions peak in the second year and then decline; hallucinations are relatively stable in prevalence and persist moderately (Holtzer et al., 2003).

GENETICS AND AD

Genetics can play a role in some cases of AD. In 1992, researchers discovered a link between familial AD and a gene on chromosome 14. The defective gene on chromosome 14 was called presenilin 1. Later, researchers discovered that families

TABLE 2-1: STAGES OF ALZHEIMER'S DISEASE

I. Early

- Confusion and loss of recent memory
- Disorientation and getting lost in familiar surroundings
- Inability to learn or retain new information
- Language problems
- Mood swings and personality changes
- Inability to care for oneself and perform activities of daily living (ADLs)

II. Intermediate

- Increased memory loss
- Wandering or pacing
- Sleep disturbances
- Inability to recognize family and friends
- Behavioral changes (such as agitation, aggression, psychosis)
- Increased risk of falls or accidents due to confused state

III. Severe or Terminal

- Often bedridden
- Incontinent
- Remote and recent memory loss
- Loss of speech
- Loss of appetite or significant weight loss
- Total dependence on caregivers

(Allen, 2003; Andrews & Andrews, 2003)

ApoE4, a protein that is found at the surface of cholesterol molecules, assists in the transport of blood cholesterol throughout the body. It is found in the neurons of healthy brains and is also detected in the amyloid plaques and neurofibrillary tangles associated with AD. ApoE4 is even found in AD patients who have no familial links. The presence of this protein appears to increase the risk of AD. However, because it is not specific to AD, it cannot be used as a diagnostic biological marker for the disease.

As previously noted, genetic factors can play a role in familial AD. The discovery of several mutated genes, that cause AD in families, does not seem to occur frequently. The frequency has been observed to have an onset prior to age 50, which is a relatively early age for AD onset. Because of the relatively small number of families involved in gene mutation, it is believed that this is an influence versus actual development of the disease.

In recent years, researchers have identified more than 70 genetic mutations capable of generating the clinical manifestations of AD. In the near future, additional mutations will surely be identified. These findings will likely point to polymorphism of genes as the cause of AD. With the current level of understanding, one thing remains clear: an inherited ApoE4 gene cannot predict who will acquire AD. Some people who have the disease also have the gene; however, up to 90% of people who have the gene do not have AD. This indicates that multiple risk factors, the presence of ApoE4 being one, may be responsibe for AD. Research on genetic and physiological changes associated with AD continues.

with a mutated gene on chromosome 1 had a much higher incidence of AD. The responsible gene was called presenilin 2. Researchers have indicated that only a small percentage of individuals develop AD if they have a presenilin 2 gene; however, the presence of presenilin 1 and 2 mutant genes accounts for 50% of cases of early familial AD.

Also in 1992, researchers discovered that, although everyone has two apolipoprotein Es, people with AD have an increased incidence in the presence of the apolipoprotein E4 (ApoE4) allele on chromosome 19. These discoveries have lead to increased interest and research into apolipoproteins.

DIFFERENTIATING DEMENTIA, DELIRIUM, AND DEPRESSION

The importance of differentiating dementia, delirium, and depression cannot be overemphasized. These three illnesses, which are manifested by cognitive, emotional, and behavioral signs and symptoms, are extremely common in health care facilities, hospitals, and nursing homes. Found in patients in all areas of nursing, including occupational health, medical offices or clinics, and home care, these illnesses can exact a price on the individual, the family, and society.

The price society pays is a concern because services designed for, and needed by, the elderly are rapidly increasing. In 1997, the estimated annual cost of AD was $80 to $90 billion. According to the Alzheimer's Association (Koppel, 2002), the cost in the United States is currently $100 billion per year. This number includes the costs of lost productivity as well as the costs of care.

More than 7 out of 10 persons with AD live at home, with almost 75% of home care provided by family and friends. Half of all nursing home residents suffer from AD or a related disorder. The average cost per patient for nursing home care is $42,000 per year, but costs can exceed $70,000 per year in some areas of the country. The average lifetime cost per patient is estimated to be $174,000.

Because treatment of dementia, delirium, and depression depends on recognizing the underlying disease, accurate assessment of a patient's illness is imperative. Nurses are in a unique position to observe and document cognitive, emotional, and functional changes. Dementias are physical illnesses, but the manifestations are often behavioral. As a person loses self-control and control of his or her environment, signs occur, such as outbursts of anger; irritability, and aggressive behavior, both physical and verbal. As the disease progresses, other common behavioral problems, including wandering, resisting care, yelling, rummaging through others' belongings, and hostile actions toward caregivers, may also occur. These increasingly severe behavioral indications are what bring families to the attention of health care providers. The progression of dementia can vary as the disease advances.

The diagnosis of dementia is warranted only if memory impairment is severe enough to interfere with social or occupational function and to cause at least one of the following impairments: agnosia, aphasia, apraxia, or disturbance in executive function. The persistence of signs of impaired intellectual function over a period of months, in a relatively stable form, suggests dementia rather than delirium (see Tables 2-2 and 2-3). Exclusion of all other specific causes of dementia is vital.

The Four A's of Dementia

Another way of approaching cognitive impairment that has been helpful to health care providers is recognition of the four A's, which indicate areas of loss:

1. **Agnosia:** Inability to recognize familiar faces, objects, or surroundings. Patients see and hear with acuity but may interpret inaccurately. They may not recognize familiar faces; may not be able to distinguish where they are; may not realize what belongs to them or to others; and may not recognize common objects, such as a toothbrush, or how they are used. Eventually, some people do not even recognize themselves in a mirror.

2. **Amnesia:** Loss of the ability to learn new information or recall old information that appears as forgetfulness. Behaviors that may be viewed as combative or resistant are often caused by frustration with forgetting information, repeated questioning, and inability to find misplaced objects. Well-meaning reward systems intended to change these behaviors may backfire because the new system cannot be learned.

3. **Aphasia:** Difficulty comprehending or expressing language. Patients who are aphasic may be unable to follow directions, express their needs, or converse with other people. Frustration with inability to express needs and wants can lead to withdrawal and anger. As a result, people with aphasia may be labeled difficult or moody rather than aphasic.

4. **Apraxia:** Loss of ability to perform learned motor skills or familiar, purposeful movements,

TABLE 2-2: DIAGNOSTIC CRITERIA FOR DEMENTIA OF THE ALZHEIMER'S TYPE

A. The development of multiple cognitive deficits manifested by both
   1) memory impairment (impaired ability to learn new information or to recall previously learned information)
   2) one (or more) of the following cognitive disturbances:
      a) aphasia (language disturbance)
      b) apraxia (impaired ability to carry out motor activities despite intact motor function)
      c) agnosia (failure to recognize or identify objects despite intact sensory function)
      d) disturbance in executive functioning (i.e., planning, organizing, sequencing, abstracting)

B. The cognitive deficits in Criteria A1 and A2 each cause significant impairment in social or occupational functioning and represent a significant decline from a previous level of functioning.

C. The course is characterized by gradual onset and continuing cognitive decline.

D. The cognitive deficits in Criteria A1 and A2 are not due to any of the following:
   1) other central nervous system conditions that cause progressive deficits in memory and cognition (e.g., cerebrovascular disease, Parkinson's disease, Huntington's disease, subdural hematoma, normal-pressure hydrocephalus, brain tumor)
   2) systemic conditions that are known to cause dementia (e.g., hypothyroidism, vitamin B12 or folic acid deficiency, niacin deficiency, hypercalcemia, neurosyphilis, HIV infection)
   3) substance-induced conditions

E. The deficits do not occur exclusively during the course of a delirium.

F. The disturbance is not better accounted for by another Axis I disorder (e.g., Major Depressive Disorder, Schizophrenia).

Code based on type of onset and predominant features:
With Early Onset: if onset is at age 65 years or below
   290.11 With Delirium: if delirium is superimposed on the dementia
   290.12 With Delusions: if delusions are the predominant feature
   290.13 With Depressed Mood: if depressed mood (including presentations that meet full symptom criteria for a Major Depressive Episode) is the predominant feature. A separate diagnosis of Mood Disorder Due to a General Medical Condition is not given.
   290.10 Uncomplicated: if none of the above predominates in the current clinical presentation

With Late Onset: if onset is after age 65 years
   290.3 With Delirium: if delirium is superimposed on the dementia
   290.20 With Delusions: if delusions are the predominant feature
   290.21 With Depressed Mood: if depressed mood (including presentations that meet full symptom criteria for a Major Depressive Episode) is the predominant feature. A separate diagnosis of Mood Disorder Due to a General Medical Condition is not given.
   290.0 Uncomplicated: if none of the above predominates in the current clinical presentation

Specify if:
   With Behavioral Disturbance

Coding note: Also code 331.0 Alzheimer's disease on Axis III.

Note. From *Diagnostic and Statistical Manual of Mental Disorders*, Fourth Edition, Text Revision. Washington, DC, American Psychiatric Association, 2000. Reprinted with permission.

TABLE 2-3: DIAGNOSTIC CRITERIA FOR DELIRIUM DUE TO MULTIPLE ETIOLOGIES

A. Disturbance of consciousness (i.e., reduced clarity of awareness of the environment) with reduced ability to focus, sustain, or shift attention.

B. A change in cognition (such as memory deficit disorientation, language disturbance) or the development of a perceptual disturbance that is not better accounted for by a preexisting, established, or evolving dementia.

C. The disturbance develops over a short period of time (usually hours to days) and tends to fluctuate during the course of the day.

D. There is evidence from the history, physical examination, or laboratory findings that the delirium has more than one etiology (e.g., more than one etiological general medical condition, a general medical condition plus Substance Intoxication or medication side effect).

Coding note: Use multiple codes reflecting specific delirium and specific etiologies, e.g., 293.0 Delirium Due to Viral Encephalitis: 291.0 Alcohol Withdrawal Delirium.

Note. From *Diagnostic and Statistical Manual of Mental Disorders*, Fourth Edition, Text Revision. Washington, DC, American Psychiatric Association, 2000. Reprinted with permission.

such as opening a door, dressing, or using utensils for eating. When a person no longer remembers what a bathroom is for, the sight, smell, and temperature of the room can be terrifying.

Understanding that the four A's are neurological losses that a patient experiences can help you plan care and decide what aspects of the patient's environment need to be changed and what new approaches to try.

Dementing Illness Case Example

Although no clinical tests specific to the diagnosis of AD are currently available, a thorough clinical work-up increases the accuracy of the diagnosis by ruling out other illnesses and conditions. The following example illustrates the various signs that suggest dementing illness:

Mrs. Naismith was observed sitting quietly in an examination room before an interview at the memory disorder clinic. Her son, who accompanied her, was outgoing and told her story. He said that she had a history of weight loss and had become isolated in her small apartment. In addition, she had chronic obstructive pulmonary disease and hypertension. Her medications included methyldopa (Aldomet) and cime-

tidine (Tagamet), taken daily. Recently, she had begun to have angry outbursts toward her son when they were talking on the telephone, and she refused to accept assistance with shopping or personal care from her son and a neighbor. Her son brought her to the clinic to find out if she had the beginning signs of AD.

A history was obtained, a physical examination was done, and after a series of laboratory tests, arrangements were made for psychological testing. One of the psychological tests was the Cornell Scale for Depression (see Table 2-4). The test is easily administered by the health caregiver and is considered reliable, particularly for persons with dementia.

Although weight loss is common in patients with dementia and AD, in Mrs. Naismith's case, the loss was attributed to clinical depression. The medications she took and her living environment contributed to the biological process of depression, which could have been mistaken for AD. Furthermore, the use of cimetidine (Tagamet) has been associated with the development of delirium (CMS, 2002d). Differentiation of delirium, depres-

TABLE 2-4: CORNELL SCALE FOR DEPRESSION (1 of 2)

Cornell Scale

Name:_____

Age:_____Sex:_____Wing:_____Room:_____

Date of This Assessment:_____

SCORING SYSTEM: Physician:_____

a = Unable to evaluate   Assessor:_____

0 = Absent   Ratings should be based on symptoms and signs occurring

1 = Mild to intermittent   during the week before interview: No score should be given

2 = Severe   if symptoms result from physical disability or illness.

a   0   1   2

A. MOOD-RELATED SIGNS

1. Anxiety: anxious expression, rumination, worrying
2. Sadness: sad expression, sad voice, tearfulness
3. Lack of reaction to present events
4. Irritability: annoyed, short tempered

a   0   1   2

B. BEHAVIORAL DISTURBANCE

5. Agitation: restlessness, hand wringing, hair pulling
6. Retardation: slow movements, slow speech, slow reactions
7. Multiple physical complaints (score 0 if gastrointestinal symptoms only)
8. Loss of interest: Less involved in usual activities

a   0   1   2

C. PHYSICAL SIGNS

9. Appetite loss: eating less than usual
10. Weight loss (score 2 if greater than 5 pounds in one month)
11. Lack of energy: fatigues easily, unable to sustain activities

a   0   1   2

D. CYCLIC FUNCTIONS

12. Diurnal variation of mood: symptoms worse in the morning
13. Difficulty falling asleep: later than usual for this individual
14. Multiple awakening during sleep
15. Early morning awakening: earlier than usual for this individual

a   0   1   2

E. IDEATIONAL DISTURBANCE

16. Suicidal: feels life is not worth living
17. Poor self-esteem: self-blame, self depreciation, feelings of failure
18. Pessimism: anticipation of the worst
19. Mood congruent delusions: delusions of poverty, illness or loss

Notes/Current Medications: _____

_____

_____

TABLE 2-4: CORNELL SCALE FOR DEPRESSION (2 of 2)

SCORING OF CORNELL DEPRESSION SCALE

1. Clinician interviews the patient using this scale.
2. Family member/caregiver observes the patient for approximately seven days. Based on observations, caregiver rates the various categories.
3. Scores are reviewed by clinician. Any discrepancy, clinician interviews both patient and caregiver for various categories.

IN RATING THE SCORE OF THE CORNELL DEPRESSION SCALE, THERE IS NO REAL CUT OFF POINT FOR DEPRESSION. HOWEVER, GUIDELINES FOR SUSPECTED DEPRESSION THAT ARE USED ARE AS FOLLOWS:

- For persons with suspected dementia, a score below 6 suggests the person is likely NOT depressed.

- For person with suspected dementia, a score of 6-9 is suggestive of minor depression.

- For person with suspected dementia, a score of 9-18 is suggestive of minor to moderate depression.

- For person with suspected dementia, a score of 18-20 is suggestive of moderate to severe depression.

- For person not suspected of having dementia, a score of 16 or above is suggestive of depression.

Note: From "Cornell Scale for Depression in Dementia," by G.S. Alexopoulos, R.C. Abrams, R.C. Young, & C.A Shamoian, 1988, *Biological Psychiatry, 23*:271-284. Reprinted with permission.

sion, and dementia is vital so that vigorous approaches can be implemented.

Dementia

Multi-infarct dementia is caused by one or more strokes that damage or destroy brain tissue. The net result is a change in cognition. The degree to which strokes are responsible for dementia is not clear, but it has been noted that a number of individuals over age 60 who have had a stroke develop dementia within 1 year (American Psychiatric Association, 2000).

The onset of vascular dementia may occur anytime in later life but is less common after age 75. It is important for a practitioner to realize that a complex interaction exists between the two diseases, stroke and vascular dementia, and the vascular component of either disease may be treatable.

Lewy body dementia has been recognized as a major cause of cognitive impairment and dementia during the past 12 years, accounting for about 15%

to 25% of individuals with dementia (Wesnes et al., 2002). Cognitive impairment that fluctuates, recurrent visual hallucinations, and parkinsonism are common. Falls, delusions, sleep disturbances, and auditory hallucinations other are clinical signs. One disturbing feature is that the use of neuroleptics may worsen extrapyramidal signs and accelerate cognitive decline. They can also trigger severe neuroleptic sensitivity reactions (hyperthermia and rapid pulse rate), sometimes with life-threatening consequences. These drugs are likely to be used because of the prominent psychiatric symptoms. Therefore, drug therapy must be tailored to the individual after investigation for causative pathology (Luggen, Miller, & Jett, 2003).

Other less common, progressive degenerative dementias include:

- Korsakoff's psychosis or syndrome (related to chronic alcoholism and vitamin B deficiency)

- Parkinson's disease

- Huntington's chorea

- Pick's disease, a disease that is clinically similar to AD, accounts for up to 5% of dementias, and usually has an earlier onset (between ages 40 and 60); typically, the first symptoms are behavioral, such as changes in social behavior and personality

- Creutzfeldt-Jakob disease, a rapidly progressing spongiform encephalopathy associated with a slow-growing virus. This transmissible encephalopathy is associated with other diseases affecting the prion protein, a cellular glycoprotein. Iatrogenic transmission has been linked to the use of contaminated growth hormone, dura mater, corneal grafts, and neurosurgical equipment. Because new sterilization techniques have been implemented, no new cases have been reported. Since 1996, increasing evidence has linked the causative agent for bovine spongiform encephalopathy (BSE), or mad cow disease in cattle and a new variation of Creutzfeldt-Jakob disease in humans (Centers for Disease Control and Prevention [CDC], 2002). Both disorders are invariably fatal brain diseases with long incubation periods of several years. From 1986 through August 2000, more than 99% of cases of BSE were reported in the United Kingdom. It is still uncertain what specific foods or food products transmit the causative agent from cattle to humans. Cattle remain the only known food animal species with BSE. According to the CDC (2002), public health measures instituted to prevent the spread of BSE have been highly effective in the United Kingdom.

- Acquired immunodeficiency syndrome (AIDS)–related dementia (10% of patients with AIDS are older than age 50, and dementia can be a sign of AIDS in any patient).

Psychosis and Agitation: What We Know

Both psychosis and agitation are common problems in AD and other dementing illnesses. These become major sources of caregiver distress and contribute to premature institutionalization and increased cost of care.

Delusional thought content (such as paranoia) is common among people with AD, with an incidence of greater than 30% (see Table 2-5). Common delusions can include:

- marital infidelity

- other patients and staff are trying to hurt the patient

- staff and family members are impersonators

- theft

- lack of recognition of home

- strangers living in the home

- misidentification of people

- people on television are real

TABLE 2-5: BEHAVIORAL AND PSYCHOLOGICAL SYMPTOMS OF DEMENTIA	
Psychosis	**Agitation**
• Delusions	• Aggression
• Paranoia	• Combativeness
• Hallucinations	• Hyperactivity (including wandering)
	• Hypervocalization
	• Disinhibition

Case Study

Mrs. T., a 94-year-old woman, was brought to the hospital emergency room experiencing headaches, temporary incontinence, and falls. She has been living with her daughter and taking no medications. Her appetite was not very robust. A diagnosis of hypertension was made (170/90 mm Hg). She was placed on a daily dose of ramipril (Altace), an angiotensin-converting enzyme (ACE) inhibitor, and sent to a skilled nursing facility for strengthening by physical therapy. She was alert and oriented upon admission. However, within 2 to 3 days, her family told staff that she "wasn't herself." She complained of weakness and chest pain and was heard coughing frequently. Mrs. T. was now confused at times and unable to participate in her therapy. The daughter questioned her blood pressure medication, but no modifications were made and no report was given to the physician or documented. After 10 days, Mrs. T. fell again and lost the small appetite she had. The nursing facility transported her to the hospital for evaluation. When reviewing the medications, a nurse noted that the dose of the ACE inhibitor was correct for a once-daily dose, but an error in transcription led to Mrs. T. receiving this dosage QID (four times a day) instead of QD (every day). Mrs. T. apparently experienced medication-related delirium.

Delirium

Delirium in older adults is associated with high mortality rates; however, most of the causes are preventable and treatable. Distinguishing between delirium and dementia can be difficult. Confounding the diagnosis is the fact that the diseases can coexist; dementia is a risk factor for delirium. Misdiagnosis due to changing levels of confusion and consciousness unfortunately lead to poor outcomes. Therefore, it is imperative that delirium be recognized early and medically managed to reduce the associated high mortality rates.

Delirium is characterized by changes in attention and cognition. Sensory deficits (such as vision and hearing loss) can mimic delirium. Delirium can be caused by metabolic disorders, such as hypothyroidism, diabetes, and nutritional deficiencies. These disorders can be detected using laboratory tests. Other common causes of delirium include minor problems, such as rectal impaction, bladder infection, tooth abscess, and alcohol abuse or overuse. These widespread causes must be ruled out before a condition can be accepted as irreversible. In most instances, treating the underlying medical problem can reduce delirium (see Table 2-6).

Inappropriate use of medications with anticholinergic effects (see Table 2-7) may lead to delirium, delusions or hallucinations and agitation. If the older adult is exhibiting any of these behavioral

TABLE 2-6: COMMON CAUSES OF DELIRIUM
• Medications
• Exogenous toxins
• Primary psychiatric disease
• Degenerative neurologic disorders with or without focal neurologic sign
• Infections
• Sleep and respiratory problems
– Changes in sleep patterns
– Obstructive apnea
• Endocrine disorders
– Deficiency syndromes (Vitamin B_{12} and thiamine)
• Primary demyelinating disease
• Vascular dementia
• Primary and metastatic brain tumors
• Recurrent seizures

TABLE 2-7: COMMONLY PRESCRIBED MEDICATIONS WITH CHOLINERGIC EFFECTS IN OLDER ADULTS	
• Cimetidine	• Nifedipine
• Prednisolone	• Isosorbide
• Theophylline	• Warfarin
• Digoxin	• Dipyridamole
• Furosemide	• Codeine
• Ranitidine	• Captopril
• Triamterene with hydrochlororthiazide	

problems it is important to take a quick inventory of medications and remember to limit the use of medications with anticholinergic effects because delirium can be induced by even mild anticholinergic medication effects.

Mild Cognitive Impairment

In recent years, much attention has been paid to what is termed the "transitional period of cognitive impairment." Mild cognitive impairment (MCI), which is a common prodrome of AD, is a state between normalcy and dementia. What is different between normal aging and early AD? Remember that the changes associated with AD are qualitative changes, such as changes in memory and behavior. The changes associated with MCI, on the other hand, only relate to memory and are therefore quantitative. Measures of neuropsychological testing are conducted to distinguish between normal aging and disease onset.

Recent research suggests that people with MCI are six times more likely to develop AD than those without MCI. Because of this high incidence of conversion to AD, it is important to be able to evaluate for MCI. The criteria for MCI include:

- memory complaints
- low performance on standardized memory tests
- normal participation in ADLs
- lack of cognitive dysfunction in domains other than memory
- lack of dementia.

Once patients have been identified as having MCI, it is important that they be routinely monitored for decline of cognitive function. It is also important to remember that all individuals with complaints of memory dysfunction should be evaluated with a complete history and physical examination and valid and reliable cognitive testing (Bieber, 2003).

DIFFERENTIATING BETWEEN AD AND DEPRESSION

Depression is common among older adults and is most frequently associated with cognitive decline. For quite some time research has suggested that an association exists between a history of depression and risk for AD. Other common conditions, such as cerebrovascular disease and parkinsonism, are also associated with depression. Hopelessness and help-lessness are common symptoms of depression and are associated with both MCI and AD. Older patients may not report the typical weight loss and sleep disturbances that are also associated with depression. First-time depression in a patient age 65 or older should be investigated as possible dementia.

AD and MCI can coexist with depression. Depression is sometimes one of the early symptoms of AD. It can be difficult to tell if depression is a result of cognitive decline, the anxiety and dysphoria that accompany a diagnosis of AD, or the effect of chemical changes that occur in the brains of AD patients.

Early stage differentiation is difficult but can be assisted by treating the depression. When depression has been successfully treated, the pure character of cognitive dysfunction of AD is visible. This then becomes the time to reevaluate cognitive function. Remember that any treatment for depression in people with AD should not include medications that have an anticholinergic action. Significant cholinergic distribution deficiencies may be present in different brain regions of AD patients. Anticholinergic medications can induce memory and behavioral abnormalities, such as delirium, delusions, and hallucinations.

The Geriatric Depression Scale (GDS) is a successful screening tool for patients with and without cognitive impairment. It is effective for cognitively impaired individuals as long as the score on a MMSE is higher than 12. The scale consists of a 15- or 30-item questionnaire (Table 2-11 shows the 15-item scale) that requires only yes-or-no responses. The scoring system is important to understand because it provides insight into levels of functional decline longitudinally and an objective means of defining the course of the individual's deficits. The maximum score for the 30-item scale is 30. Depressed individuals without dementia usually score between 24 and 30. A score of 20 or less is found in patients with dementia, delirium, schizophrenia, or an affective disorder. The scoring system for the 15-item scale is found in Table 2-8.

TABLE 2-8: GERIATRIC DEPRESSION SCALE (SHORT VERSION)

Choose the best answer for how you have felt over the past week.

1.	Are you basically satisfied with your life?	YES / **NO**
2.	Have you discontinued many of your activities and interests?	**YES** / NO
3.	Do you feel that your life is empty?	**YES** / NO
4.	Do you often get bored?	**YES** / NO
5.	Are you in good spirits most of the time?	YES / **NO**
6.	Are you afraid that something bad is going to happen to you?	**YES** / NO
7.	Do you feel happy most of the time?	YES / **NO**
8.	Do you often feel helpless?	**YES** / NO
9.	Do you prefer to stay at home, rather than going out and doing new things?	**YES** / NO
10.	Do you feel you have more problems with memory than most people?	**YES** / NO
11.	Do you think it is wonderful to be alive now?	YES / **NO**
12.	Do you feel pretty worthless the way you are?	**YES** / NO
13.	Do you feel full of energy?	YES / **NO**
14.	Do you feel that your situation is hopeless?	**YES** / NO
15.	Do you think that most people are better off than you are?	**YES** / NO

TOTAL GDS: _____   (GDS maximum score = 15)

Answers in **bold** indicate depression. Each bold response counts as 1 point.

Scoring

0–4 points	Normal, depending on age, education, complaints
5–8 points	Mild
9–11 points	Moderate
12–15 points	Severe

Retrieved June 18, 2004 from http://www.stanford.edu/~yesavage/GDS.html

DIAGNOSING AD

Emerging diagnostic methods that use biochemical markers and imaging of disease-specific pathology hold the potential for accurately diagnosing AD at the earliest stage of the illness the time when disease-modifying treatment can be most effective (Clark & Karlawish, 2003; Kennedy, 2001).

First, remember that the only way we have found to date to diagnose AD is at autopsy (Kennedy, 2001; Wengenack, Curran, & Poduslo, 2000). Keeping this in mind the only way to diagnose AD is to rule out other disease processes by evaluating the cause of symptoms.

The diagnosis of AD is not merely a diagnosis of exclusion. Although there is no definitive test yet to diagnose AD, AD deficits unfold in a characteristic order. These deficits can reflect the principal causes of the disease. Therefore diagnosis of AD can be said to be a diagnosis of inclusion based on the history and clinical presentation. Early diagnosis is based on:

- clinical findings
- patient history
- physical, neurological, and psychiatric examinations
- laboratory studies
- cognitive testing
- informant reports.

(Griffith, 2002)

Questioning family members about their loved one's personality changes, losses in memory, or altered behavior can help the primary provider differentiate between the normal process of aging and disease processes. Correct and early diagnosis of dementia is important.

DEMENTIA Mnemonic

The process for diagnosing AD can be remembered by using the mnemonic DEMENTIA.

Drugs and alcohol

Eyes and ears

Medical disorders

Emotional and psychological disorders

Neurological disorders

Tumors, trauma, and toxic effects

Infections

Arteriosclerosis

The following delineates each of the parts of the mnemonic.

Drugs and Alcohol: During an evaluation for dementia, be sure to evaluate all medications, including over-the-counter drugs. Keep in mind that older adults commonly borrow their friends' medications without understanding their intended use or adverse effects, and confusion is a common adverse effect of many medications in older adults. Older adults also frequently abuse alcohol. Be sure to review their alcohol use history.

Eyes and Ears: Sensory deficits contribute to disorientation and confusion. In many cases, older adults are self-conscious or embarrassed and do not seek help for these deficits. Rather, they attempt to respond to conversations and, because they do not understand other people's input, they respond with inappropriate responses. Vision loss can cause older adults to trip over or bump into objects, which appears to others that they are disoriented, demented, or confused.

Medical Disorders: Many medical disorders can attribute to confusion and disorientation. Two common disorders to consider are uncontrolled diabetes and hypothyroidism. Vitamin B_{12} deficiency and other nutritional deficiencies can also lead to confusion and mental derangement.

Emotional and Psychological Disorders: Psychiatric illnesses are commonly confused with AD. These illnesses can include mood disorders or paranoia.

Neurological Disorders: Multi-infarct dementia must be differentiated from AD.

Tumors, Trauma, and Toxic Effects: Magnetic resonance imaging (MRI) and computed tomography (CT) scans are effective tools for differentiating between AD and pathological causes of changes in memory and behavior. Even mild head injuries can lead to confusion. Toxicity can occur as a result of overexposure to such substances as carbon monoxide and methyl alcohol.

Infections: Urinary tract infections and upper respiratory infections are common causes of confusion. When an older person presents to the emergency department with acute onset of confusion, one of the first assessments performed is a urinary sample for infection.

Arteriosclerosis: As a heart fails, it loses its ability to pump blood to the lungs for oxygenation. Arteriosclerosis can lead to heart failure, and insufficient blood supply to the brain can result in confusion.

(Smith, 2002)

Diagnostic Screening Tools

Most of the screening tools for differentiating AD from other disease processes involve cognitive assessment. Cognitive function consists of processes by which we perceive, store, retrieve, and use information. In older adults, cognitive function can decline in the presence of illness. A nurse's ability to assess cognitive function is critical to maintaining an individual's cognitive status or identifying particular states that affect cognitive function, such as dementia, delirium, and depression. Nursing assessment is also imperative to establishing clinical goals and the effectiveness of medical regimens.

Diagnosing AD can be an overwhelming task because there are so many likely causes of the signs exhibited. The first step in the diagnosis process is assessment, which needs to include a thorough and complete history, physical examination, laboratory tests such as blood chemistries, thyroid-stimulating hormone levels, electrolytes, and electrocardiogram testing aimed at ruling out other causes of dementia (see Table 2-9). Early on, the history is by far the most important component of the examination. #19

The second step in the diagnosis process is the evaluation of cognitive function. Diagnostic tools must provide precise information about the individual's ability to function. They must address the nature and cause of the impairment as well as any evidence of lingering cognitive function.

When selecting an instrument to assess cognitive function, nurses should determine the purpose of the assessment. Is it for screening, monitoring, or diagnosing, or is it multipurpose? Different tools address each of these areas. For evaluation of AD, the provider should know which of the wide array of screening instruments are brief and reliable.

Some tests must be serial (repeated assessments at set intervals of time) to provide monitoring of activities and functions. Serial assessments allow comparison of functional ability that can be used to evaluate changes in cognitive function over time. For example, at an initial assessment, a man indicates that he forgets to take his medicine once per week. In a subsequent assessment, he reports that he forgets daily. These assessments could indicate a decline in cognitive function.

Methods of Assessment

Each method of assessment has advantages and disadvantages. A nurse must choose an assessment tool based on the desired outcome from the use, the time involved, and the demands on the examiner and patient. The following outline provides important considerations in cognitive assessment.

Formal and Informal Methods of Assessment

A. Formal methods are those that assess cognitive function through the use of standardized instruments.

  1. Advantages: Standardized assessments provide for comparison across individuals and nurses.

  2. Disadvantages: There are individual influences on performance, such as pain, education, fatigue, time of day, culture, perception, and physical abilities.

B. Informal methods of cognitive assessment are structured observations and nurse-individual interactions (such as assessing for apraxia).

TABLE 2-9: BASIC LABORATORY TESTS FOR CAUSES OF POSSIBLE DEMENTIA	
Test or Study	**Common Problems Detected**
Complete blood count	Anemia, infections
Blood chemistry	Kidney or liver disorders, diabetes
Electrolyte screen	Electrolyte imbalances
Thyroid function studies (thyroid-stimulating hormone, thyroxine, triiodothyronine, ratios)	Hypothyroidism or hyperthyroidism
Assays of vitamin B_{12} and folate levels	Vitamin deficiencies
VDRL test	Syphilis
HIV tests	AIDS-related dementia
(APA, 1994)	

1. Advantages: These observations may more accurately indicate an individual's cognitive ability and performance.

2. Disadvantages: It can be difficult to judge individual changes in condition, and there is a risk of variability of interpretation by different examiners.

C. Other considerations for assessment

1. Characteristics of the environment in which the assessment is conducted

   a. The physical environment should be a comfortable temperature. It must have adequate, but not glaring, lighting and be free from distractions. Other people should not be in the room, if possible. Position the patient appropriately to make good eye contact and to maximize the individual's sensory abilities.

   b. The interpersonal environment of the examiner and patient should allow the patient to set the pace for the assessment. The assessment must be emotionally nonthreatening.

2. Timing considerations

   a. The timing should take into consideration the actual cognitive abilities of the individual and not extraneous factors.

   b. Times of the day to avoid are immediately upon waking, immediately before meals, and immediately before or after medical diagnostic or therapeutic procedures. Also avoid times when a patient may be in pain or discomfort.

D. Outcomes of assessment

1. Individual

   a. Detection of deviations must be prompt and early.

   b. Appropriate care and treatment must be instituted in a timely manner.

   c. Plans of care should appropriately address corrective and supportive cognitive functions.

2. Health care provider

   a. Assessment and documentation of cognitive function is timely.

   b. Appropriate strategies are developed to address any deviation in cognitive function.

   c. Competence is present in cognitive assessments.

   d. Evidence of ability to discriminate among the different types of cognitive changes or decline must be provided.

3. Institution

   a. Documentation of cognitive function increases.

   b. Referral to appropriate advanced practitioners or psychiatric specialists increases.

(Fulmer, Mezey, Bottrell, et al., 2002)

Mini-Mental Status Examination

The Mini-Mental Status Examination (MMSE) is the most widely used screening tool for cognitive function. Table 2-10 provides some sample items from the Mini-Mental Status Exam. The scoring system for the MMSE is important to understand. A maximum of 30 points can be scored on the test. Individuals with mild impairment score between 24 and 29 points. A score of less than 24 is the benchmark for cognitive impairment. Individuals with a moderate level of impairment score between 14 and 24. Moderately severe impaired individuals can score from 5 to 14, while those with severe AD can score as low as 0. As a user of the MMSE, it is important to understand that individuals with less than a ninth grade level of education may score less than 17. Use of the MMSE on a regular basis can be beneficial for assessing possible declines in cognition over time. The average decline on the MMSE of AD patients is 2 to 4 points per year (Folstein, Folstein, & McHugh, 1975; Ebersole & Hess, 2001).

TABLE 2-10: MINI-MENTAL STATUS EXAMINATION

Orientation to Time

"What is the date?"

Registration

"Listen carefully, I am going to say three words. You say them back after I stop. Ready?

Here they are...HOUSE (pause), CAR (pause), LAKE (pause). Now repeat those words back to me."

[Repeat up to 5 times, but score only the first trial.]

Naming

"What is this?" [Point to a pencil or pen.]

Reading

"Please read this and do what it says." [Show examinee the words on the stimulus form.]

CLOSE YOUR EYES

Reproduced by special permission of the publisher, Psychological Assessment Resources, Inc., 16204 North Florida Avenue, Lutz, Florida 33549, from the Mini Mental Status Examination, by Marshal Folstein and Susan Folstein. Copyright 1975, 1998, 2001 by Mini Mental LLC, Inc. Published 2001 by Psychological Assessment Resources, Inc. Further reproduction is prohibited without permission of PAR, Inc. The MMSE can be purchased from PAR, Inc. by calling (800) 331-8378 or (813) 968-3003.

Clock Drawing Test

Another commonly used cognitive assessment tool is the Clock Drawing Test (CDT). This is the easiest and fastest screening tool to use, usually taking less than 5 minutes to administer. Simply ask the patient to draw the face of a clock with all its numbers and hands and then state the time as it was drawn. Successful administration of this test relies on a patient having good visuospatial ability, judgment, planning, and other skills.

Scoring of the CDT, with a total of 6 possible points:

Number 12 on top of the clock?	3 Points
Numbers on clock present?	1 Point
Both clock hands present?	1 Point
Time correct?	1 Point

A score less than 4 indicates impairment. When used in conjuction with the MMSE, the CDT provides adequate sensitivity and specificity for screening.

Mini-Cog Exam and Memory Impairment Screen

Two additional screening tools are the Memory Impairment Screen (MIS) and the Mini-Cog Exam. The Mini-Cog combines parts of the CDT and MMSE into one test (see Table 2-11). Both the Mini-Cog and the MIS are easy to administer (Borson, Scanlan, Brush, Vitaliano, & Dokmak, 2000). As with the MMSE and CDT, these tools can be used in serial assessments.

MOSES Scale

The purpose of the MOSES Scale is to measure the quality of life of elderly people who are unable to communicate. It is a standardized measure of residents' physical, cognitive, and emotional functioning. Properly assessing the functional status of residents of long-term care facilities is important for a number of reasons: placement decision, care plan development, and resident status screening over periods of time. Reliabilitiy of this instrument is particularly good for easily observable behaviors, such as self-care activities and disorientation, and is somewhat lower for behaviors indicative of depression, irritability, and withdrawal. The MOSES Scale is also a tool that can systematically measure the associations between environmental design features of nursing home special care units and the incidence of aggression, agitation, social withdrawal, depression, and psychotic problems among people living there who have AD or a related disorder. It can also provide the assessment information of changes in intellect occurring in the person with a cognitive disability. See Appendix A.

To test for apraxia, simply ask the patient to put on an examination glove or pantomime an everyday task, such as making a cup of tea, brushing teeth,

TABLE 2-11: ADMINISTRATION OF THE MINI-COG

1. Please repeat and remember these three words: Apple–Table–Penny.

2. Please draw a clock with all 12 numbers and place the hands at 2:30.

3. Now please recall the three words.

Scoring

1. Recall after the clock drawing
   a. 0 = impaired
   b. 1-2 = possibly impaired; evaluate the clock
   c. 3 = unimpaired

2. Normal clock = all numbers present and in correct sequence, time displayed as requested (no partial credit)

3. Abnormal clock = impaired

Note. From "The Mini-Cog: A Cognitive 'Vital Signs' Measure for Dementia Screening in Multi-Lingual Elderly." by S. Borson, J. Scanlan, M. Brush, P. Vitaliano, & A. Dokmak, 2000. *International Journal of Geriatric Psychiatry, 15*(11), 1021-27. © John Wiley & Sons Limited. Reprinted with permission.

putting a key in a lock, or washing a dish. Observe the behavior.

Global Deterioration Scale

Another recommended tool is the Global Deterioration Scale and Clinical Dementia Rating for measures of dementia-related dependency. This is another scoring scale that provides information regarding dementia-related dependency.

Remember that a person cannot always remember what he or she has forgotten. When the patient is unable to fully participate, you need collateral informants, such as family members or caregivers. Investigate the following topics with these informants:

- Memory complaints

- Signs of dementia

- Language problems

- Changes in personality

- Disorientation

- ADLs

- Hygiene

- Financial, property, and household care.

(Glaser, 2001)

Early diagnosis of AD is beneficial for several reasons. It provides time for reversible causes of cognitive impairment to be ruled out. It also permits patient participation in the decision-making process for such issues as living arrangements for the remaining years of life and choice of long-term care facilities and caregivers (Glaser, 2001).

Novel treatments can provide symptom relief and can slow the progression of AD if initiated early enough in the disease progression, while the patient is still at a high level of functioning. These treatments can provide additional time for patients and families to make crucial medical, legal, and financial decisions. The additional time also allows for family and caregiver support, training, and planning before the disease progresses so that they do not find themselves ill-equipped to deal with the day-to-day problems of AD or unable to cope with the disease because they had not identified support systems or care providers for their loved one.

DIAGNOSTIC TESTING FOR AD

Because biochemical changes that reflect the disease-related pathology take place in the bodies of AD patients, it is likely that a combination of biochemical profiles and quantitative neuroimaging, in conjunction with clinical and neurobehavioral assessment, will soon be used to detect and monitor AD and its associated conditions. There has been, and continues to be, a concerted effort to identify biochemical markers that can function as diagnostic tests at the earliest point of the disease. Two of the potential sources of markers are urine and cerebrospinal fluid (CSF) (Black, 1999).

So far, the biochemical marker most studied is CSF levels of the tau protein. Almost all dementias, strokes, and head trauma produce elevated levels of the tau protein. The tau levels in CSF can be as much as 10 times higher in patients with AD compared to those without the disease. Along with elevated levels of tau are reduced CSF levels of beta-amyloid. Neither CSF levels of tau nor beta-amyloid are related to the duration of the patient's symptoms or degree of disease.

When clinical features of AD are ambiguous, imaging studies such as CT and MRI can be used to identify brain lesions and quantify brain atrophy associated with AD. Through the use of single-photon emission computed tomography (SPECT), bilateral or asymmetrical temporal or parietal lobe hypoperfusion can be identified in patients suspected of having AD. As evidenced in a limited amount of research studies, the positive identification of these findings can raise the probability that AD will be found at autopsy to approximately 90%. A normal SPECT scan reduces the likelihood of AD to 70%. Recent studies suggest that MRIs of specific brain regions yield information about neuronal changes that may herald prodromal AD (Killiany et al, 2000).

Most clinicians who suspect dementia screen for thyroid dysfunction and vitamin B_{12} deficiency. These levels are tested along with miscellaneous electrolytes and a complete blood count — not so much to identify AD, but rather to rule out other contributors to dementia.

Delayed Diagnosis

Uncertainty in mild cases can lead to a delay in diagnosing AD. Some practitioners ask, "Why cause unnecessary anxiety and inappropriate life choices in many elderly who never get AD?" (Crystal, 2001). However, these delays are no longer acceptable because current treatments can alter the course of AD. There are drugs with palliative effects on cognitive function, in both early and more advanced stages of AD. These medical therapies may delay onset or slow progression of the disease. Early treatment also has the potential to impact the costs associated with AD. Patients, caregivers, and society share the benefits of not delaying diagnosis.

SIGNS AND SYMPTOMS OF AD

The onset of AD is insidious, with a decline in function that is smooth but accelerates during the middle stage. It is during this stage that behavioral disturbances emerge. None of the signs or symptoms that develop in AD patients are unique to the disease at its various stages.

Listed here are the 10 warning signs of AD published by the Alzheimer's Association, along with the expression of each in the daily lives of individuals with AD.

1. *Recent memory loss that affects job skills.* Problems with memory affect recent or short-term memory. At first, the memory loss may affect only those skills that are associated with very specific tasks. The chemist cannot recall a key formula and attributes it to "getting older;" another person forgets a colleague's name and cannot remember it later either. Later, the memory problem becomes a bit more severe and individuals forget or have failure of recall. For example, they may forget to turn off the oven or fail to recall when they are supposed to take medications or cannot recall the days of the week.

2. *Difficulty performing familiar tasks.* We can all be so busy or stressed that we forget common tasks. We might forget the potatoes in the oven and only remember to serve them at the end of the meal. However, individuals with AD might prepare a whole meal and forget they prepared it.

3. *Problems with language.* Who has not searched to find the right word? With AD, the problem is that not only are simple words forgotten but incongruous words are substituted for the word

that was forgotten. Many times, it is not just one word that is forgotten or replaced, but an entire sentence that is unintelligible.

4. *Disorientation to time and place.* Have you ever been in the middle of doing something and then asked, "gosh, do I have the right day?" If so, you are likely to quickly be able to come up with the right day. AD makes it difficult for individuals to distinguish not only the day but also where they are and how they got there.

5. *Poor or decreased judgment.* Individuals with AD find it difficult to handle problems. An example might be difficulty driving due to increased cautiousness or difficulty making decisions. They may also inappropriately dress — for example, they may wear several layers of clothing on a very warm day.

6. *Misplacing items.* Surely you have heard stories about the person who could not find their glasses only to realize that they were on top of their heads the whole time. AD patients do not simply misplace their glasses but they may put them in the freezer or a cereal box.

7. *Changes in mood or behavior.* We all have days where we get moody or have some form of mood swing. However, the moods of people with AD can instantly change. They may quickly go from sitting quietly and reading a book to being sad or even crying uncontrollably.

8. *Changes in personality.* With mood or behavior changes may also come mild personality changes, such as loss of spontaneity, apathy, or withdrawal from social interactions. For example, for no apparent reason, people with AD may become instantly agitated, exhibiting irritability, confusion, and suspicion. These changes generally occur early in the disease progression.

9. *Loss of initiative.* When it is a bright, sunny spring day outside and you are inside doing housework, engaging in business activities, or performing a social obligation, you become tired and disinterested in what you are doing. Individuals with AD can become so passive that they need constant cues to become engaged in any type of activity.

10. *Problems with abstract thinking.* Although many people have a dislike for doing such activities as balancing their checkbooks or paying monthly bills, individuals with AD do not even remember what the numbers are or what to do with them.

FUNCTIONAL ASSESSMENTS

Nurses play a central role in any setting where there are older adults. They can assess functional abilities through direct observation during routine care as well as through gathering information from colleagues, family members, and patients. Functional assessments provide a point of reference for patient progress. Serial functional assessments provide a dialogue for health care providers, caregivers, and family members and provide outcome measures of nursing interventions and medical care.

Functional assessments are really assessments of daily function, or the capacity to safely perform ADLs. A comprehensive functional assessment supplies a systematic means of assessing the abilities of individuals and comparing them to a baseline functional status. Functional assessments can be sensitive indicators of health or illness. When a nurse finds a discrepancy from the baseline, he or she has the opportunity to immediately explore possible causes. All instances of functional decline must be assessed in a timely manner. Assess for acute illness and musculoskeletal or neurological decline.

The purpose of standardized functional assessments is to identify maximum patient autonomy. Standardized assessment instruments can include:

1. ADLs

   a. Feeding, bathing, dressing, mobility, and toileting

2. Instrumental ADLs

   a. Shopping, cooking, housework, transportation, and finance and medication management

3. Sensory capacity (the impact of vision and hearing ability on the performance of ADLs)

4. Informant-based tool to assess dimensions of function (a means of gathering information from caregivers and family members)

5. Functional activities questionnaire

COMPLICATIONS OF AD

Some patients who discover they have AD and know about or realize the eventual mental and physical decline in store for them may attempt suicide. This is especially true in the early stages. Others may not take such drastic steps but may use alcohol or substance abuse to cope with their diagnoses. The behavioral complications and manifestations of AD are numerous and have serious implications for treatment, family, and costs. Chapter 8 discusses these behaviors at length as well as the interventions used in their treatment.

SUMMARY

More questions than answers have been raised by the various theories that attempt to explain aging. All areas of the body are affected by aging, but no single cause of aging has been found. Genetic factors are implicated in some disorders that commonly occur with age, such as hypertension, coronary artery disease, malignant neoplasms of the breast and stomach, and now AD. AD may have several fundamental genetic causes.

AD is the most frequently occurring type of dementia in older adults. The relationship between the biological (pathological) and the biochemical (neurochemical) changes seen in AD is complex. Determination of neurochemical deficits in AD has focused on the neurotransmitters of the cholinergic system. Risk factors for AD include increased age, female gender, head trauma, and family history. Research on genetic and physiological changes associated with AD continues.

Currently, no test exists to definitively diagnose AD; autopsies are the only means of definitive diagnosis. However, the presence of memory deficits and other characteristics in a person's history and clinical presentation are included among the criteria for a positive diagnosis of AD. Therefore, diagnosis of AD can be said to be a diagnosis of inclusion. Understanding and differentiating among delirium, dementia, and depression also assist in the diagnosis of AD as well as the treatment of behavioral symptoms.

Although numerous diagnostic tools have been developed to identify AD and support practitioners in their care of older adults, the most reliable and sensitive tests remain the MMSE and the CDT. The MOSES Scale is another beneficial tool for measuring the behaviors of people with dementia or potential dementia. Imaging studies assist practitioners in identifying brain atrophy and brain lesions.

EXAM QUESTIONS

CHAPTER 2
Questions 11-20

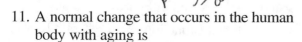
Not sure of d, I picked the best answer

11. A normal change that occurs in the human body with aging is

   a. neurons in the CNS show signs of regeneration. *degeneration*

   b. brain weight decreases by as much as 40% by age 80. *decreases by 17%*

   c. intelligence decreases markedly.

   (d.) simple recall declines, but learning skills remain the same.

12. To understand causes of brain deterioration in people with AD, it is helpful to recognize mechanisms of cell damage, which include

   a. neuritic plaque and beta-amyloid plaque.

   b. abundant acetylcholine and beta-amyloid plaque.

   c. abundant acetylcholine and tangles of tau.

   (d.) beta-amyloid plaque and tangles of tau.

13. The neurotransmitters first found to be deficient in people with AD is

   a. dopamine.

   b. adrenaline.

   (c.) acetylcholine.

   d. glutamate.

14. Early diagnosis of AD is important because this is the time when

   (a.) treatment for AD is most effective.

   b. a practitioner can differentiate among depression, delirium, and dementia.

   c. evidence of memory impairment is apparent.

   d. behaviors are at their worst and are easily corrected.

15. A diagnosis of dementia is correct only if there is

   a. accurate interpretation of impaired functional status.

   b. acute memory impairment and gait disturbances.

   c. ability to perform new motor skills and forgetfulness.

   (d.) memory impairment that is severe enough to interfere with social functioning and difficulty comprehending or expressing language.

16. The four A's of cognitive impairment are

   a. affect, amnesia, aphasia, and apraxia.

   b. aphasia, affect, ability, and agnosia.

   c. amnesia, attitude, agnosia, and aphasia.

   (d.) agnosia, amnesia, apraxia, and aphasia.

17. Your patient wanders during the night when you expect him to be sleeping. Sometimes, the wandering actually resembles agitation rather than purposeful movement. The stage of AD you would expect this patient to be in is

    a. late stage.

    b. early stage.

    c. intermediate stage.

    d. denial stage.

18. A helpful mnemonic used to diagnose AD by evaluating symptoms and ruling out other disease processes is

    a. AGITATION.

    b. PARANOIA.

    c. PSYCHOSIS.

    d. DEMENTIA.

19. A correct statement regarding formal and informal assessment as a means of diagnosing AD is:

    a. the history is by far the most important component of any examination with regard to providing a diagnosis of AD.

    b. individual observations by nurses are accurate across different observers.

    c. standardized assessment tools do not demonstrate accuracy across individuals and nurses.

    d. the environment and timing of any assessment is of little significance to the accuracy.

20. Recent research suggests that individuals with mild cognitive impairment (MCI) are six times more likely to develop AD than those without MCI. The characteristics you would expect to see in people with MCI include

    a. memory complaints but normal performance on standardized memory tests.

    b. normal participation in ADLs with no complaints of memory loss.

    c. cognitive dysfunction and low participation in ADLs.

    d. low performance on standardized memory tests.

CHAPTER 3

COMMUNICATION AND HUMOR THERAPEUTICS

CHAPTER OBJECTIVE

After completing this chapter, the reader will be able to discuss the nursing process, including best practice interventions, for treating communication concerns of patients with Alzheimer's disease (AD).

LEARNING OBJECTIVES

After studying this chapter, the reader will be able to

1. formulate interventions intended to improve communication with patients with AD.

2. discuss narrative story telling and translate this intervention into practice.

3. describe interventions for handling repeated questions.

4. discuss the importance of touch as a form of communication with older adults and AD patients.

5. specify the importance of humor in therapeutic interventions.

INTRODUCTION

This chapter discusses techniques for communicating with older adults with AD. It also addresses the nurse's role in the use of therapeutic activities for AD, such as humor and touch.

COMMUNICATION

Patients with dementia experience life "in the moment," and being in the moment is often the key to communicating with, and understanding, them. According to the *Male Caregiver's Guidebook,* published by the Alzheimer's Association in 1990, communication is the most important quality in enhancing a loving relationship, and lack of communication is most destructive to a loving relationship. These facts are not surprising to family caregivers or nurses. Obstacles to communication when caring for someone with dementia can be difficult, overwhelming, and frustrating.

A common question asked of family members and caregivers of persons with AD is "What is the biggest problem in caring for people with AD?" You can probably guess the answer: communication breakdown. As AD progresses, patients become unable to speak and understand less and less. Communicating with them poses two problems. One problem is the difficulty these patients have expressing themselves to others; another is the difficulty they have understanding what others say to them (Head, 2003).

In the early stages of AD, communication difficulties involve short-term memory loss or loss in the ability to give objects in the environment their proper name, such as calling a cat a cat and not a spoon. Understanding humor, following complex directions, and understanding complex conversations becomes difficult (see Table 3-1). Patients may have trouble figuring out what they want to say and take longer to think about things. In the middle stages, as the neurological condition progresses, disorientation and confusion increase and increasing difficulty understanding and responding to language can cause people with AD to withdraw from social situations. In the latter stages, patients may not speak at all or may use repetitive phrases and are usually extremely disoriented.

TABLE 3-1: AD STAGE-RELATED COMMUNICATION PROBLEMS	
Early Stage	Short-term memory loss; difficulty "naming" things; difficulty following directions; difficulty understanding complex conversations
Middle Stage	Increasing disorientation and confusion; increased difficulty understanding and responding to language can lead to social withdrawal
Late Stage	Use of repetitive phrase or progression to complete loss of speech; extreme disorientation

Failure to understand what a patient is trying to communicate can lead to catastrophic reactions. Some basic principles and strategies can help caregivers improve their communication. First, slow down and calm down. A slow, calm approach can defuse a potentially escalating situation. No more than one person should attempt communication with the patient. If a patient becomes increasingly restless and agitated while attempting to communicate, nonverbal skills should be used to enhance the communication. Look directly at the patient, and maintain good eye contact when speaking. Some patients try to hide their problems with finding the right words by saying, "I don't want to talk about it." Others who have not used curse words in the past may start cursing (Haak, 2002).

If possible, stay on the same positional level with the patient. If the patient is sitting, sit with him or her; if the patient is standing, stand. Verbal and nonverbal messages need to match. If a disparity exists, patients with dementia are more likely to respond to the unspoken, or nonverbal, message. Remain aware of your facial expressions, and be alert to the patient's expressions. Gestures can be used to help with what you are trying to say. Point at what you are describing, or use nonverbal cues such as simulating holding a glass and drinking (Alzheimer's Association, 2004).

As the disease progresses and memory loss increases, language abilities and reading comprehension diminish. When a person with AD is still able to remain at home, you may notice that his or her mail goes unopened or is left lying around, and the newspaper is still rolled up or neatly organized; you can tell that it has not been read. These are clues to the fact that the person with AD is losing the ability to use language.

Another clue is the use of words when speaking. The individual may stumble over words and have increasing difficulty understanding spoken word. The person may even start to make up words or use words that do not make sense. When this occurs, caregivers must pay closer attention to what is being said. Bits and pieces of the conversation can be used to figure out what is being communicated. This occurs because people with AD can be totally in touch with the world around them but still lose the ability to express themselves. When speaking to people with AD, slow down and give these individuals time to evaluate and respond to what is being communicated to them.

When patients have trouble expressing a desire or explaining what they want, try guessing. Professional and family caregivers use this best practice creatively and effectively. By slowing down and considering both verbal and nonverbal cues, you may pick up on what the patient is trying to say. Ask if you are guessing correctly. Stay relaxed, and repeat or rephrase what you think is being said. A patient's gestures or signals may indicate that you have guessed correctly or incorrectly. Try responding to the underlying meaning of what a confused patient wants rather than to the specific words said (Haak, 2002; Pietro, 2002). This practice promotes the dignity of the patient and helps isolate and meet unmet needs (Mariano, Gould, Mezey, & Fulmer, 1999).

Difficulties With Expression

You may suspect that a patient with AD is having difficulty communicating if he or she begins:

- Having difficulty finding the right words
- Using familiar words repeatedly
- Inventing new words to describe familiar objects (confabulation)
- Frequently losing train of thought
- Experiencing difficulty organizing words logically
- Reverting to speaking in a native language
- Cursing or using offensive words
- Speaking less often
- Relying on nonverbal gestures.

Optimizing General Communication with AD Patients

Here are some suggestions for improving communication with patients with AD:

- Rule number one: keep it simple.
- Use neutral tones that are gentle and relaxed.
- Approach the person from the front.
- Speak slowly and clearly.
- Use an auditory level that the person with AD can clearly understand.
- When having difficulty with communication, reduce environmental distractions.
- Break tasks and instructions into clear, simple steps.
- Ask one question at a time.

- Allow enough time for a response.
- Avoid interrupting, criticizing, correcting, and arguing.
- Do not talk about the person as though they are not there.
- Use nonverbal communication, such as pointing and touching.

Narrative Approach

Dementia causes misunderstandings that lead to communication difficulties. These misunderstandings frustrate the caregiver and the person with AD. Remember that processing information becomes more difficult as AD progresses. Because of the communication misinterpretation on the part of the person with AD, communication with caregivers gets harder and harder as the disease progresses. Changes in the tone of the voice normally used with others to emphasize a point can easily make the caregiver appear to be angry or shouting (Geldmacher, Heck, & O'Toole, 2001).

As formal caregivers, nurses must become more proficient in communicating with AD patients by selecting interactive methods to help construct meaning with individuals who have diminished capacity to communicate. Failure to take part in conversation among family members contributes to the overall stress of caregivers.

As cognitive difficulties progress, the ability to carry on the normal give-and-take of conversations diminishes, too. Remember that the mind does not record the entire world; rather, it creates its own world based on the individual's environment, experiences, and expectations. Think about the stories you have told to others about an event in your life. You "wrote" this story by putting it into a narrative form for others to understand; you rehearsed it and performed it. If you have lived with another person for a long period, you have probably heard stories repeated. People with AD are no different, they tell their stories to others. Repetitions of narratives help caregivers understand who people with AD are and what they are trying to convey. However, as the dementia of AD progresses, the stories they have written and tell become fragmented; they lose bits and pieces of the stories.

Remember that conversation requires give-and-take, or turn-taking. The problem with AD is that individuals get lost in the story and, as a result, the story loses coherence. The story becomes vague. Instead of the normal flow of conversation, with each participant contributing, turn-taking by the AD individual becomes more frequent with little elaboration and relevance to the subject matter. Nurses have to recognize the fragments of the story, and in order to do that they need to know the story.

In normal storytelling, we use strategies to help our listeners "listen" to our story; however, people with AD are unable to signal the beginning of the story, provide the context of the story, identify when the listener needs additional information for clarification and, most importantly, stay on tract with the story while providing an ending to the story (Moore & Davis, 2002).

Moore and Davis (2002) have likened these story fragments to blocks of a quilt, with each block having a beginning and an end. All of the blocks must be pieced together in order for the quilt (the story) to be complete. Many of the blocks are repeated in the quilt, so too is the repetition of the story. Caregivers just have to help build the blocks in order to complete the quilt and understand the story.

The nurse is able to help construct the story by paying close attention to what is being said. "If the AD speaker presents what sounds like part of a story that the nurse has heard or another part of it either from the AD speaker, another caregiver, or a family member, the nurse repeats the utterance, waits to see if the AD speaker adds anything new, and then speaks a phrase about the other part of the story" (Moore & Davis, 2002, p. 263). Understanding of the narratives helps family members comprehend what the person with AD is trying to communicate.

Guidelines for Giving Reminders to AD Patients during Conversation

- Listen carefully to the AD speaker, and try to place yourself within the framework of the story (the speaker's reality).

- Repeat the speaker's full phrase slowly, and pause.

- Always look for the beginnings and endings of stories.

- Repetition suggests that there is more of the story to come or that there is another story. Look for the "new event" in the conversation.

- Record the details in a notebook or on a file card and keep it with the treatment records for other providers.

- Introduce a topic on file in your future conversations.

   – Phrase it as a statement.

   – If the AD patient recognizes the statement, he or she is likely to access other details of the life story and share it in the conversation.

- Keep the conversation on track and end it with an evaluation of the story events.

- Suspend your expectations of how an AD patient will handle a narrative. You can expect to see the following characteristics during conversations

   – Vague or empty speech

   – Turn-taking during conversations becomes more frequent but with few elaborations on the topic and more irrelevancies.

Your efforts can have a positive calming effect, that prevents such behavior eruptions as agitation and anxiety (Small, Gutman, Makela, & Hillhouse, 2003).

Repeated Questions

Many nurses and other staff personnel find it distressing when a patient with dementia asks the same question or repeats the same statement over and over again. However, fear or worry may cause repetition. For example, Mrs. Turner asked repeatedly when her daughter was coming. Staff members would sometimes tell her that her daughter lived out of state and visited just last month. The question would then be repeated in a few minutes. This behavior may be a sign of the fear and insecurity Mrs. Turner is experiencing, or it may be an indication that she cannot remember things for even brief periods and does not realize that she received an answer a short time ago (Tappen, Williams, Barry, & DiSesa, 2001).

Several different strategies may be useful for dealing with repetitive questioning or statements. For some patients, ignoring the statement or question may work. For others, this strategy makes the situation worse and upsets them. Sometimes, distraction helps. Take the patient for a walk or offer a snack or juice. For some patients, rather than answering repeated questions, reassuring them that everything is fine and that things will be taken care of is effective. For example, Mrs. Turner worried that not being in her own home would make her miss her daughter's visit. Reassuring her that everything is okay could allay that fear. Remember, though, as with all interventions, what works today or this morning may not work the next time; be flexible.

This list of recommendations can help you be in the moment to communicate with patients with AD:

- Listen to what is said and seek out what is unspoken.

- Always treat the patient like an adult. Do not talk down to him or her.

- Speak slowly in a low-pitched voice, and identify yourself during each interaction. Do not ask if the patient remembers your name.

- When you ask a question, wait for an answer. If the patient does not answer, repeat the question. For example, point to the patient's arm and say "Does your arm hurt?"

- If the patient is stuck on a word, try guessing. Use words, gestures, pictures, pointing, and facial expressions to help.

- Be consistent, and use simple language. Do not use figures of speech, such as "hop into bed" or "let me give you a hand."

When supervising or managing other staff members who must communicate with patients with dementia, nurses need to remind them that verbal and nonverbal strategies can be taught and learned. Some caregivers seem to have an innate awareness of how to communicate with patients with dementia. Others appear to be incapable of communicating with these patients or unwilling to learn the methods for effective and compassionate communication.

Many studies speculate that some staff members may lack insight into how their behaviors affect others. They also cite lack of training as a contributing factor to decreased communications (Pietro, 2002). These staff members refuse to alter their style to accommodate others and continue to talk loudly and hurry through tasks in an abrupt and controlling manner. Any staff member who continues to behave in this manner after documented evaluations and ongoing in-service training should be informed that he or she is unsuited for working with patients with dementia and should be dismissed or transferred to another unit. Nurses who supervise and manage other staff members must demonstrate proper communication skills to the staff and must make decisions for the benefit of patients.

Although all of the above content has been directed at all caregivers, certified nursing assistants (CNAs) are the individuals who make up 85% of nursing staff and provide 80% to 90% of a resident's care. One can immediately understand that these professionals have a critical impact on the quality of life of their residents. Because of this, one might ask, "Does their education match their ability to influence outcomes of residents?" The answer is, "No." CNAs receive 70 to 100 hours of basic education and are only required to have approximately 1 hour of continuing education per month. A study conducted by Harrington et al. (2000) indicated that inadequate training was one of two basic explanations why nursing homes in the United States do not provide high-quality care. As a group, CNAs are undertrained, underappreciated, underpaid, and overworked; all of these factors impact the quality of care of residents.

Unfortunately people who train CNAs fail to provide them with consistent strategies for communicating with people with AD. Furthermore, CNAs who have received training on communication strategies commonly fail to use them, most likely because of the training methods that were employed. Research indicates that the best methods for improving communication between CNAs and people with AD are "doing methods," such as demonstrations, role playing, and case studies. Visualization and active participation assist in removal of many learning barriers (Pietro, 2002). Unlike real life, role-playing can always be repeated or redone to improve performance. Training must be ongoing and positively reinforced.

TOUCH THERAPY

Touch has been considered a fundamental component of nursing care for centuries. Think about how many times you physically touch someone and how many times someone else may physically touch you as part of performing your routine nursing activities. Each of these physical encounters may hold a different meaning to you, based on who touched you, where you were touched, where the touching took place, and your state of mind at the time of being touched.

When you touch a patient as part of your caring, each incidence carries with it some meaning. Physical touch in caring can have meaning on several different levels: spiritual, physical, emotional, and social. For example, to the patient, it may convey the meaning "I am being comforting" or "I am relating to you." Touch may also be used to gain someone's attention.

Touching older adults generally produces positive feelings. Touch is a form of communication between the participants and is the most frequently used behavior in relationships between people (Chang, 2001). Older adults commonly respond to touch when there have not been any shared vocalizations, and many times they respond more to touch than to verbal communications (Butts, 2001).

In communicating with a patient with AD, touch becomes even more meaningful and significant (Butts, 2001). As people grow older, they long to be touched by other caring people. When verbal skills are impaired or changed, touch becomes even more important. Proper touching should follow these guidelines:

- Before touching a patient, the patient must see the person making the contact.

- The patient should not be startled with a sudden touch. Touch gradually while looking for a reaction. It should be noted whether the patient pulls away or changes position. This reaction may indicate that the touch is not pleasurable.

- A light touch is usually considered a stimulant.

- A firm touch is calming and can be reassuring.

- Touching is more agreeable on certain areas of the body than on other areas. One area that is easily touched and on which touching is calming is the upper arm, between the shoulder and elbow.

Touching patients who have dementia can also produce unexpected reactions. They may become angry or even sexually aroused. This reaction does not mean that the touching was wrong. The caregiver must remain calm and distract the patient. When disease involves the brain, as with AD, misinterpretations can occur, but do not avoid touching simply because it might be misunderstood. Touching builds trust and communication, prevents feelings of isolation and loneliness, and enhances older adults' senses of well-being and self-regard (Butts, 2001; Gwyther, 2001).

HUMOR THERAPY

Laughter is like changing a baby's diaper; it doesn't permanently solve any problems, but it makes things more acceptable for a while.

—*Ashleigh Brilliant* (1981)

The medical and educational worlds have been relatively intolerant of humor. According to one story, a nurse-educator was walking down a hallway one day outside a classroom full of nursing students. The students burst out laughing and continued laughing for several minutes. The instructor commented to another much younger nursing instructor, "There can not be anything productive going on in there; listen to them laugh." However, the attitude of health care and education toward humor has another side, an openness and flexibility that have been recognized since ancient times.

The Humor Project, Inc. (www.humorproject.com) has been taking humor seriously since 1977 (Goodman, 2001). The creator of this organization's website suggests four tips for helping people take humor "seriously:"

1) Put humor into the physical environment. Use posters and other visual displays.

2) Use humor as a tool rather than a weapon. One teacher put it this way, "You don't have to blow out my candle to make yours glow brighter." Humor can be appropriate, timely, and tasteful.

3) Build humor into the workplace. Be creative and model humor.

4) Humor's bottom line: Work should not be boring or dull; it should be fun. If it is not fun, what a waste that is. Set the tone by "telling stories on yourself." Some people have the ability to tell stories about some event that could have been serious but, because of the way the story is told, it becomes obvious that the storyteller was able to "roll with one of life's punches."

Probably the most dramatic and well-documented event in recent history that brought humor into the spotlight for health care was the illness of Norman Cousins (Dossey, 1996). In 1964, after being diagnosed with ankylosing spondylitis, a crippling and painful disease that causes severe inflammation of the spine and joints, Cousins checked out of the hospital and into a hotel. He spent the time in the hotel studying the relationship between psychological stress and certain diseases and watching Laurel and Hardy films, the Marx Brothers, and clips from the television show *Candid Camera.* In 1989, in his book *Head First: The Biology of Hope,* Cousins speculated on how he literally laughed himself back to health. As a result, a new specialty — humor therapy — was born.

Patty Wooten (1996), a nurse who is an expert in the field of therapeutic humor and the founder of *Jest for the Health of It Services,* has researched the role of humor, specifically how it can be used to help nurses develop a greater sense of control to overcome professional burnout. After a 6-hour humor training course, she found, "If one is encouraged and guided to use humor, one can gain a sense of control in your life."

Because of the seriousness of their work, nurses may have difficulty staying in touch with the playful, childlike nature within themselves. Caring for patients with AD is often stressful. Feeling out of control is a natural tendency. Although nurses cannot always control the situations presented to them, they can control their reactions to the situations (Laurenhue, 1996).

One of the goals of humor therapy for nurses is to try to understand where other people are coming from. First, nurses must understand themselves and become aware of the choices they make every day. This is the first step in taking responsibility. Being conscious of what they are doing brings people's values and actions into congruence (see Table 3-2). Developing a sense of humor is easier when people feel good about themselves.

The most important part of understanding another person's perspective is to realize that all

TABLE 3-2: 50 EXCUSES FOR A CLOSED MIND (OR HOW TO KILL AN IDEA!)

1. We tried that before.
2. Our place is different.
3. It costs too much.
4. That's beyond our responsibility.
5. We're too busy.
6. That's not my job.
7. It's too radical a change.
8. Not enough time.
9. Not enough help.
10. That will make our equipment obsolete.
11. Our organization is too small.
12. Not practical.
13. The staff will never buy it.
14. It's against company policy.
15. We've never done it before.
16. Runs up our overhead.
17. We don't have the authority.
18. That's too ivory tower.
19. Let's get back to reality.
20. That's not our problem.
21. If it ain't broke, why fix it?
22. You're right but...
23. You're 2 years ahead of your time.
24. We're not ready for that.
25. We've always done it this way. Why change now?
26. No room or equipment.
27. Not enough staff.
28. No budget.
29. Can't teach an old dog new tricks.
30. Good thought, but impractical.
31. Let's give it more thought.
32. Let's hold it in abeyance.
33. Put it in writing.
34. They will laugh at us.
35. Not that again.
36. Where did you dig that one up?
37. That's what to expect from staff.
38. We did all right without it.
39. It's never been tried before.
40. Let's form a committee or task force.
41. Has anyone else tried it?
42. I don't see the connection.
43. It won't work.
44. What you're really saying is...
45. Maybe that will work in your department, but not mine.
46. Let's all sleep on it.
47. I know a fellow who tried it.
48. Too much trouble to change.
49. It's impossible.
50. Your own excuse!!!

Note. From *Stepping Out: Stepping Out of the Box – Jump Starting Your Creativity,* by S. Boyd (susan-boyd.com), 1999. Retrieved September 20, 2004 from http://www.fluidpowerjournal.com. Reprinted with permission from Susan Boyd.

behavior has meaning. Nurses can use their senses of humor to add enjoyment to the lives of patients who have AD. For patients who have dementia, body language and tone of voice carry more importance than do words.

Here are some suggestions for incorporating humor into your life and your care:

- Turn off the television and socialize. People laugh 30 times more often in a social setting than they do alone.

- Learn something new. Try an activity, such as in-line skating, that you may not excel at, and try it with someone you like.

- Choose your friends carefully. A friend you laugh with is a treasure. Unload the duds and cultivate the gems.

- Do not be lazy. It is not a bother to make the extra effort to be silly or funny. Make wisecracks or use puns.

- Cultivate running jokes. When you find yourself in a moment of shared hilarity, make the most of it. Repeat it, and keep laughing.

- Master the art of comic complaining. Exaggerate and overstate. Poke fun at yourself.

- Share the joke. When you hear or read something funny, pass it along and laugh all over again.

- Get a pet. Stupid pet tricks launched David Letterman's career. Cats and dogs crack people up and do not have to be trained to be funny.

- Start the day with a laugh. Fifteen minutes of cartoons can set the silliness mood for the rest of the day.

- Avoid humor that might offend others, such as off-color jokes or humor targeted at a person's race, illness, or ethnicity.

- Avoid tasteless and morbid humor.

- Avoid slang terms or expressions that might not be understood.

Preschoolers laugh an average of 400 times per day. Adults laugh an average of 15 times per day. Many nurses are their own worst enemies, constantly ridiculing themselves for real or imagined mistakes as they enter a "serious" profession such as nursing. Studies have shown that most people say four times as many bad things as good things about themselves. People who are in control can control their reactions to behavior that is bizarre or not easily understood, even when the situation cannot be controlled. People's thoughts, feelings, and behaviors are all within their control. As Ashleigh Brilliant (1981) said, "We have only two things to worry about: either things will get back to normal, or that they already have."

Older people and those with dementia have the capacity to appreciate and respond to humor (Bethea, Travis, & Pecchioni, 2000; Davidhizar & Bowen, 1992; Ewers, 1983; Williams, 1986), and small-group humor therapy has been shown to reduce agitation in nursing home residents with dementia (Watson et al., 1997).

The use of humor by spousal AD caregivers and adult children of frail older adults is an interesting phenomenon. They frequently include smiles, jokes, and "punch lines" in their stories of behavioral problems. They also use humor to describe the role rever-sal that so frequently accompanies caring for parents with dementia (Bethea, Travis, & Pecchioni, 2000).

Pollmann (1999) found:

- humor is an essential and energizing force in AD caregiving

- humor is not perceived as appropriate in early stages of AD but, as adaptation occurs, humor is valued

- a positive attitude and a sense of humor create joy of the moment

- humor enables caregivers to approach difficult situations with a feeling of being in control.

From a scientific perspective, no one has ever satisfactorily explained why humans have the capacity to laugh. Nevertheless, humans do laugh, and laughter appears to have physiological benefits for nurses, patients, and their family members and caregivers. Since Florence Nightingale first started nursing, humor has been a vital part of the nursing practice. More studies are needed to understand how laughter works; to determine if it affects the immune system or longevity, as has been suggested; and to measure the significance and efficacy of humor as a therapeutic approach. One truth that is known about laughter is that it produces physiological affects such as endorphin release which, in turn, decreases levels of pain. (Jech, 2002; Mooney, 2000; Orhon, 2002; Roach, 1996; Southam, 2003).

SUMMARY

Patients with dementia experience life in the moment and being in the moment is often the key to communicating with and understanding them. Communication is the most important technique for enhancing a loving relationship, and lack of communication is destructive to a loving relationship. Obstacles to communication when caring for someone with dementia can be difficult, overwhelming, and frustrating. As the functional status of people with AD declines, their ability to express themselves decreases. Nurses must find strategies to enhance communication with these patients.

An ever-increasing body of knowledge allows us to understand the subjective experiences of people with AD. Interestingly enough, one of the lingering characteristics of people with AD is their value and use of humor and hope. This offers nurses another area to explore for enhancing communication. Humor is also an effective therapeutic tool for nurses who deal with the stress of working with people with AD.

EXAM QUESTIONS

CHAPTER 3
Questions 21-30

21. Communication problems during the early stage of AD include

    a. short term memory loss and difficulty naming things.

    b. short term memory loss and complete loss of speech.

    c. long term memory loss and use of a repetitive phrase.

    d. extreme disorientation and social withdrawal.

22. Communication with patients with AD can be optimized if you

    a. use neutral tones and a gentle, relaxed pace.

    b. speak quickly to avoid distractions.

    c. do not touch patients with AD.

    d. ignore questions.

23. Recent research has likened communication with people with AD to "building" a quilt. Important strategies to use in building a conversation are

    a. listening to the stories the person is trying to tell, envisioning them, and keeping thorough records of the stories.

    b. not waiting for the person to finish their story if you know a part of it and can add to it.

    c. making up stories so all staff members know the same stories.

    d. ignoring the stories because they change all the time.

24. Your patient with AD has repeatedly asked you when her husband will be coming to visit. Your best response to these questions is to

    a. tell her that her husband died 2 years ago and will not be coming to visit.

    b. take her for a walk and talk about the flowers and trees outside.

    c. call her daughter so she can inform the patient that her husband is not coming.

    d. always use the same intervention for repeated questions.

25. A helpful intervention when communicating with patients with AD is to

    a. use figures of speech such as "hop into bed" to simplify language.

    b. listen to what is said and seek out what is unspoken.

    c. ask the patient if they remember your name with each interaction.

    d. avoid guessing, if the patient is stuck on a word.

26. Touching an older adult has been shown to

    a. instill negative self-esteem.

    b. produce negative feelings.

    c. replace verbal communication.

    d. be a stimulant or calming influence.

27. A correct statement about humor as therapy is

    a. no one can explain why humans laugh.

    b. most people say more good things than
       bad things about themselves.

    c. people should not repeat things that poke
       fun at themselves.

    d. nurses do not need to worry about the
       meaning of behaviors.

28. Patty Wooten, a nurse humorist, has done
    research on the use of humor and

    a. caring for patients with AD.

    b. overcoming burnout in nursing jobs.

    c. the relationship between stress and cardiac
       illnesses.

    d. controlling the values a nurse takes into an
       intensive care unit.

29. One appropriate way that a nurse can
    incorporate humor into one's life is to

    a. read about and increase one's morbid
       humor.

    b. increase knowledge of humor slang.

    c. avoid using humor directed at oneself as it
       can be offensive.

    d. start the day with a laugh.

30. Research on the use of humor with people
    with AD shows that

    a. humor increases agitation in nursing home
       residents with dementia.

    b. humor enables caregivers to feel in-control
       during difficult situations.

    c. people with dementia do not have the
       capacity to appreciate or respond to humor.

    d. humor is associated with underlying
       depression and should be avoided.

CHAPTER 4

NUTRITION AND INCONTINENCE

CHAPTER OBJECTIVE

After completing this chapter, the reader will be able to discuss the nursing process for incontinence and nutritional concerns in patients with Alzheimer's disease (AD).

LEARNING OBJECTIVES

After studying this chapter, the reader will be able to

1. indicate the importance of interpreting the nutritional status of people with AD and recognize barriers to adequate nutrition in nursing facilities.

2. recognize the types of malnutrition found among older adults and evaluate the influence of each on the outcomes of people with AD.

3. summarize how the four A's of AD influence nutrition.

4. discuss the prevalence and risk factors of urinary incontinence.

5. identify the types of persistent urinary incontinence, their associated signs and symptoms, and their impact on quality of life.

6. discuss treatment options for urinary incontinence.

INTRODUCTION

What nurses do evolves from the nursing process, the problem solving process that forms the basis for nursing actions. Once a problem is clearly delineated, the solutions become evident. The nursing process is holistic and does not represent a simple cause-and-effect relationship. One need or concern affects every other need or problem. The nursing process does not deal simply with the physiological or psychological needs of patients with dementing conditions. Needs are overlapping and involve the whole person.

This chapter describes best practice interventions that can be used to meet nutritional and incontinence needs of patients with dementia. The strategies discussed are not all-encompassing but indicate what has worked best for others.

NUTRITION

Food is more than just something to eat. It turns a meal into a sensory and social transaction that brings quality to the life of any person, especially one with dementia. According to estimates, 85% of elderly patients in nursing homes and hospitals are malnourished. No one is deliberately starving these individuals, but elderly people may forget to eat or may be too tired to eat without some kind of intervention. Malnourishment results in fatigue; increased confusion; greater risk of infections; mus-

#31

cle wasting; skin breakdown due to thinning, shearing, or tearing; and poor wound healing.

Nutritional Status of Older Adults

Here are some statistics related to the nutritional status of older adults:

- An estimated 31% of males and 61% of females older than age 65 have incomes of $10,000 or less annually. This low income adversely impacts access to food and food choices.

- Among people age 75 and older, 40% of men and 30% of women are at least 10% underweight.

- Nearly half of people age 65 and older are clinically malnourished at the time of admission to a hospital, and two-thirds are malnourished at the time of discharge.

(Allen, 2002)

Evaluating Nutritional Status

As AD progresses, the need for assessment of nutritional status and for assistance with eating increases. Nutritional assessment includes keeping a diary of food intake, a weight history (including the patient's previous usual body weight, not just weight related to height), and monitoring weight and height during a specified interval. For example, Mr. Wheeler was 6' (1.8 m) tall and weighed 155 lb (70 kg) at the time of his assessment. Conversations with his wife revealed that although this weight was below the norm for his height, he had weighed between 155 and 165 pounds (70 and 75 kg) for the previous 15 years, making this weight his usual body weight.

Physical assessment should focus on tracking weights and changes in those weights, to include skin turgor, skin lesions (especially pressure and non-healing ulcers), changes in skin color, thin or brittle hair, muscle wasting, oral status (including loose teeth or poorly fitting dentures), fissures around the mouth, enlarged, smooth, or beefy red tongue, and poor hygiene.

The nurse must also pay special attention to cultural, ethnic, or religious preferences. In many care settings nutritional assessments consist primarily of obtaining a 24-hour dietary recall with patient or caregiver, and these by themselves are insufficient in the assessment process. Remember that families determine traditions and rituals that surround eating. It is very helpful for caregivers to understand these rituals and traditions and then try to work within these individual practices. These can include: a) rituals used before meals; b) religious rites or prohibitions; and cultural or special cues to eating.

In clinical settings, the serum level of albumin is a useful indicator of a patient's protein status; less than 3.5 mg/dl is considered indicative of depletion of visceral protein storage (Morley & Omran, 2001). Although hemoglobin level and hematocrit are typically used to measure iron status, they are also useful indicators of anemia caused by folate or protein deficiency. Hemoglobin levels less than 12 g/dl and hematocrit less than 35 ml/dl indicate severe anemia in elderly women (more common in women than in men). These measures do not present a complete nutritional picture, yet they are easy to evaluate. If a specific nutrient deficiency is suspected, additional studies can be done. Because patients with AD are at high risk for nutritional deficiencies, additional evaluation by a registered dietitian may be indicated.

Even though 55% of geriatric inpatients have protein-calorie undernutrition, most cases of this condition are never diagnosed or treated (Sarkisian & Lachs, 1996). Protein-calorie malnutrition, which is associated with famine in developing countries, can occur in institutionalized elderly people who take in too little protein, too few calories, or both for too long (Womack & Breeding, 1998).

Several studies have looked at the barriers to adequate nutrition for residents in nursing facilities (Abbasi & Rudman, 1994; Crogan, Shultz, Adams, & Massey, 2001). The findings suggest that food service issues, such as residents not liking the food served or the food not looking good to eat, may also play a role. In addition, lack of assistance from nursing assistants, lack of time to assist, and poor education on methods of helping residents negatively impact the nutritional status of residents. According to the research, nurses rely on nursing assistants to identify and report problems with eating, chewing, and swallowing; however, nursing assistants do not feel they are qualified or have time to communicate this type of information.

All nutritional deficiencies are less easily detected in elderly people than in younger people. Diseases and the medications used to treat them, plus the process of aging itself, can modify biochemical standards used to assess nutritional status. (See Figure 4-1.) For instance, kidney or liver damage can potentially affect albumin levels and diminish the value of albumin assays as a tool (although measurement of serum albumin level remains the most practical laboratory test to evaluate body reserves of protein).

Change in body weight, loss or gain, is still the most significant indicator of nutritional status in the elderly, particularly in patients with dementia who wander. In one study, loss of weight was judged to be a substantial concern for patients with AD. Those with AD lost 21% more weight than patients without dementia (Thomas, 1995). Calorie depletion is high during wandering, and patients who wander are less able than other patients to sit still long enough to eat a meal. Thus, weight loss is critical.

Weight loss is a common finding among residents in long-term care facilities (LTCFs). It is associated with higher rates of death, length of hospitalization, infections, and falls. Keller, Gibbs, Boudreau, Goy, Pattillo, and Brown (2003) conducted a study to determine whether body weight can be maintained or improved in dementia residents of special care units (SCUs) using a comprehensive nutrition intervention strategy. The intervention, which included consulting a dietitian and individual menu changes, significantly promoted weight gain in comparison with standard treat-

ment. Factors such as pacing, type of dementia, sex, age, number of comorbid conditions, and medications were significant predictors of weight change. Weight gain or maintenance, regardless of facility site, was associated with survival. Body weight can be maintained in residents of SCUs regardless of pacing and other clinical characteristics.

According to the Centers for Medicare and Medicaid Services (CMS) (2002b), formerly the Health Care Financing Administration, weight loss among nursing home residents is significant when it reaches the following levels of loss: 5.0% of body weight in 1 month, 7.5% in 3 months, or 10.0% in 6 months. These losses may reflect changes in diet, activity, metabolism, or ability to eat or swallow food. Obesity can also be a sign of malnutrition. Weight that is 20% above or 10% percent below desirable values for height may be associated with poor nutritional outcomes. However, recent studies have documented that the best or ideal body weight for older adults older than age 65 may be 10% to 20% above the weights listed on standard height and weight tables. According to the Nutrition Screening Initiative from the Administration on Aging (2002), older people whose weights were 30% above the listed weights had better outcomes if they became ill than those who were 10% below the average. This finding reflects a growing awareness of the impact of adequate nutrition and body weight on health consequences.

Causes of Malnutrition in Older Adults

Many older people live alone or with a dependent spouse and are unable to get around as easily as they once did. This can prevent them from meeting their nutritional needs. Financial problems also lead to nutritional deficits and malnutrition. Malnutrition has been reported to affect as much as 60% of the older adult population in the United States, including those who live in the community, nursing homes, and hospitals. Malnutrition worsens frailty and loss of function in older adults. This can lead to greater worry and apprehension by family

FIGURE 4-1: EVALUATION OF THE OLDER ADULT WHO IS FAILING IN THE COMMUNITY

Systematic Identification and Measurement of Commonly Impaired Domains

Impaired Physical Functioning	Malnutrition	Depression	Cognitive Impairment
• Activities of daily living • Instrumental activities of daily living • Performance measures	• Weight • Weight trend • Albumin • Cholesterol	• Geriatric Depression Scale • Center for Epidemiologic Studies Depression Scale • Geropsychiatry evaluation if warranted	• Mini-Mental Status Examination • Exclude delirium • Diagnostic algorithms

Contributors Unique to Each Domain

• Specific neurologic and visual disorders • Specific musculoskeletal disorders • Shoes or podiatric problems • Environmental obstacles • Caregiver ability • Comorbid conditions • Medications	• Changes in food preference • Ill-fitting dentures • Other dental problems • Speech or swallowing problems • Financial or social problems	• Bereavement • Decreasing socialization • Shrinking social network • Depressive history • Response to illness	• Specific causes of dementia • Risk factors for delerium • Attention to reversible causes

Contributors Common to All Domain

- Impairments in any or all of the other three domains
- Established chronic diseases that are decompensating
- New, unrecognized medical illness (infection, cancer, endocrine disease, cardiovascular disease)
- Medications
- Visual and/or hearing impairment
- Pain
- Environmental factors
- Elder abuse and neglect
- Social dysfunction

Consider the Interaction of Impairments at All Levels

Note. From "'Failure to thrive' in older adults." by C.A. Sarkisian & M.S. Lachs, 1996, *Annals of Internal Medicine, 124*(12), 1072-78. Reprinted with permission.

members as well as additional time and energy spent on the care of older adults (Abbasi & Rudman, 1994; Seiler, 2001)

Malnutrition among the elderly in nursing homes and other LTCFs can lead to death or chronic disability. Specifically, research shows evidence of widespread protein-calorie malnutrition, which implies that many nursing home residents have inadequate food intake. Dementia, depression, social deprivation, and loneliness can contribute to the lack of desire to eat or prepare food.

Malnutrition in elderly people is defined as an inadequate nutritional status or undernourishment, characterized by insufficient dietary intake, poor appetite, muscle wasting, and weight loss. In the elderly, malnutrition is an ominous sign. Malnutrition can be brought on by such personal issues as loss, dependency, loneliness, and chronic illness, which commonly impact morbidity, mortality, and quality of life. Elderly patients with unintentional weight loss are at higher risk for infection, depression, and death. The leading causes of involuntary weight loss are depression (especially in residents of LTCFs), cancer (lung and gastrointestinal malignancies), cardiac disorders, and benign gastrointestinal diseases. All of these conditions can lead to decreased immunity against diseases. Management is directed at treating underlying causes and providing nutritional support. Consideration should be given to the patient's environment and interest in and ability to eat food. Nutritional deficits have also been shown to contribute to diseases in which memory failure is a major symptom (Lutz & Przytulski, 2001).

Failure to Thrive

Weight loss in older adults is often associated with failure to thrive (FTT). A comprehensive evaluation should include exploration of physical, functional, social, and emotional problems, and initial treatment should focus on eradicating any identified problems. In addition, it is essential to evaluate

motivation to eat and, if necessary, implement interventions to strengthen motivation and thereby improve oral intake.

The term "failure to thrive" was exported from pediatrics in the 1970s and is used to describe older adults with various concurrent chronic diseases, functional impairments, or both. Despite this heterogeneity, FTT has had its own International Classification of Diseases, Ninth Revision, (ICD-9) code since 1979 and has been approached as a clinically meaningful diagnosis in many review articles. Lonergan (1991) reported that in 1991 the National Institute on Aging described FTT as "a syndrome of weight loss, decreased appetite and poor nutrition, and inactivity, often accompanied by dehydration, depressive symptoms, impaired immune function, and low cholesterol" (Lonergan, 1991). This conceptual framework, however, can create barriers to proper evaluation and management. The most worrisome of these barriers is the reinforcement of both fatalism and intellectual laziness. These concepts need to be balanced with a deconstructionist approach, wherein the major areas of impairment are identified and quantified and their interactions are considered.

The evaluation and management of individuals with FTT is extremely challenging. In the elderly, FTT is characterized by a gradual decline in physical or cognitive function (Resnick, 2001). Typically, the patient's decline comprises deteriorating social competence, weight loss, loss of appetite, increasing frailty, and diminishing initiative, concentration, and drive. This general failure of older people is all too commonly blamed on "old age" or senility or is regarded as a dementing process and, therefore, the physical basis is overlooked.

Some contributors to FTT are unmodifiable, some are easily modifiable, and some are potentially modifiable but only with the use of resource-intensive strategies. Factors that contribute to FTT include protein-energy undernutrition, loss of muscle mass (sarcopenia), problems with balance and endurance, declining cognition, and depression. It occurs near the end of life in older adults whose independence is declining. FTT is associated with morbidity and, in some cases, imminent mortality (Verdery, 1995; Sarkisian & Lachs, 1996).

Poor nutritional status is an essential feature of FTT. The presence of malnutrition is one of four elements upon which a diagnosis of FTT is based (Osato, Stone, Phillips, & Winne, 1993; Sarkisian & Lachs, 1996). Serum albumin levels of patients with FTT averaged 3.2 g/dl (range 2.1 to 4.2 g/dl) on hospital admission (Osato et al., 1993). Many clinicians indicate that the presence of FTT mandates an aggressive search for the cause. Obviously, the diagnosis of FTT is not made unless all other potential underlying causes for the condition have been systematically eliminated.

Leading geriatric authorities have expressed that the term FTT should be abandoned as a diagnostic entity because this label can be stigmatizing and, at the least, distracts the clinician from a systematic evaluation of the combination of interacting deficits known to be prevalent in patients who are said to have FTT, including: impaired physical functioning, malnutrition, depression, and cognitive impairment. Like many problems in geriatric medicine, FTT is more clinically approachable when broken down into measurable domains.

As previously mentioned, FTT can eventually lead to death. As Sarkisian and Lachs (1996) noted, "a high proportion of all deaths in old age were preceded by a period of 'pre-death,' during which the patient was unable to care for himself in consequence of loss of mobility, incontinence, or mental abnormality... It seems that many of those who survive into old age enter a phase of 'pre-death,' in which they outlive the vigor of their bodies and the wisdom of their brains" (Sarkisian & Lachs, 1996, p. 1073). It is therefore helpful to review the synonyms associated with pre-death (see Table 4-1).

TABLE 4-1: PREDEATH SYNONYMS
• The individual dwindles and fails to maintain current status
• Failure of the physical person and the psychosocial person
• Biopsychosocial failure
• Asthenia-cachexia syndrome
• Person wastes away
• End-stage frailty
• Taking to their bed
(Sarkisian & Lachs, 1996)

Physiological Changes and Nutrition

One of the normal physiological changes of aging is a decline in the senses of taste and smell. These senses help protect us from noxious agents found in foods and the environment. Chronic diseases and acute conditions, such as Parkinson's disease, diabetes mellitus, AD, and others, can affect ability to taste and smell. Some medications can also interfere with these senses as well as decrease appetite.

People with AD have a reduction in saliva, the vicid fluid that carries the enzymes that break down foods, assists in tasting and smelling foods, and starts the digestive process. Sensitivity to taste and smell usually decreases with age. About one-third to one-half of a person's taste buds stop functioning by age 70. As a person ages, sensory receptor cells in the nose and on the tongue are replaced less often. Reduced taste and smell sensations can also be the result of dental problems and treatments, including oral trauma, dry mouth, periodontal (gum and bone) disease, burning mouth syndrome, and denture-related inflammations.

Everyday items associated with a decrease in taste, smell, and appetite include full or partial dentures, over-the-counter preparations such as toothpastes, denture adhesives and cleansers, and mouthwashes. The taste loss some individuals experience may be the result of their life experiences, such as smoking or eating spicy foods.

Anorexia, which is characterized by a disinterest in eating, can have multiple causes in older adults. One of the main causes of anorexia in the older adult population is medications. Anorexia in older adults can be a direct result of medications. It is important to understand the side effects of medications, which can include dehydration, early satiety, loss of appetite, nausea and vomiting, and altered sense of taste. Commonly prescribed medications that cause these effects include most diuretics, digoxin, selective serotonin reuptake inhibitors, antidepressants, chemotherapeutic agents, and certain antibiotics.

Attention to food preferences is critical in revitalizing appetite and improving eating skills. Overeating, not eating at all, or taking food from others is not uncommon for people with AD. Patients with dementia may have delusions about food and eating, including fears related to shapes and consistencies, and nurses must be aware and tolerant. Loss of appetite can be due to medical causes of anorexia, such as dental problems and nausea. Always suspect depression when you cannot explain anorexia in an older adult. Anorexia is the hallmark sign of depression in older adults and should always be investigated. Start by simply asking the person if he or she feels sad. A number of geriatric depression scales can also be used. One that is frequently used is the Geriatric Depression Scale by Sheikh and Yesavage (1985). (See pg. 25.)

More than 250 drugs have been implicated in decreased taste sensations. These include:

- cholesterol-lowering drugs
- antihistamines
- anticancer medications
- asthma medications
- antihypertensives
- certain cardiac medications
- muscle relaxants
- antidepressants
- anticonvulsants.

Comparisons of healthy elderly individuals and their younger counterparts show that the threshold (minimal amount of stimulation) in each taste category is higher in the older subjects. The threshold for sweet taste is 3 times higher; salt detection, 11 times; acid detection, more than 4 times; and bitter tastes, almost 7 times. Also keep in mind that the threshold rises as disease processes interfere with normal functioning; for example, an older person might not be able to smell or taste mashed potatoes with satisfaction but might be able to taste lemon meringue pie.

Poor nutrition also affects fluid and electrolyte balance. Adequate intake of fluid is important in patients with dementia. Dehydration can be caused by excess loss of water, failure to recognize the need for water, or inability to drink or swallow water. Older people are at increased risk for dehydration due to normal physiological changes of aging, including increased fat and decreased lean body mass associated with decreased total body water (DiMaria-Ghalili, 2002). Early signs of dehydration are weight loss and dark or concentrated urine. Signs of increased confusion, agitation, or lethargy may also be present. Observable signs include a dry cracked tongue or lips, sunken eyes, and increased pulse rate.

Fluids should be offered often during the day, because active patients with dementia may forget to drink. The methods used to administer fluids to patients in hospitals and nursing homes can be problematic. Pitchers or jugs at the bedside are inconvenient and are often too heavy or bulky for frail elderly people to handle. Some nursing facilities are now setting up systems of best nursing practices to offer and give fluids in ways that more closely resemble how most people get fluids at home and at work using smaller, individual water bottles that are refilled frequently.

In patients with serious protein loss, fluids can shift into the tissues, causing edema. Edema increases the risk of pressure ulcers. Anemia reduces the amount of oxygen available to the tissues for metabolism and, therefore, also impairs healing. This situation is not good for anyone but is especially dangerous for people with AD who cannot follow instructions or assist in their care.

Pica activity is common in AD. Patients with this condition place objects of all kinds in their mouths, such as beads, flowers, and hearing aides. They may even swallow the objects. Patients who exhibit pica behavior should be checked often for foreign objects in the mouth or throat.

Signs and Symptoms of Nutritional Deficiencies and Dehydration

The following signs and symptoms may indicate the presence of a nutritional deficiency or dehydration:

- decreased skin turgor (elasticity)
- furrowed tongue
- elevated temperature
- elevated pulse
- weakness
- confusion.

Four A's of AD and Nutrition

You may recall from chapter 2 that another way of looking at cognitive impairment that has been helpful to health care providers is the four A's: apraxia, agnosia, aphasia, and amnesia. These areas of loss also influence nutrition. Aphasia keeps the person from being able to verbally express food preferences. Apraxia (inability to carry out voluntary muscular activities) makes manipulation of utensils and swallowing difficult. When agnosia is present, individuals cannot recognize familiar items because sensory cuing is limited. Lastly, amnesia causes people with AD to forget that they have eaten or reduces the ability to recognize the need to eat (Amella, 2003).

Plan care to maximize improving nutritional intake and self-feeding for older adults while identifying contextual factors that contribute to optimal dining experiences. Plan mealtime care for an older individual with cognitive or physical impairments. As health care providers, nurses must assist with increasing food intake in people who are currently malnourished or who are at high risk for decreased nutritional intake.

Physical and Cognitive Limitations

Individual assessment must include observation of eating habits. As a patient's ability to perform the activities involved in eating declines, supervision of eating and reassessment is necessary. Patients in the advanced stages of AD have difficulty remembering the steps needed to bring food to the mouth, chew it, and swallow it. Be sure to assess the types of foods eaten, when eating occurs, and what utensils are able to be manipulated. Many individuals have physical limitations, and numerous methods and cues can be employed to assist in the mechanics of eating. You can cue individuals by placing your hand over their's and reminding them of a self-feeding routine. Pantomime or gestures can also be valuable tools.

Self-feeding can be encouraged by honoring food preferences and by providing finger foods (make sure that these items truly are finger foods). Restrictive diets should be avoided. Proper eating should not be expected. If patients want to eat dessert first, allow them to do so. High-calorie foods that are nutrient dense (have more nutrients in a smaller amount of food), such as a super cereals and fortified puddings or soups, should be offered. Patients should be encouraged to eat at their own pace, and one-to-one supervision should be provided if necessary. Several small feedings per day may increase intake. A brainstorming care conference can be a wonderful venue to come up with creative ways of improving nutrition.

An early sign of being unable to chew or swallow is the holding of food in the mouth. Studies have helped to define the broad range of issues related to individuals with dementia and swallowing or chewing (Kayser-Jones & Pengilly, 1999; Micelli, 1999). Dysphagia that goes unrecognized by nursing staff can lead to:

- improper positioning at mealtimes (such as eating while partially reclined in bed)

- inappropriate feeding, such as large bites of food and rapid feeding

- food and liquids of the wrong consistency being offered

- labeling of the patient as "difficult," "combative," "uncooperative," or "noncompliant" when food is refused.

Pureeing or chopping food and slowing down and feeding smaller amounts may help. In the advanced stages of AD, patients may completely lose the ability to chew or swallow. At this time, critical decisions must be made about providing nourishment through feeding tubes. Available data have failed to show that tube feeding is effective in thin, ill, demented people (Newsview, 2001). There have been no increases in overall survival rates of AD patients after placement of a feeding tube. A decrease in aspiration pneumonia and pressure ulcer healing have not proven to be positive effects of placing feeding tubes in demented elderly patients. A Newsview article (2001) stresses that other factors; including administrative convenience, reimbursement, and liability issues are more likely to affect feeding tube placement. Patience, skill, consistency, and an awareness of the patient's needs can have a significant impact on how soon, or if, the decision must be made.

Suggestions for Feeding Patients With AD

Here are some tips that can help improve your success with feeding patients who have AD:

- Patients should be in a sitting position to facilitate swallowing and prevent choking.

- Give patients finger foods to enable independent feeding, and allow patients who pace to eat while walking.

- Provide foods that are preferred and well-liked by the patient. A restrictive diet is unnecessary.

- Serve foods with strong flavors hot or cold, rather than tepid, to increase appeal.

- Enrich foods with fortified milk (powdered milk mixed with whole milk).

- Offer liquid supplements to increase calories. Instant-breakfast drinks mixed with ice cream are commonly more appealing than commercial types.

- Evaluate patients for other illnesses, responses to new medications, or depression if a change in appetite is noted.

- Increase the amount of personal assistance available by using volunteers or other family members.

- Decrease distractions and make the surroundings pleasant and calming. Feed patients as soon as they are seated and play their favorite music.

- Offer courses separately with only the needed utensils to avoid overwhelming patients.

As the person with AD develops difficulty swallowing, follow these guidelines:

- Stimulate opening of the mouth by brushing the spoon against the lips.

- Place food and fluids well into the mouth.

- Give only small boluses of food at one time.

- Offer frequent reminders of the expected behavior (for example, say, "Open your mouth, chew the food, and swallow.") because people with AD can forget that they are eating.

- Use facilitation techniques, such as gently brushing the cheeks and neck, to encourage swallowing.

- Encourage patients to cough gently after each swallow to assure the throat is clear.

- Have food ready after each swallow.

If you discover insufficient caloric intake in your nutritional assessment, you must then devise a plan to increase calorie intake. You may find that some older people are unable to express their individual preferences. In this case, ask family members and other staff members about the patient's likes and dislikes for particular foods. An additional reason for insufficient caloric intake is that memory losses may cause older adults to forget they have eaten. These memory losses may also lead to frequent inquiries about when they will eat by some of those who have forgotten when they last ate.

Many older adults suffer a tremendous amount of pain throughout the day. Offer pain medications prior to meals to improve functioning and thus increase nutritional intake. Never use a syringe to feed an individual. If the person requires a syringe feeding to bypass a swallowing or chewing problem, he or she most likely has a neuromuscular deficit in need of intervention from a specialist.

Because patients with AD cannot realistically perceive the environment, some modifications must be made. For example, to prevent burns, food should not be served too hot to put into the mouth. This problem is more likely to occur in the home. A quiet, well-lit setting for meals should be provided. Fewer distractions increase the likelihood of food consumption. Because darker colors are often perceived as a "stop" signal, white or light-colored plates and bowls with little or no pattern should be used.

Other suggestions for meal preparation and serving include:

- deboning meats
- not using individual packets for condiments or small containers of cream or butter
- pouring milk into a glass rather than leaving it in the carton and not providing straws unless specifically indicated
- serving rolls rather than slices of bread
- serving soup in cups or mugs rather than in bowls.

- unwrapping napkins if they are wrapped in plastic.

In later stages of the disease, the following practices are recommended:

- Serve decaffeinated coffee unless the patient specifically requests regular coffee.
- Use forks and spoons only. For patients in the last stages, use only spoons and cut all food before serving it.

Nutrition Assistance Programs

The Older Americans Act provides nutritional services and other services to older people who are in social and economic need. According to the U.S. Administration on Aging, which administers the Older Americans Act, the nutrition programs were set up to address dietary inadequacy and social isolation among older people. Home-delivered meals and congregate nutrition services are the two primary nutrition programs of this Act. For those who qualify, food stamps are another aid for improving nutrition. Under this program, a one-person household can receive up to $115 a month in food stamps to buy certain grocery items.

Government Officials Comments Regarding Older Americans Act Nutrition Program

"If the Older Americans Act Nutrition Program was a restaurant, the sign out front would say, 'Six billion served.' For 30 years, this program not only has provided nutritious, healthy meals to older Americans, but also has touched their lives by linking them to community services that allow them to remain independent." — *Department of Health and Human Services Secretary Tommy G. Thompson (2004).*

"The [Older Americans Act] Nutrition Program is a proven success story. It effectively targets older adults who are poorer, more likely to live alone, and are at higher nutritional risk." — *Assistant Secretary for Aging Josefina G. Carbonell* (AOA, 2004).

In different areas of the country, community organizations provide grocery-shopping assistance for the homebound, especially older adults. These organizations shop for and deliver groceries to people at their request, with the recipient paying for the groceries. Some agencies tack on a small service fee. The Elderly Nutrition Program (ENP) is the nation's oldest framework for providing community- and home-based preventive nutrition and health-related services to older persons. The ENP program currently provides congregate and home-delivered meals and other nutrition- and health-related services to about 7% of the older population, including an estimated 20% of the nation's poor elderly.

Nutritional Evaluation and Outcomes

Basic nutritional assessment includes a diet history and nutritional status, with special attention to cultural, ethnic, or religious preferences. In many care settings, nutritional assessments consist primarily of obtaining a 24-hour dietary recall from the patient or caregiver.

In summary, nurses must evaluate their plans of care. Listed here are some of the areas for evaluation and outcomes that should be considered.

1) Individual
   a) Weight
   b) Corrective or supportive strategies
   c) Quality of life issues and social aspects
2) Health care provider
   a) Mealtime disruptions
   b) Educated in special needs of AD patients
   c) Maintenance of adequate intake in care plans
3) Institution
   a) Documentation of nutritional status
   b) Frequency of nutritional assessments
   c) Referrals to appropriate professionals
   d) Modifications to nutritional program

INCONTINENCE

For many older adults, even those with AD, losing the ability to control elimination is a source of great concern and embarrassment. Incontinence, the inability to control the elimination of urine and feces, can lead to social isolation and lessen the quality of life for many older adults. #38

Incontinence occurs in 15% to 30% of elderly people in the community and in up to 50% of elderly people who are institutionalized (Ebersole & Hess, 2001). These percentages are much higher for patients with dementia and are a significant factor in the decision to institutionalize patients with AD. Family and professional caregivers react strongly to toileting problems and incontinence (Gwyther, 2001; Hutchinson, Leger-Krall, & Skodol Wilson, 1996).

"Functional incontinence" is the term used to describe the incontinence that most often occurs during the course of AD. This type of incontinence occurs when urine or feces are lost because the patient is unaware of the need to urinate (impaired cognition) or cannot reach a toilet because of immobility or some other barrier. Urinary problems usually occur before bowel problems in patients with AD. #39 Medications and the environment can also cause functional incontinence. It is common for people to urinate more often as they become older, but incontinence should be manageable (Gwyther, 2001).

Managing incontinence involves looking for the underlying causes and attempting corrective action. The update of the Omnibus Budget Reconciliation Act mandated that residents in nursing homes must be assessed and plans of care developed. Urinary incontinence was one of the major issues focused on as clinical practice guidelines evolved. In patients with functional incontinence, efforts must be made to implement a toileting program (U.S. Department of Health & Human Services, 2001).

As caregivers, nurses can address the problem of incontinence. Most types of incontinence can be improved with interventions. Among the most effective interventions is behavior modification. However, certain medications and surgical interventions may be needed for some individuals. All interventions must be directed at lessening the psychological and social effects of incontinence, thus improving an individual's quality of life.

Many people attempt to hide their incontinence from their family members, doctors, and nurses. However, as their problem worsens or as the disease progresses, it is difficult to conceal. People may deny having urinary incontinence or leakage but admit to having "problems with my bladder."

Maintaining dignity and privacy are two of the major issues related to incontinence. Best practices include being discreet when talking to a patient about toileting. Whispering when discussing toileting needs (although acting natural) and avoiding embarrassment are keys. Another best practice involves not using pads for incontinence when the person is only intermittently incontinent. Simply applying a brief or pad encourages the patient to rely on the device and lose toileting abilities, thus becoming humiliated and degraded. In addition, staff members generally attend first to patients who do not wear pads or briefs for incontinence.

The characteristics of the incontinence should be noted, including the onset, frequency, and severity as determined through the person's description of the problem and the pattern of incontinence behavior. As problems occur with incontinence, families and residential caregivers begin to look for cues from the patient so they can recognize when toileting is needed. Cues may be verbal or nonverbal, and their presence should be part of the assessment for incontinence. The nurse should talk to the family, if the patient is at home, or to the hands-on caregiver to find out how the patient signals the need to go to the bathroom. Cues may be behavioral, such as becoming restless or fidgety, trying to get up without help, or wandering at night. Experienced staff and caregivers can tell when toileting is needed by reading the eyes or facial expressions of patients.

It is important to ask the following questions of your patients if they have the ability to discuss the problem (if they have significant communication problems, your observation skills are extremely important in answering these questions):

- Do you leak urine when you cough, laugh, or sneeze?

- Do you leak urine when you exercise?

- Do you leak urine on the way to the bathroom?

- Do you find yourself always rushing to the bathroom?

- Do you awaken during the night to use the bathroom?

- Do you frequently limit your fluid intake when you are away from home so that you won't have to worry about finding a restroom?

- Do you avoid trips or going certain places because you may not know where the bathroom is?

- Do you have to stop frequently to urinate when taking car or bus trips?

- Do you often have strong, sudden urges to urinate that you cannot control?

- Do you wear pads in your underwear or diapers to protect your clothes from getting wet?

If individuals answer "yes" to any of these questions, they may have urinary incontinence.

Treatable Causes of Urinary Incontinence

DIAPPERS is a mnemonic that can help you remember the treatable causes of urinary incontinence:

Delirium

Infection

Atrophic urethritis/Vaginitis

Pharmaceuticals

Psychological factors

Endocrine conditions

Restricted mobility/Restraints

Stool impaction

Alternatively, consider the mnemonic **DRIP**:

Delirium or **D**rugs

Restricted mobility or **R**etention

Infection or **I**nflammation or **I**mpaction of stool

Polyuria (diabetes, hypercalcemia, hypothyroidism, congestive heart failure).

Other causes of urinary incontinence include constipation and inflammation from atrophic vaginitis or atrophic urethritis.

Types of Persistent Urinary Incontinence and Associated Signs and Symptoms

Urinary incontinence can be a short-term problem that responds to treatment, or it can be a persistent problem. Several types of persistent incontinence exist, each with its own signs and symptoms.

Urge incontinence: Associated with a strong urge to void. Caused by an overactive detrusor muscle. Leads to excessive involuntary bladder contractions. Can be caused by a number of neurological conditions, including stroke, spinal cord lesions, and multiple sclerosis

Stress incontinence: Due to pelvic muscle weakness. Associated with actions that increase intra-abdominal pressure, such as:

- coughing
- sneezing
- lifting
- bending
- laughing.

Overflow incontinence: Associated with overdistention of the bladder muscle. Can be present with stress or urge incontinence. This condition is due to an underactive bladder muscle or a bladder obstruction and can be caused by:

- medications (adverse effects)
- radical pelvic surgery
- diabetic neuropathy
- low spinal cord injury
- benign protatic hyperplasia.

Functional incontinence: Physical or psychological impairment leads to impaired urinary function, even with an intact urinary system.

In the early stages of AD, incontinence is unusual. Incontinence in early stages may be caused by other problems that require detection and treament. Later in the disease progression, it is common for people with AD to experience loss of bladder or bowel control. Other illnesses, such as diabetes and stroke, and medication side effects may also trigger incontinence. (See Table 4-2 for a list of risk factors associated with incontinence.) Possible problems include:

- *Urinary tract infections.*
- *Other acute illnesses.*
- *Fear:* The person may fear that an embarrassing accident will occur. This fear may cause him or her to visit the bathroom more times than necessary.
- *Fluids that act as diuretics, such as coffee, tea, and cola.*
- *Abrupt movement:* Urine release may be caused by a sneeze, laugh, or cough. Weak pelvic muscles in women can also cause uncontrollable loss of urine.
- *Fecal impaction:* As the urethra is pinched off by stool, bladder control is lost, and urine is released in spurts and trickles to prevent rupture.
- *Dehydration:* Inadequate fluid intake can lead to overconcentrated urine that irritates the bladder and causes difficulties with bladder control. Dehydration can also cause urinary tract infections that lead to incontinence. Withholding fluids when a person starts to lose bladder control may compound the problem.
- *Out-of-control chronic illness, such as diabetes or congestive heart failure.*
- *Enlarged prostate.*
- *Clothing:* Zippers and buttons on clothing can make it difficult for a person to undress in time

to use the toilet.

- *Environment:* The person may have trouble finding the bathroom or getting to it in time because it is too far away.

- *Drugs:* Drugs that diminish a person's ability to feel body sensations, such as the urge to urinate, should be evaluated, including sedatives, hypnotics, antidepressants, anticholinergics, diuretics, and antianxiety agents.

TABLE 4-2: RISK FACTORS ASSOCIATED WITH INCONTINENCE

• Immobility	• Low fluid intake
• Impaired cognition	• High impact physical activities
• Medications	
• Morbid obesity	• Diabetes
• Fecal impaction	• Stroke
• Smoking	• Estrogen depletion
• Delirium	• Pelvic muscle weakness
• Environmental barriers	• Childhood nocturnal enuresis

Assessment of Urinary Incontinence

Urinary symptoms usually provide clues to the possible causes of the problem. It is important to conduct a thorough physical exam and history and then combine this information with the urinary symptoms. The following content applies to individuals with or without AD.

History

Significant past medical history includes the number of births, recurrent urinary tract infections, bladder repair surgeries, urethral dilations, pelvic radiation and cystitis in females, and prostate surgery in men. The history should also include an assessment of memory impairment and environmental barriers. A mental status assessment can help to determine if the person has memory loss. A functional assessment should also be conducted to determine if the individual has difficulty walking, thus impeding his or her ability to gain access to a toilet.

Symptoms

Symptoms can be classified as obstructive or irritative. Obstructive symptoms include hesitancy, dribbling, intermittency, impaired trajectory, and sensation of incomplete emptying. Irritative symptoms include nocturia, frequency, urgency, and dysuria. Obstructive symptoms often require referral to a urological specialist, whereas irritative symptoms can often be controlled by behavioral interventions.

Patients with urinary retention, or incomplete emptying of the bladder, may complain of lower abdominal pain and a strong desire to urinate. Remember that people with neurologic injuries (such as spinal cord injury) may experience minimal to no pain. Additional questions to ask the person to determine voiding dysfunction secondary to outlet obstruction include:

- Do you experience dribbling after voiding?

- Do you void in small quantities?

- Do you have difficulty initiating urination?

- How often do you urinate?

- How many times do you awaken at night to go to the bathroom?

Urinary retention is noted by determining the amount of urine left in the bladder 10 to 15 minutes after voiding. This is known as the postvoid residual volume (PVR). Normal PVR is less than 200 ml unless infection is present. In elderly patients, a PVR of 200 ml may be considered normal. Retention may be caused by neurologic damage, bladder atonia from medications, or fecal impaction. If abnormal PVR is found, the person should see a urologist.

Environmental Barriers

Certain environmental barriers, such as the location of the toilet, may also contribute to incontinence. This is especially true in older persons. In these cases, incontinence may improve with the use of catheters, urinals, or other urinary assistive or collective devices. Assistive devices include raised toilet seats, bathroom grab bars, toilet seat arms, and clothing that facilitates toileting. Collective devices include male and female urinals, bedside commodes, bed pans, and more easily accessible bathrooms.

Bladder Records

As part of the assessment process, good bladder records or diaries can often provide enough information to guide interventions (see Table 4-3).

TABLE 4-3: BLADDER RECORD EXAMPLE				
Date & Time				
Voided In Toilet				
Urine Leakage* S M L				
Activity with Leakage				
Liquid Intake				
* Code for S-M-L: S=Slightly damp M=Mildly wet, underwear or protective pad is definitely wet L=Large urine loss, even outer garments are wet				
Place an X next to "Voided In Toilet" each time the patient empties his or her bladder in the toilet.				

Problem areas and their correlation with urine leakage, frequency, pattern of the incontinence episodes, and voiding patterns can be obtained from the record. Excellent urinary and bowel incontinence assessment forms are available and can easily be ordered and adopted. However, each nurse should seek out and implement the assessment format that works best for him or her, within the limits of the employing agency or facility. Interestingly, in practice, bowel incontinence is not considered as much of a problem as urinary incontinence because it occurs less frequently, approximately every 1 to 2 days (Hutchinson et al., 1996). The best way to treat urinary incontinence is to detect the underlying cause and then, if possible, treat it. Keep in mind

that urinary tract infection or pneumonia can occur concurrently with urinary incontinence.

Daily fluid intake should also be recorded. Because drinking enough liquids is important, the patient should be encouraged to drink at least 2 L per day. Liquids should not contain caffeine or be alcoholic in nature, because these substances are bladder irritants.

Assessment of each patient's pattern of urinary incontinence is critical. The pattern can be assessed during a 3- to 4-day period. The patient is monitored every 1 to 2 hours for incidents of incontinence or voiding, and the findings are recorded. At the end of the assessment period, the record shows when the patient should be toileted on the basis of the patient's individual schedule, not a pre-established idea of toileting every 2 hours, as is done in some facilities. The key to a toileting program is to individualize it to the patient's schedule for urinating. For example, Mr. Jackson needs to urinate several times in the morning and then only once in the afternoon and once after the evening meal. He does not like to get out of bed at night, so he needs to have a urinal placed by his bed at night where he can see it. Occasionally, Mr. Jackson needs to be reminded what the urinal is for.

Toileting Programs

Patients with dementia require both physical and cognitive assistance to meet their toileting needs. Factors that affect toileting programs in a facility are the size and weight of the patient and the patient's need for assistive devices. Toileting becomes more time-consuming and potentially dangerous with larger or heavier patients. Practices for toileting that incorporate recognition of physical and cognitive needs are listed here (Hutchinson et al., 1996; Lancaster, 1998):

- Follow routines that fit the patient's schedule.

- Provide visual cues. Signs may assist an individual in finding the bathroom. Placing colored rugs on the bathroom floor and lid covers on the toilet may help the bathroom stand out. Avoid having items nearby that can be mistaken for a toilet, such as a trash can.

- Monitor incontinence. Identify when accidents occur and plan accordingly. For example, if they happen every 2 hours, get the person to the bathroom before that time. To help control incontinence at night, limit intake of liquids after dinner and in the evening.

- Remove obstacles. Make sure clothing is easy for the individual to remove. Clothing with Velcro™ may be easier to remove than clothing with buttons.

- Provide reminders. Because AD can cause forgetfulness, you may need to periodically remind a patient with AD to use the bathroom. Also, watch for visible cues, such as restlessness, or facial expressions that may indicate the need to use the bathroom.

- Be supportive. Help a person with AD retain a sense of dignity despite incontinence problems. A reassuring attitude helps lessen feelings of embarrassment.

- Have the patient drink six to eight glasses of fluids each day.

- Be observant and read verbal and behavioral cues.

- Respond to the cues.

- Communicate regularly with the patient's family members or other caregivers as conditions change.

- Be consistent and make toileting each patient a priority. When professional or family caregivers get busy, the first routine to suffer is toileting.

The goal of any program for patients with AD or other forms of dementia is to encourage the patient's functional abilities as long as possible and to enhance the quality of life.

Case Study

One afternoon, Mr. Sloan, an elderly man with dementia who lives in a nursing facility, was observed trying to crawl over his bed rails. His sheets were wet from top to bottom. When a nurse approached, Mr. Sloan explained, although confused, that he had finished his nap and wanted to get up now. He also pointed to his wet sheets and said, "I sweat a lot when I sleep." Although this gentleman could not make many of his needs known verbally, he wanted to retain his sense of personal dignity by explaining the wet bed as he wished the nurse to see it. This knowledge underscores the care and services nurses provide to manage the needs of patients with dementia who are incontinent.

Managing Urinary Incontinence

Managing urinary incontinence is important. To do this, you need to understand the different devices and products that can be used to contain urine that leaks (see Table 4-4). This table provides a brief review of products available through local pharmacies, through medical equipment dealers (DMEs), or directly from manufacturers. Medicare and other major insurers pay for most of these products in a limited monthly number. Health maintenance organizations and other managed care insurers do not routinely pay for these products.

Absorbent products (such as pads and adult diapers) that can be found in drug stores are considered personal hygiene products and are not paid for by insurers. Be sure you understand the products authorized by your institution for the treatment of incontinence as well as substitutions that can be used to meet the repayment structure of insurance providers yet still be considered effective and safe for your patients.

Treatment goals include:

- increasing bladder capacity

- increasing awareness of signals of a full bladder

- increasing the patient's ability to respond to a bladder contraction by using the outer sphincter muscle to withhold urine (pelvic exercises).

TABLE 4-4: URINARY INCONTINENCE TREATMENT & PRODUCTS

Urge incontinence

Bladder relaxants such as oxybutynin
   (Ditropan) or imipramine
Estrogen
Biofeedback
Bladder training
Surgical removal of bladder irritants or release
   of the outlet obstruction
Diapers
Regularly timed toileting

Stress incontinence

Alpha-adrenergic agonists, such as imipramine,
   pseudoephedrine, or phenylpropanolamine
Pelvic floor exercises
Biofeedback
Bladder training
Surgical bladder neck suspensions if needed
Estrogen
Diapers

Overflow incontinence

Decompression of the bladder with intermittent
   catheterization
Surgical removal of obstruction
Alpha-adrenergic blockers, such as prazosin or
   terazosin
Indwelling catheterization, if needed
Diapers
Bladder training
Functional incontinence
Adaption of environment to patient's needs
Diapers
Bladder training and regularly timed toileting,
   if possible

Incontinence products

Individual protection
   Light to moderate protection
      Pads, shields, and guards
   Moderate to heavy protection
      Belted undergarments, disposable pads, pants
   Heavy protection
      Briefs & protective underwear

Bed & furniture protection
   Washable and disposable pads

Reusable products
   Pants, pads, undergarments

Cleansing products
   Wash cloths, cleaning solutions, gloves

Attempt therapeutic trials designed to change behavior or pharmacological treatments. Maintain bladder control records to evaluate the effectiveness of interventions.

SUMMARY

Nutritional deficiencies occur with unfortunate frequency in older adults and can be the result of medications, disease, or accessibility. Malnutrition in older adults can be a significant problem but is not easily identifiable. Because so many older individuals have nutrition problems, nurses must be particularly skillful in nutritional assessments, interventions, and follow-up for older adults. They must also be knowledgeable about the physiological declines that can contribute to poor nutrition. At the same time, understanding the alteration in homeostasis created by poor nutrition and the various nutritional assistance programs available assists in developing plans to provide maximal nutritional intake and feeding programs for individuals with AD.

FTT is a diagnosis that needs to be rethought. Quantifying the nature and level of the patient's impairments, recognizing that deficits interact in mutual and complex ways to create further impairment, and treating the easily remedied contributors may be a more rational approach.

Incontinence occurs in 30% to 50% of all older adults. This percentage is greater in patients with AD because of mental and physical declines caused by the disease. Nurses must be able to recognize treatable causes and symptoms of incontinence, such as medications, urinary tract infections, low fluid intake, fecal impaction, mobility difficulties, and delirium, and direct their efforts at lessening the psychological and social effects of incontinence, thus improving quality of life.

EXAM QUESTIONS

CHAPTER 4
Questions 31-40

31. The nutritional status of people with AD is a serious concern because

    a. approximately 85% of older adults in hospitals or nursing homes are malnourished.

    b. most older adults who are hospitalized with malnutrition, leave the hospital in an improved nutritional state.

    c. nutritional deficiencies are more easily detected in elderly people with AD.

    d. interventions for malnutrition have not been successful in people with AD.

32. In the clinical setting, a good indicator of an individual's protein status is

    a. blood urea nitrogen.

    b. serum creatinine.

    c. serum albumin.

    d. serum potassium.

33. The most common type of malnutrition among institutionalized elderly people is

    a. protein-calorie.

    b. non-nutrient-dense.

    c. carbohydrate.

    d. muscle-sparing.

34. "Failure to thrive" (FTT) is a term used to describe older adults with various concurrent chronic diseases or functional impairments. Characteristics of FTT include

    a. weight loss, inactivity, and an intact immune system.

    b. weight loss, decreased appetite, dehydration, and depression.

    c. decreased appetite but satisfactory nutrition.

    d. dehydration, poor nutrition, and high cholesterol.

35. Mr. Miller has malnutrition and, despite nursing efforts to increase his intake, he remains 30% underweight. When you assess Mr. Miller, you would expect to find

    a. edema in his upper extremities only.

    b. increased wound healing.

    c. impaired wound healing.

    d. pink and moist conjunctivae and good skin turgor.

36. A behavior that represents one of the four A's influence on nutrition is when the person with AD

    a. says, "I want cereal to eat."

    b. can use their fork and knife to eat.

    c. can identify the potatoes on their plate

    d. keeps asking when it will be time to eat, just after eating.

37. The condition that would not be considered a barrier to adequate nutrition in a nursing home is

should be accurate

a. inaccurate reports of residents' abilities to chew and swallow.

b. residents dislike of the food served or unappetizing appearance of the food.

c. lack of assistance from nursing assistants, lack of time to assist, and poor education on methods of helping residents.

d. lack of kitchen facilities to prepare proper nutrition.

38. The percentage of elderly people in the community who experience incontinence is

a. 5% to 10%.

b. 15% to 30%.

c. 35% to 50%.

d. 60% to 75%.

39. An accurate statement about the relationship between incontinence, AD, and aging is

increases

a. the frequency of urination decreases as a person ages.

b. in the early stages of AD, incontinence is a normal part of the disease.

c. medications are rarely the cause of incontinence.

d. if incontinence develops, urinary problems usually occur before bowel problems do.

40. The best practice intervention for prevention of incontinence is

a. place all patients on a 2 hour toileting schedule.

b. do not use pads for incontinence if the patient is only intermittently incontinent.

c. when caregivers are busy, use incontinence briefs to prevent accidents.

d. try not to read too much into a patient's nonverbal language about toileting.

CHAPTER 5

FALLS AND RESTRAINT USE

CHAPTER OBJECTIVE

After completing this chapter, the reader will be able to discuss falls and identify the need for safety interventions for patients with Alzheimer's disease (AD).

LEARNING OBJECTIVES

After studying this chapter, the reader will be able to

1. describe demographics related to falls in older adults.

2. identify risk factors for falls in older adults.

3. identify interventions for fall prevention and minimization of injury in older adults, especially those with AD.

4. identify components of a fall evaluation.

5. specify the nurse's role in the proper use of physical restraints.

6. recognize the extent of the use of various forms of restraints on older adults and their influence on patient outcomes.

INTRODUCTION

One of nursing's major goals is to maintain the safety of the patient. Nurses must be aware of potential accidents and injuries even with the most functional of patients. As people age or when people have AD, this goal becomes harder to attain. Optimizing an individual's functional ability, reducing the risk of falls, and reducing the need for physical or chemical restraints can help nurses achieve this goal. Nurses must examine the reasons people fall, learn to predict when falls may occur, and design and implement the proper interventions for falls.

FALLS

A fall is defined as an event that results in part of the patient's body coming to rest inadvertently on the floor or on another surface lower than the patient, including an event where a patient is found on the floor unable to account for his or her situation.

As an individual ages, the likelihood of experiencing an injury from an accident increases. With every injury, the possibility of the injury becoming disabling also increases. Among people older than age 65, accident-related injuries are the fifth leading cause of death. In addition, falls are the leading predictor of morbidity and mortality in the elderly population (Mariano, 1999; Better ElderCare, 2002). Falls can result in decreased physical functioning, disability, and reduced quality of life. Decreased confidence and fear of falling can lead to further functional decline, depression, feelings of helplessness, and social isolation.

Approximately 50% of older patients who fall report that they, "tripped and fell." In many cases, patients report that they tripped over a curb or an uneven sidewalk or stumbled while carrying groceries up stairs. Most individuals view falls as accidents that are unpredictable and, therefore, unavoidable. However, this is not the case. Falls are one of several geriatric syndromes that deserve careful evaluation and treatment. Most falls in the elderly are caused by complex interactions of several factors particular to the person and within his or her environment (Allen, 2003).

Some research has been conducted to evaluate the role that human factors play in home safety, particularly in regard to warning labels and falls. For example, cognitive decline impairs the ability to comprehend warning signs that may be posted to inform of hazards. Memory loss also impairs comprehension of warning symbols and warning information (Rogers & Fisk, 2000).

Approximately one-half of falls in the elderly can be attributed to factors in the environment, such as slippery floors and loose rugs; the remainder can be attributed to individual causes, such as lower extremity weakness, gait disorders, effects of medications, or acute illness. Medications play an important part in falls. Drugs such as sedatives, antidepressants, and antihypertensives that can cause postural hypotension, sedation, decreased reaction time, and decreased cognitive ability may directly lead to falls (Allen, 2003).

As care providers, nurses are responsible for providing safe environments for older adult patients to optimize their functional status. The key indicators of baseline functional status are the basic activities of daily living (ADLs), with emphasis on transfers and mobility for nursing home patients and on independent ADLs, including transportation and meal preparation, for people living at home. A nurse must understand how falls occur, how falls impact older patients, how falls can be prevented, and how to identify patients at risk for falls. (Better ElderCare, 2002; Fuller, 2000; Fulmer, Mezey, Bottrell, et al., 2002; Abraham, Bottrell, Dash, et al., 1999; Yardley & Smith, 2002).

Fall Statistics

For many elderly people, falls and their associated injuries can cause significant disability. It is helpful to review the following facts to understand the seriousness of the problem:

- Older adults are hospitalized for fall-related injuries five times more often than they are for injuries from other causes.

- Approximately 30% of older adults who live independently in their own homes fall at least once per year.

- Falls are the leading cause of injury deaths among people age 65 and older.

- The annual incidence of falls is approximately 30 percent in persons over age 65.

- One-half of adults over age 75 who fracture a hip as a result of a fall die within 1 year of the incident.

- The risk of falls is greater in older persons, with the annual incidence increasing to 50% in people over age 80.

- Women are more likely to sustain fractures as a result of falls because of their increased risk of osteoporosis.

- Approximately 85% of falls in the home occur in the afternoon and early evening.

- Of those who fall, 20% to 30% suffer moderate to severe injuries that reduce mobility and independence and increase the risk of premature death.

- Falls are a major cause of severe nonfatal injuries and a common cause of hospital admissions for traumatic injuries among older adults.

- A fall with fracture is a frequent precursor to long-term residence in a nursing home.

- Of the 1.5 million nursing home residents nationwide, approximately 50% fall at least once each year.

- About 1,800 fatal falls occur each year in U.S. nursing homes.

- Among people 85 years and older, 20% of fall-related deaths occur in nursing homes.

- The strongest predictors in the risk profile for recurrent falls are previous falls, urinary incontinence, visual impairment, and functional limitations.

- Fear of falling is a prevalent experience among community-living elderly persons.

(Mariano, 1999).

Fear of falling and loss of self-confidence, which can occur after approximately half of all falls, are associated with functional decline, increasing depression, decreased quality of life, and further fall risk (Tideiksaar, 2003). Fear of falling also limits participation in many types of beneficial activities. In a study that assessed fear of falling, Yardley and Smith (2002) recognized two particular fears about falling: (1) the expectation of physical harm and consequent functional incapacity as well as loss of independence and (2) the expectation of embarrassment, which might lead to decreased confidence and social identity. Concern about loss of identity was found in the surveys but was not mentioned in the discussions. This finding is consistent with other indications that suggest elderly people do not want to discuss concerns about the fear of falling. This fear can keep older adults from engaging in healthy behaviors, such as exercising and socializing. Interventions that incorporate balance training as well as confidence building have been shown to be effective in reducing both fear of falling and the number of falls (Allen, 2003).

Nursing Homes and Falls

An estimated 40% of older adult admittances to nursing homes are related to falls and instability (thus placing these patients at risk for another fall). Many times, the facility is unfamiliar, which leads to confusion and fear. Furthermore, patients in nursing homes or extended care facilities tend to be frailer than older adults living in the community. They also tend to be older and more cognitively impaired, and they have greater limitations in their ADLs.

Common Causes of Nursing Home Falls

- Weakness and gait problems are the most common causes of nursing home falls. Together, they account for approximately 24% of all falls in nursing homes.

- Environmental hazards account for 16% of nursing home falls. Such hazards include wet floors, poor lighting, lack of bed rails, clutter, improper bed height, and improperly maintained or fitted wheelchairs.

- Medications, especially psychotropic drugs, can increase the risk of falls and fall-related injuries.

- Other causes of falls include difficulty transferring and poor foot care.

Prediction of Falls

Prediction of falls is associated with identification of a set of existing risk factors (see Table 5-1). These factors are placed in one of three categories: extrinsic (contributing factors outside the person), intrinsic (anticipated physiological), and intrinsic (unanticipated physiological).

Extrinsic factors

Environmental factors are the most common causes of falls. Wet floors, throw rugs, electrical cords, pets, toys, and bathtubs can all lead to slips and falls. Furnishings such as unstable tables or furniture that is too low or too high and use of step stools (especially if unstable) are additional contributors to falls. Bed rails are commonly considered safety devices that decrease the risk of falls. However, confused or demented individuals frequently attempt to climb out of bed over raised bed rails and fall. Clothing that is too long, such as a long bathrobe, can catch on doorknobs or railings.

Foot problems and ill-fitting and inappropriate shoes and clothing are occasionally contributing factors to falls in older people. For example, some older women insist on wearing shoes that are fash-

TABLE 5-1: RISK FACTORS FOR FALLS IN OLDER ADULTS

Age-related
- Decreased muscle tone and strength
- Impaired mobility, gait, or balance
- Decreased proprioception
- Poor balance
- Vision problems
- Previous history of falls

Disease-related
- Arthritis
- Sensory deficits
- Alterations in bladder function
- Stroke
- Postural hypotension
- Hip fractures
- Peripheral neuropathies
- Dementia
- Parkinson's disease or parkinsonian syndrome

Environment-related
- Poor lighting
- Slick or irregular floor surfaces
- Loose rugs
- Shoes in poor repair or with slippery soles
- Sidewalks in poor repair
- Steep or unsafe stairways
- Objects in pathways
- Long bathrobes or other loose clothing
- Bathroom fixtures that are too low or too high or do not have arm supports

ionable even though they are not safe or functional. Failure to put on shoes or slippers also contributes to falls. Shoe soles that are too slippery or too sticky can also cause a person to stumble and fall. Poor lighting, low toilet seats, and unlocked wheels on beds or chairs can also contribute to falls.

Unsafe activity is another reason people fall. For the general population, these activities can include climbing on ladders, wearing slippers out in the snow, climbing up on a roof to repair it, carrying too many things, and failing to turn on lights to see at night. Because dementia impairs the judgment of those who have it, these people may partake in unsafe activities without any consideration to the risk of harm.

Assistive devices have long been contributors to falls. Older adults have either not been properly educated on the use of walkers and canes or fail to follow the teaching on how to use these devices. Improper maintenance of assistive devices can also contribute to falls. These devices need to be evaluated frequently to assure that they are in proper repair. For example, it is not uncommon to find the rubber tips missing from canes and walkers. These rubber tips provide the devices with nonskid surfaces that can help to prevent falls. Lastly, some older adults with dementia demonstrate poor judgment through refusal to use recommended assistive devices.

Among community-dwelling older adults, alcohol use and abuse can lead to personal neglect, abnormal gait, and tremors, which all increase the risk of falling.

Intrinsic factors (anticipated physiological)

Recent history of a fall is the most significant risk factor for falling. Gait and balance disturbances, dizziness, confusion, weakness, and visual disturbances predispose older adults to falls. Aging contributes to impaired gait, decreased stride length and step height, prolonged reaction time, and decreased visual acuity and depth perception. These disturbances in mobility are enhanced when an older adult is demented. Judgment, visual-spatial perception, and the ability to orient oneself to the surroundings are more difficult for an individual with dementia (Greubel, Stokesberry, & Jelley, 2002).

The cognitive decline in AD alone is a predictor of falls and is associated with a striking rise in the sequelae of severe falls. When older adults with AD must move quickly to avoid a hazard, the incidence of falls increase. Because their ability to make quick adjustments in their posture is impaired, they often trip or stumble. If they do fall, the incidence of severe fractures is tripled or quadrupled and fall-related mortality is tripled. The increased incidence of mortality and injury is the direct result of inability to compensate in posture or body position and lack of strength and motor control to keep from falling and control falling (Hauer, Pfisterer, Weber, et al., 2003).

Researchers have indicated that a link also exists between postural instability and attention. As people age, the mental speed of processing input that comes to the attention of the brain decreases. This processing ability is called executive function. Decline in executive function is seen early in AD. Decreasing attention coupled with the changes in balance and coordination associated with AD has been linked to increased falls (Hauer et al., 2003; Sheridan, Solomont, Kowall, & Hausdorff, 2003; Verghese, Lipton, Hall, et al., 2002). Divided attention also decreases gait speed and causes variations in stride and gait timing. Simply stated, when older adults with dementia have to simultaneously conduct a task and walk, their postural stability is negatively impacted and their risk of falling is significantly increased.

Using or attempting to use a commode, urinal, or bathroom increases the risk of falls. Many older adults cannot sense that they need to urinate until it is almost too late and, therefore, they hurry to the bathroom. Because of decreased motor ability, environmental elements, and decreased cognition, their risk of falling during these times is increased.

Some medical equipment can also contribute to falls. Indwelling urinary catheters and I.V. tubing and poles are risk factors for falls because they are associated with spills and trips. Urinary catheters can lead to urinary tract infections or incontinence after removal, which also increase the risk of falls. Nasogastric tubes can interfere with vision, especially for people with vision problems who are unable to wear their glasses.

Medications also increase the risk of falls. The variety of drugs taken, improper dosing, and changes in individual physiology can influence the pharmacodynamics and pharmacokinetics of medications.

Medications can lead to significant blood pressure drops that are enough to compromise cerebral blood flow and bring about syncope. (Kamel, Phlavan, & Malekgoudarzi, 2001; Rubenstein, Powers, & MacLean, 2001; Better ElderCare 2002). The adverse effects of medications may include induced or increased confusion and disorientation.

The following drugs are among those that may contribute to falls:

- psychotropics
- benzodiazepines
- antihistamines
- anticholinergics
- narcotics
- sedative-hypnotics.

Additionally, withdrawal from alcohol or benzodiazepines can lead to falls.

Many individuals with AD become depressed and require phamacologic management. Selective-serotonin reuptake inhibitors (SSRIs) are considered relatively safe drugs to administer because their reduced adverse effects decrease the risk of falls.

Additional factors, such as dizziness, vertigo, and syncope, can all be associated with physiological hypotension that is medication induced. Ear infections and Ménière's disease are disease inducers of dizziness.

Intrinsic factors (unanticipated physiological)

Cardiac arrhythmias decrease cardiac output and thus blood flow to the brain and peripheral tissues. Lack of perfusion to the brain can lead to dizziness and syncope. Lack of perfusion to the peripheral tissues can lead to neuropathies and gait disturbances. Seizure activity with tonic-clonic involvement and loss of balance induces falls and increases mortality in older adults. Transient ischemic attacks are intermittent interruptions in blood flow to the brain that generally indicate blockage of a carotid artery or occlusion of blood flow to the cerebrum. With decreased blood flow, loss of balance, weakness, dizziness, and syncope can occur.

Fall Risk Assessment

Patients must be assessed for the potential risk of falling at the time of admission using a rating guideline or risk assessment for falls. When a person is identified as being at risk for falls, interventions include:

- assignment to a room that is closer to the nursing station

- an identifier placed on or in the person's medical chart and treatment records

- notification of family and staff of the appropriate activity level

- establishment of a toileting schedule for incontinence (should be posted)

- physical therapy (PT) and occupational therapy referrals, if necessary, for gait and functional assessment

- initiation of standardized patient safety plans.

Remember that individuals who take medications or have cardiovascular disease may suffer from orthostatic hypotension and conditions such as hypoglycemia and vertigo induce dizziness that may increase the incidence of falls. These patients require closer monitoring and follow-up.

PT should include range-of-motion (ROM) exercises. Ambulation must be supervised, and staff must instruct the patient on fall prevention. When AD progresses to the point that patients are unable to follow instructions, these individuals must be supervised directly.

Being well informed about why falls occur and what risk factors are associated with falls in elders and, in response, developing fall prevention guidelines are insufficient to prevent falls. The ability to reduce falls depends on understanding evidence-based fall prevention strategies and, more importantly, on turning evidence-based strategies into best practices under real-world conditions. For example, in one study, exercise advice delivered by a physio-

therapist in the home to increase physical activity reduced the risk of falling in women over age 80 (Thorogood, Hillsdon, & Summerbell, 2003).

Fall Interventions and Considerations

Falls are not just the result of getting older. Because falls are caused by the interaction of a number of different factors, fall prevention requires a combination of medical treatments, rehabilitation, environmental modifications, and technological interventions. Although these strategies are applicable to all older adults, they can be easily modified for people with AD:

1) Physical conditioning or rehabilitation, such as exercise, to improve strength and endurance; PT; gait training; or walking programs should be initiated. Exercise can improve endurance, strength, gait, and function in chronically impaired, fall-prone elderly people. Walking and weight programs can improve leg power. Leg power is a strong predictor of self-reported functional status in elderly women. For clients who are bedridden, it is important to obtain bedside therapies to maintain muscle strength and ROM. Many long-term care facilities (LTCFs) have walker clubs that promote socialization and participation in physical activities and, thus, functional independence.

2) The major risks and benefits of exercise are important considerations when evaluating, preventing, and treating common ailments of older adults. Cardiovascular disease remains a significant risk factor in older athletes. However, with appropriate medical screening and moderate levels of exercise, cardiovascular risks generally are minimized. The most common ailments among older athletes are musculoskeletal. Osteoporosis-related falls and fractures, osteoarthritis, tendon injuries, and meniscal tears are among the most prevalent injuries. Osteoporosis risks and osteoarthritis symptoms are both improved with regular physical activity. Most older women

should also take calcium and vitamin D supplements to slow osteoporosis.

3) Regular aerobic exercise, even when started as late as age 55, is associated with a 1 to 2 year increase in life expectancy as well as with increased functional independence.

4) Sensory (hearing and vision) deficits can be managed by ensuring that eyeglasses and hearing aids work, are clean, and have been updated in a timely manner. Make sure that individuals use their aids as designed. Also, make sure that lighting is adequate for vision, without producing glare. In people with AD, glare can contribute to confusion and agitation. Install and maintain nightlights in bathrooms to assist with night vision.

5) The ideal footwear is a comfortable, flat-soled shoe. Older patients should be encouraged to wear practical footwear, such as sneakers, crepe-soled shoes, or slippers with nonskid treads for walking on tile floors or similar surfaces. When older adults experience significant changes in their gaits, such as shuffling, or have difficulty with the height of their step, leather-soled shoes are recommended because they do not stick to the floor, which can cause the individual to stumble and fall.

6) Environmental assessments should be performed and modifications instituted to improve mobility and safety (such as installing grab bars, adding raised toilet seats, lowering bed heights, and installing handrails in the hallways). Ensure that the home or facility is free from clutter, throw rugs, and dangerous electrical cords. Check that floors and stairs are in good repair. Be sure that any new admission to the facility is oriented and reoriented as needed to the surroundings. Promote the arrangement of furniture to enhance visibility and mobility. If a piece of furniture is hard to distinguish from its surroundings, try to change the fabric pattern or place a contrasting item of color on it to help distinguish it from the surroundings.

7) Review prescribed medications to assess their potential risks and benefits, especially as associated with possible falls. If you detect a change in the individual's mental status, an immediate review of medications is imperative.

8) Use technological devices such as alarm systems that activate when patients try to get out of bed or move unassisted and protective hip pads to reduce falls or associated injuries.

9) Monitor nutritional status. Poor nutrition can lead to decreased protein and albumin in the body as well as mineral and electrolyte problems. Poor nutrition can also enhance adverse reactions to medications by impacting the pharmacokinetics and pharmacodynamics. The sense of thirst is decreased in older adults, and reliance on it to detect the need for hydration is not appropriate. Encourage people with dementia to drink frequently, unless otherwise medically indicated. Small, frequent feedings that include finger foods and foods high in fiber are advised. For people unable to tolerate oral feedings, it may be necessary to include parenteral nutrition. If poor nutrition is the result of reduced finances or inability to obtain food, it is important to have the counsel of a social worker to find alternative means of obtaining proper nutrition.

10) Perform patient and family teaching to increase their involvement. This can range from emphasis on the importance of muscle strength training and proper nutrition to removal of environmental hazards. Many community-dwelling elderly individuals consider falls to be preventable and understand the importance of fall-related risk factors, but they do not consider themselves at risk for falls.

11) Increase staff awareness of fall risk factors. Inservices that review and remind staff of the obstacles that can lead to falls and removal of those obstacles can reduce falls.

12) Assist with elimination. For people who remain in

their homes, ensure that bathroom facilities are in working condition and that the individuals are able to get to them. Raised toilet seats are beneficial to individuals with reduced ROM and strength as well as those with poor balance. Install grab bars to assist with lowering the body to the toilet and the tub and rising up from them. Encouraging a regular routine of elimination can decrease the incidence of hurried visits to the bathroom, which are likely to result in trips and falls.

13) Ensure that assistive devices are the correct height for the individual and are in working order.

14) A fall risk index or questionnaire may be available at your facility. If not, develop one so that that fall risk can be calculated based on individual mobility factors, living conditions, unsafe behaviors, ADLs, and medication use.
(Gruebel, Stokesberry, & Jelley, 2002; Jensen, Lundin-Olsson, Nyberg, & Gustafson, 2002; National Center for Injury Prevention and Control, 2002)

Fall outcome indicators for nurses that should be monitored include:

1) Fall rate injury index developed by the facility

2) Classification of injury into one of the following categories
   a. No injury
   b. Minor injury
   c. Moderate injury
   d. Major injury
   e. Death

3) Analysis of when falls occur
   a. By classification of falls

Evaluating a Fall

Evaluating the well-being of a person who fell is the first step in assessing a fall. Airway, breathing, and circulation (ABCs) are the first part of any evaluation. If the person has an injury that is affecting any of the ABCs, alert EMS. If you determine that the person is not in immediate danger, move on in your assessment of the patient and the situation.

Look for changes from the individual's baseline functional status.

Assess for symptoms that occurred prior to the fall, such as lightheadedness, palpitations, chest pain, vertigo, and incontinence. Ask witnesses about the fall to gain more information. In this part of the evaluation, look for changes in mental status that may have caused the fall or resulted from it. Evaluation of mental status commonly requires verification with one or more of the following references: a family member, a friend, a caregiver, or the patient's medical records.

Review the medication regime. Look for drugs that can cause orthostatic hypotension or sedation, such as benzodiazepines. Assess alcohol use, but keep in mind that it may be difficult to get an accurate history of use. One example of falls induced by medications can be demonstrated by the story of an older adult who was taking sleeping medications at night. She awoke with a need to use the bathroom during the night and her room was very dark. She was so sedated from the medication that her gait was unsteady and as she attempted to get up, she fell, hitting the nightstand on the way to the floor. She arrived in the emergency department with face fractures, numerous abrasions, and broken bones.

Lastly, document your findings, including patient physical assessment; assessment of the scene (including suspected reasons for the fall, such as a wet spot on the floor or an electrical cord in the aisle); use, lack of use, and condition of protective devices and shoes; and analysis of patient risk factors.

RESTRAINT USE

The Centers for Medicare and Medicaid Services (2002a) defines physical restraints as: "Physical restraints are defined as any manual method or physical or mechanical device, material, or equipment attached or adjacent to the resident's body that the individual cannot remove easily which restricts freedom of movement or normal access to one's body.

Full Bed Rails may be one or more rails along both sides of the resident's bed that block three-quarters to the whole length of the mattress from top to bottom. This definition also includes beds with one side placed against the wall (prohibiting the resident from entering and exiting on that side) and the other side blocked by a full bed rail. Included in this category are 'veil' screens (used in pediatric units) and enclosed bed systems" (p. 2).

The DHHS (2000) definition of chemical restraints is found in their State Operations Manual includes the following: "'Chemical Restraints' is defined as any drug that is used for discipline or convenience and not required to treat medical symptoms. 'Discipline' is defined as any action taken by the facility for the purpose of punishing or penalizing residents. 'Convenience' is defined as any action taken by the facility to control a resident's behavior or manage a resident's behavior with a lesser amount of effort by the facility and not in the resident's best interest" (p 44).

Use of physical restraints and psychoactive medications (chemical restraints) can have hazardous and adverse outcomes. Anything that inhibits movement is considered a restraint, including vests, geri-chairs, bars, belts, psychotropic medications, and bed rails that keep a person from getting out of bed (see Table 5-2 and Table 5-3). Loss of autonomy, humiliation, and fear epitomize the experience of being restrained. Other consequences are skin breakdown, incontinence, constipation, fecal impaction, depression, social isolation, behavioral problems, and decline in function, such as decreased mobility. The ultimate consequence is death. When a physically restrained person falls or slips out of a wheelchair, the injuries can be much more serious than a fractured hip.

Many individuals feel that restraints are one of the best methods of keeping individuals from falling. Some nurses rationalize using restraints on people with AD to reduce wandering and safety for confusional states (Gallinagh et al., 2002). This is

far from the truth. Most studies indicate that no association exists between restraint use and reduction of falls (Gallinagh et al., 2002).

On any given day, one-half million patients are physically restrained in hospitals and nursing homes in the United States, more so than in any other Western country. Most patients who are restrained are older adults (Strumpf, Evans, & Bourbonniere, 2001). A decade of concentrating on restraint reduction in LTCFs has resulted in a significant decline in use. Many facilities are now restraint-free environments or allow only minimal use of restraints after intensive assessment and failure of alternatives. As a result, recently the focus has shifted to reducing the use of physical and chemical restraints in acute care hospital settings. For example, the Centers for Medicare and Medicaid Services (CMS) enacted an additional condition for participation in the Medicare program for hospitals entitled "Patient Rights." Many of the standards mandated by CMS are similar to long-term care restrictions on restraint use.

The Joint Commission on Accreditation of Healthcare Organizations (JCAHO) has issued similar standards for acute care settings. The standards require education of staff on safe and proper application and use of restraints, trials of less restrictive alternatives, and on-site individualized assessment by the patient's clinician as well as hospital clinicians. The successful reduction of both physical and chemical restraints in LTCFs highlights the need to promote further reduction in acute care settings.

The Omnibus Budget Reconciliation Act of 1987 mandated a drastic reduction in the use of physical and chemical restraints in LTCFs. In 2001, JCAHO issued guidelines to significantly reduce the use of restraints. According to these new recommendations, restraints are to be used only in emergencies that could lead to patients harming themselves or others. In addition, restraints should be used as a last resort only after other interventions have failed.

TABLE 5-2: RESTRAINTS: CONSUMER INFORMATION SHEET (1 OF 2)

WHAT ARE RESTRAINTS?

Physical Restraints: Any object or device that restricts movement or the ability to get to a part of the body. Usually a specialty device is used. Examples include vest or jacket restraints, waist belts, geri-chairs, hand mitts, and lap pillows.

Chemical Restraints: Psychoactive drugs used to treat behavioral symptoms in place of good care.

WHY ARE RESTRAINTS USED?

- Facilities or family members believe (usually mistakenly) that they ensure safety;
- As a substitute for adequate numbers or levels of staff;
- Facility fear of liability.

WHO IS USUALLY RESTRAINED?

- A resident with a history of falls, aggression, or wandering;
- A resident with a pre-existing injury or medical condition which makes walking or standing unsafe.

WHAT ARE THE *GOOD* OUTCOMES OF RESTRAINT USE?

Physical Restraints: In rare instances a restraint may enable a resident to do more, for example, a half bed rail may allow a partially paralyzed person to turn over; a seat belt may help double amputees to remember that they cannon walk on missing legs (they may have the feeling that their legs are still there).

Chemical Restraints: A resident's distressing behavioral symptom, such as depression, might be treated with a psychoactive drug when measures such as increased activities or talking with a social worker do not work.

WHAT ARE THE *POOR* OUTCOMES OF RESTRAINT USE?

Accidents involving restraints which may cause serious injury.

Changes in body systems which may include: Poor circulation, chronic constipation, incontinence, weak muscles, weakened bone structure, pressure sores, increased agitation, depressed appetite, increased threat of pneumonia, increased urinary infections, or death.

Changes in quality of life which may include: Reduced social contact, withdrawal from surroundings, loss of autonomy, depression, increased problems with sleep patterns, increased agitation, or loss of mobility.

CURRENT LAWS and REGULATIONS WHICH GOVERN RESTRAINT USE

- The Nursing Home Reform Act of 1987 states the resident has the right to be free from physical or chemical restraints imposed for purposes of discipline or convenience and not required to treat the resident's medical symptoms.

- This law also includes provisions requiring:
  — quality of care — to prevent poor outcomes of care;
  — assessment and care planning — for each resident to attain and maintain her highest level of functioning;
  — residents be treated in such a manner and environment to enhance quality of life.

STRATEGIES FOR REDUCING RESTRAINT USE

Although reducing restraint use can be frightening for some families and staff members, there are many facilities that have successfully committed to a restraint-free environment without an increase in resident injuries. Committed families and staff members working together to follow an individualized care plan can make this a reality which can benefit both residents and caregivers. In fact, research confirms that non-restrained residents require fewer minutes of direct nursing care when compared to similar residents who are restrained. However, a Federal government report notes that in order to be effective, restraint reduction activities must involve the whole facility, including "administrators, nursing directors, physical and recreational therapists, service delivery staff including nursing assistants, and housekeeping personnel." (p. 354) Family members and advocates should expect and insist that the facility be responsible and proactive in:

TABLE 5-2: RESTRAINTS: CONSUMER INFORMATION SHEET (2 OF 2)

- Completing a **comprehensive resident assessment:** Assessments gather information about how well residents can take care of themselves and when they need help. They identify strengths and weaknesses, plus lifelong habits and daily routines.

- Formulating an **individualized care plan:** Based on strengths and weaknesses identified on assessment, a care plan is developed for how staff will meet a resident's individual needs. It should describe what each staff person will do and when it will happen. The care plan is designed at a quarterly care-planning conference, attended by staff, residents, and their families. The care plan should change as the resident's needs change.

- Training staff to assess and meet an individual resident's needs — hunger, toileting, sleep, thirst, etc. — according to the **resident's routine rather than the facility's routine.**

- Supporting and encouraging professional caregiving staff to **think creatively** of new ways to identify and meet residents' needs.

- Providing a **program of activities** enjoyed by the resident, such as exercise, outdoor time, or small jobs agreed to and enjoyed by the resident.

- Providing the resident with **companionship,** including volunteers, family, and friends.

- Creating a **safe environment** with good lighting, mattresses on the floor to cushion falls out of bed, appropriate, comfortable seating, alarms, clear and safe walking paths inside and outside the building.

- Making permanent staff assignments and promoting staff flexibility to meet residents' individualized needs.

  If the nursing home is resistant to restraint reduction, you may want to suggest that they contact NCC-NHR for materials which provide information on specific programs for reducing restraint use including:

- Restorative care including walking, and independent eating, dressing, bathing programs;

- Wheelchair management program — to assure correct size, good condition, and appropriate seat cushions;

- Individualized seating program — chairs, like wheelchairs, should be tailored to individual needs;

- Specialized programs for residents with dementia, designed to increase their quality of life;

- Video visits — videotaped family visits when families live far away;

- Wandering program — to promote safe wandering while preserving the rights of others;

- Preventive program based on knowing the resident — to prevent triggering of aggressive behavioral symptoms and using protective intervention as a last resort;

- Toileting of residents based on their schedules rather than on staff schedules.

If you are interested in learning more, the National Citizens' Coalition for Nursing Home Reform (NCCNHR) has several publications that may be of interest. Call 202-332-2275 for a publication list or visit the website at http://www.nccnhr.org.

While the federal regulations for nursing homes define chemical restraints as drugs used for medical symptoms such as hallucinations or delusions, these medical symptoms are only those that have an adverse or frightening effect on the patient. Even in these cases the use of as-needed psychotropic medication is discouraged. If these medications are used more than twice in a 7-day period, they must be reevaluated by the prescribing clinician.

TABLE 5-3: COMMONLY USED PSYCHOACTIVE DRUGS

Antipsychotics (neuroleptics)

    Chlorpromazine (Thorazine®)

    Fluphenazine (Prolixin®)

    Haloperidol (Haldol®)

    Loxapine (Loxitane®)

    Mesoridazine (Serentil®)

    Molindone (Moban®)

    Perphenazine (Trilafon®)

    Risperidone (Risperdal®)

    Thioridazine (Mellaril®)

    Thiothixene (Navane®)

    Trifluoperazine (Stelazine®)

Antidepressants

    Amitriptyline (Elavil®)

    Bupropion (Wellbutrin®)

    Desipramine (Norpramin®)

    Doxepin (Sinequan®)

    Fluoxetine (Prozac®)

    Imipramine (Tofranil®)

    Maprotiline (Ludiomil®)

    Nortriptyline (Pamelor®)

    Paroxetine (Paxil®)

    Protriptyline (Vivactil®)

    Tranylcypromine (Parnate®)

    Trazodone (Desyrel®)

    Venlafaxine (Effexor®)

Anxiolytics (antianxiety agents)

    Short-acting benzodiazepines

        Alprazolam (Xanax®)

        Lorazepam (Ativan®)

        Oxazepam (Serax®)

        Temazepam (Restoril®)

    Long-acting benzodiazepines

        Chlordiazepoxide (Librium®)

        Clonazepam (Klonopin®)

        Clorazepate (Tranxene®)

        Diazepam (Valium®)

        Halazepam (Paxipam®)

        Prazepam (Centrax®)

Some of the drugs that can be considered chemical or pharmacological restraints are antipsychotics, anxiolytics, sedatives, hypnotics, mood stabilizers such as valproic aid (Depakote), and antidepressants (Sloane & Hargett, 1997) (see Table 5-3). In November of 2001, The Office of the Inspector General of the Department of Health and Human Services (HHS) released a report on psychotropic drug use in nursing homes. The findings indicate that 85% of psychotropic drug use in nursing home residents is considered appropriate based on guidelines established by the CMS. Another 8% of psychotropic drugs are used inappropriately. Inappropriate use of drugs include:

1) too high dose

2) lack of appropriate drug reduction attempts

3) unjustified chronic drug use

4) no documented benefit to the resident

5) wrong type of drug being given for a particular diagnosis

6) unnecessary or duplicate drug therapy.

Further investigation using survey data disclosed rates of anti-psychotic and anti-anxiety drug use in long-term care have actually been rising. However, the use for most psychotropic drugs appears to be medically appropriate.

A practical nursing approach to drug therapy, particularly the use of psychoactive drugs, is the concept of benefit versus risk. This idea helps nurses assess patients' potential drug-related problems and provides a useful framework for discussing drug information with patients' families and other care providers (Todd, 1986; Lantz & Shelkey, 2001).

Typically, nurses initiate the decision to physically restrain patients. Some nurses consider physical restraints a form of protection for patients and a protection for the nurses from litigation. The risk of falling and the need to protect tubes and intravenous lines are often given as reasons for using physical restraints. Nurses who practice in psychogeriatric wards or LTCFs have more knowledge about restraint guidelines and are less inclined to use them than nurses in acute care settings (Weiner, Tabak, & Bergman, 2003). One study examined nurses' attitudes toward, knowledge of, and practice in the use of physical restraints with older patients in acute care settings (Matthiesen, Lamb, McCann, Hollinger-Smith, & Walton, 1996). The findings showed little relationship between a nurse's amount of experience working with elderly people or education about use of restraints and the inappropriate use of physical restraints. However, significant differences in practice reflected the standard of care and philosophy of the unit or setting where the nurse worked. This finding points out the importance of role models who can show nurses and other caregivers how to solve problems and examine alternatives to the use of restraints. As role models in hospitals and other clinical settings, nurses are challenged to provide high-quality, cost-effective care for elderly and demented patients, emphasizing alternatives to restraints. Doing more with less has become a theme of hospital-based care.

Restraints and Fall Prevention

Restraints can actually contribute to fall-related injuries and deaths. Limiting freedom of movement and personal autonomy results in deconditioning and muscle atrophy that can increase functional decline.

Since new federal regulations took effect in 1990, nursing homes have reduced the use of physical restraints. Although some institutions have reported an increase in falls, fall-related injuries have decreased in most nursing homes and other LTCFs.

Alternatives to Restraints

Because agitation can lead to use of restraints, it is important to review other causes of agitation, such as inability to express one's needs (Talerico, Evans, & Strumpf, 2002), pain, overwhelming external stimuli, and physical restraints.

Before instituting the use of restraints, determine and treat underlying physiological causes of agitation or confusion. A useful mnemonic of possible causes for this behavior is the Seven I's (Stewart, 1995, 2000).

1. *Iatrogenic:* Inadvertently caused by treatment, for example, an anticholinergic agent or a sedative

2. *Infection:* Most commonly urinary tract infection or pneumonia

3. *Injury:* Such as a fractured hip

4. *Illness:* Exacerbation of a preexisting illness, such as diabetes or chronic obstructive pulmonary disease

5. *Impaction* (fecal)

6. *Inconsistency* in the environment: Any major change in routines, such as mealtimes or bedtimes

7. *Is* the person depressed?

Here are some strategies that can be used as alternatives to restraints:

1) Modify the environment to include carpeted floors and lowered beds.

2) Use positioning devices such as wedge cushions and other specialty cushions.

#44

3) Have a wheelchair or seating assessment done by a physical or occupational therapist (Rader, Jones, & Miller, 2000). As much as 80% of elderly persons experience problems with their wheelchairs, such as discomfort, restricted mobility, and poor posture (Shaw & Taylor, 1992). Patient sliding out of chairs is commonly cited as a reason for the use of restraints. Poorly fitted seating can also lead to problems with circulation, gastrointestinal and urinary tract dysfunction, and high blood pressure. Other problems include difficulty with speech, swallowing, chewing, breathing, and productive coughing. Informed nurses can make a preliminary assessment of seating and mobility needs and share it with physical or occupational therapist (see Table 5-4).

TABLE 5-4: ASSESSMENT FOR SEATING AND MOBILITY

Sitting position:	Walking:	Wheelchair:
Describe how the person usually sits.	Yes or No?	Yes or No?
• Slouched?	• With assistance?	• Transfers self?
• Leaning forward?	How much?	• Uses arms?
• Leaning to either side?	• Uses cane?	• Uses legs?
Which side?	Quad cane?	• Electric?
• Head forward?	Walker?	
• Position of legs?	Brace?	
Legs roll in?		
Legs roll out?		
Legs too high?		
Legs too low?		

(Jones, 1995)

4) Ask a family member or friend to stay with the patient.

5) Use motion-sensors or alerting devices.

6) Create a nonslip or nonskid surface to walk on. Cheaper products, such as nonslip rug backings, usually work best. Use a nonslip surface or strips on the floor by the side of the bed to avoid the use of bed rails.

7) Increase involvement of the patient in structured psychosocial activities.

8) Increase supervision and observation times, and make changes in nursing care, such as increases in assistance with toileting and ambulation.

9) Increase the use of therapeutic touch and active listening by nurses and other caregivers.

Again, it is important to remember that what works today for a patient with AD or dementia may not work tomorrow. The reality is that continual reassessment is required.

Restraints and Families

Although great emphasis has been placed on decreasing the use of restraints in health care facilities, one area that has not been addressed is the view of patients' family members. The opinions of patients' family members may be one of the biggest challenges or obstacles to decreasing the use of restraints. Families strongly believe in the use of restraints to protect their family member from falling or to safeguard the loved one in situations in which "not enough help" is available. Most family members are not informed that a hospitalized patient is going to be restrained and are not given a specific reason for the restraint or told the potential benefits or risks of using restraints (Kanski, Janelli, Jones, & Kennedy, 1996). Nurses in each practice setting should determine who is responsible for educating families about families' legal rights, the benefits and risks of the restraint use, and alternatives to restraints.

The best time to discuss the use of restraints is before or at the time of admission. Informal conferences can be held to discuss the relevant issues with other caregivers and the patient's family. Nurses should keep communication with families open and should provide family members with information, such as reprints of articles with easily understood information on the use of restraints. This information reinforces what nurses are attempting to teach and reassures patients and families that although restraint-free care is not risk free, the benefits more often outweigh the physical and emotional problems associated with the use of physical restraints.

Restraint Documentation

JCAHO has outlined documentation requirements for the use of restraints. It is imperative when using restraints to document patient behaviors that have led to the use of restraints, what other interventions were used, and why these methods failed. Also document the type of restraint used, when use was initiated, and when it was discontinued. During restraint use, it is important to document how the patient's safety, food, fluid, and elimination needs were met. Assessment of circulation, injury, skin integrity, and readiness for removal must also be documented.

SUMMARY

As care providers, nurses have the responsibility of providing a safe environment for older adult patients and optimizing their functional status. Falls are not just the result of getting older. Falls can occur as a result of functional decline, or they can induce functional decline in older adults. Falls are the leading predictor of morbidity and mortality in the elderly population. Prediction of falls is associated with identification of a set of existing risk factors. These factors are placed in one of three categories: extrinsic, intrinsic (anticipated physiological), and intrinsic (unanticipated physiological). The cognitive decline in AD alone is a predictor of falls and is associated with a striking rise in the sequelae of severe falls.

Many falls can be prevented. Because falls are caused by the interaction of numerous factors, fall prevention requires a combination of medical treatment, rehabilitation, environmental modification, and technological interventions. Although these strategies are suggested for use with all older adults, they can certainly be modified to meet the need of patients with AD.

Patients must be assessed at the time of admission for the potential risk of falling using a rating guideline for falls risk assessment. Research indicates that no association exists between restraint use and reduction in falls. Use of physical restraints and psychoactive medications can have hazardous and adverse outcomes.

EXAM QUESTIONS

CHAPTER 5
Questions 41-50

41. Falls in older adults

    a. are rarely attributed to environmental factors *50% are*

    (b.) may be directly attributed to drugs such as sedatives and antihypertensives.

    c. are the leading predictor of nursing home placements in the elderly population.

    d. are viewed by most individuals as *No* predictable and avoidable accidents.

42. The most common causes of falls in older adults are

    a. intrinsic factors (anticipated physiological).

    b. intrinsic factors (unanticipated physiological).

    (c.) extrinsic factors (environmental).

    d. inappropriate restraint use.

43. The best method for preventing patients with AD from falling when they need to urinate at night is

    a. use a nonslip surface next to the bed.

    b. restrict fluid intake after 3:00 p.m.

    c. provide increased periods of exercise.

    d. offer a snack upon awakening.

I should have known this. C doesn't make sense I been must have tired!

44. A nursing intervention that can reduce harm to patients who are at risk for falling is

    a. moving their rooms *closer* farther from the nurses station so that the patients can build endurance by walking increased distances.

    (b.) participating in care of individuals with risk of falling by using physical therapy.

    c. using incontinence products.

    d. posting warning signs throughout the facility.

45. A measure used to reduce the risk of falls is

    a. raise the height of the bed to prevent bending.

    b. institute pet therapy for protection.

    (c.) provide sneakers or slippers with a non-skid tread.

    d. assist with ladder use to climb heights.

46. When a resident experiences a fall, the proper sequence of a nurse's responsibilities are

    a. assessment of airway, breathing, and circulation; assessment of circumstances just prior to the fall; and documentation.

    b. assessment of circumstances just prior to the fall and documentation.

    c. notification of EMS; assessment of airway, breathing, and circulation; and assessment of circumstances just prior to the fall.

    d. assessment of airway, breathing, and circulation; assessment of circumstances just prior to the fall; documentation; and notification of EMS.

47. According to JCAHO guidelines, restraints should be used

    a. only in emergencies where patients may harm themselves or others.

    b. as an initial intervention for safety.

    c. anytime the patient is at risk to fall.

    d. only with permission from the patient.

48. A positive outcome from the use of restraints is that they

    a.. prevent skin breakdown.

    b. may enable a resident to do more.

    c. prevent fall-related injuries and deaths.

    d. ensure patient comfort.

49. The initial assessment following any fall should begin with

    a. how frequently the person has fallen recently.

    b. reasons the person may fall again.

    c. airway, breathing, and circulation.

    d. past injuries from previous falls.

50. In November of 2001, the Department of Health and Human Services reported that the use of psychotropic drugs as chemical restraints in nursing homes

    a. have been on the rise but were medically appropriate.

    b. have been on the decline and were medically inappropriate.

    c. were inappropriate in 85% of the cases.

    d. were causing falls in the majority of the residents.

CHAPTER 6

PAIN AND HOSPITALIZATION

CHAPTER OBJECTIVE

After completing this chapter the reader will be able to outline the prevalence of, assessment of, interventions for, and outcomes for pain in patients with Alzheimer's disease (AD) and discuss pharmacological treatment of pain in these individuals. The reader will also be able identify reasons for hospitalization of people with AD and the care they should receive while hospitalized.

LEARNING OBJECTIVES

After completing this chapter, the reader will be able to

1. summarize quality of life, how it can be measured, and how pain can impact it.

2. discuss the prevalence of pain in older adults with dementia.

3. identify inadequacies of research in pain management for older adults with dementia.

4. identify inadequacies in assessments and identification of pain in older adults with dementia.

5. discuss pain management strategies for older adults with dementia.

6. identify the major reasons for hospitalization of people with AD.

7. discuss plans that can assist in smoother transitions of people with AD into acute hospital settings.

INTRODUCTION

One of the goals of nursing is to enhance the quality of life for older adults, especially in the face of declining abilities. Remember that high functioning does not necessarily represent a high quality of life. Nurses can maximize quality of life by reducing pain, connecting with individual spirituality, enhancing the environment, and designing physical activity programs.

QUALITY OF LIFE

Nurses must change their thinking about quality of life in older adults. Although patients with AD have disabilities, nurses should focus on the function rather than the impairment. Definitions of quality of life have always focused on medical interventions and implied that health and function are vital to defining quality of life. As a result, the medical community has used health status or functional status and quality of life interchangeably. When asked, however, older adults report that their physical problems are not at all important to their quality of life (Johansson, 2003).

"Assessments of quality of life are subjective and depend on preconceived value systems" (Loefler, 2003, p. 893). Clinicians use tools that evaluate quality of life in a medicalized sense of the term that does not take into consideration the difference between quantity of life and quality of life (Loefler,

2003). Measuring quality of life for people with terminal dementia is difficult because demented individuals cannot express what they perceive their quality of life to be.

Implementation of a single scale to measure this concept is questionable because quality of life is multidimensional. For this reason, using a scale that measures "...the dimension that is most relevant in a specific situation, e.g., the dimension that is likely to be influenced by a behavioral or pharmacological intervention" (Blasi, Hurley, & Volicer, 2002) is recommended. These dimensions can include:

- social interaction
- awareness of self
- enjoyment of activities
- behavioral competence
- psychological well-being
- adequately controlled symptoms
- attention to spiritual needs
- environmental quality.

In recent literature, an 11 item observational scale called QUALID (Quality of Life in Late-Stage Dementia) was developed to combine indications of mood, comfort, and simple enjoyable interactions. The scores do not correlate with severity of dementia measured by the Mini-Mental Status Examination. Therefore, this scale may be useful for measuring quality of life for individuals with terminal dementia (Blasi, Hurley, & Volicer, 2002).

PAIN

All humans have experienced pain at some point in time. For many older adults, pain can significantly affect quality of life. For decades of research on pain, researchers failed to look specifically at the older adult population. When caring for older adults, especially those with dementia, nurses should ask themselves many questions about pain management: Which intervention is best for which

person? How much medication is dangerous or sufficient? How can I satisfactorily assess pain in an individual with cognitive impairment? How and when will I know the cognitively impaired individual has achieved relief from pain? It would be wonderful to have care plans designed that could answer these questions but, unfortunately, they don't exist. The positive side is that researchers are currently in the process of obtaining some of these answers.

Nursing's fundamental focus is the promotion of comfort and relief of pain. Although pain management for older adults, especially those with AD, is complex and challenging, it is an area that can be rewarding for the nurse.

Prevalence of Pain in Older Adults

The prevalence of pain in the general population of older adults is estimated to be between 50% and 80% (Briggs, 2003; Brummel-Smith, London, Drew, et al., 2002; Cohen-Mansfield & Lipson, 2002; Fulmer, Mion, & Bottrell, 1996; Panda & Desbiens, 2001). "Despite increased prevalence of pain in older adults, chronic pain is not a normal consequence of aging. Pain is always the result of a pathologic condition — either physical or psychological" (Panda & Desbiens, 2001, p. 1597). All types of pain affect older adults in some way: physically, socially, psychologically and, incidentally, economically. Unrelieved pain increases these effects and increases the risk of complications in people who already have pre-existing conditions.

What evidence is there to support that older demented adults (such as those with AD) are experiencing pain? Self-reports, observations of caregivers, physician reports, and initial diagnoses are indications. People with impaired communication who cannot verbalize pain also experience it. Older adults suffer from multiple disease processes that include pain among their characteristics. Chronic conditions can also cause pain, including musculoskeletal conditions, such as osteoarthritis, peripheral vascular disease, and peripheral neuropathies.

Defining Pain

Pain can be classified as acute or chronic:

- **Acute pain** is usually attributable to a consequence of tissue damage induced by injury or disease.

- **Chronic pain** is pain that lasts beyond the acute phase. Chronic pain is more challenging to treat than acute pain and can lead to physical, social, and psychological changes. The causes of chronic pain are not clearly identifiable and are most often multifaceted. Chronic pain can be further classified as nonmalignant and cancer-related pain (Briggs, 2003; Fulmer et al., 2002; Panda & Desbiens, 2001). Chronic pain that lasts longer than 6 months is associated with a high rate of depression, around 90% (Kepfer & Eisendrath, 2003). "Unremitting pain and the inability to resolve it can lead to a sense of helplessness" (Kepfer & Eisendrath, 2003, p. 1508). Coupled with the depression that can occur in AD and the feelings of hopelessness and helplessness, the outcome of chronic pain in AD is a reduced quality of life.

Pain's definition is expanded by identification of the causes of pain. Disease processes, soft-tissue injuries, and medical treatments such as surgery and other procedures cause nociceptive pain. Nociceptive pain is associated with stimulation of specific peripheral or visceral receptors that relay pain information to the brain; therefore, it is localized and responsive to treatment. An abnormal process in the peripheral or central nervous system as a result of nerve damage (diabetic neuropathies, phantom limb pain, postherpetic neuralgias, and cerebrovascular accidents) induces neuropathic pain. This type of pain is more diffuse and less responsive to treatment. These two types of pain can also be described as fast-track and slow-track pain. Descriptors for fast-track include stabbing or sharp; while slow-track is throbbing and dull. One must take care when assessing pain and remember that these types of pain can overlap.

Pain Research

Most research that has looked at pain has done so retrospectively, using charts, notes, treatment records, and medication records. Research on pain has historically disregarded people with cognitive impairments and most notably those with severe communication restrictions. Only a handful of studies have evaluated pain in noncommunicative or demented persons (Cohen-Mansfield & Lipson, 2002). This fact makes investigation of pain in older adults with some form of dementia even more pressing.

The question arises then, with all the multidimensional tools that have been developed for assessing pain, why is there a problem assessing pain in patients who are cognitively impaired? The answer lies in the patient's inability to communicate. The diminished ability to communicate leaves uncertainty for the assessor in both the ability to assess the pain and the actual pain level in the person with the impairment (Fisher, Burgio, Thorn, et al., 2002). Caregivers also experience difficulty in acceptance of cognitively impaired individuals' reports of pain (Ferrell, 2000; Parmelee, 1996). Research indicates that no evidence exists to support exaggeration or fabrication of pain by older adults with dementia (Bruce & Kopp, 2001; Parmelee, 1996).

Uncertainty leads to underidentification and, therefore, undertreatment of pain in this population of individuals (Briggs, 2003; Cohen-Mansfield & Lipson, 2002; Parmelee, 1996). In fact, research has found that only one-third of cognitively impaired individuals can report pain using one of the established pain measurement tools (Brummel-Smith et al., 2002; Sherder, 2000; Wynne, Ling, & Remsburg, 2000). Other studies indicate that approximately 50% of individuals with milder forms of impaired cognition can report pain using at least one scale, usually the Wong-Baker Faces Pain Rating Scale or the Present Pain Intensity Index of the McGill Pain Questionnaire (Briggs, 2003; Kamel, Phlavan, Malekgoudarzi, Gogel, & Morley, 2001).

Several studies have demonstrated that individuals with more advanced forms of dementia receive one-third the amount of medication for pain as do others who are more cognitively enhanced. Cohen-Mansfield and Lipson stated that, as compared to individuals with mild or moderate cognitive impairment, patients with severe cognitive impairment were classified as having less "disease" and, therefore, less pain (2002). These findings may reflect older adults' inability to remember and report pain to caregivers; inability of caregivers to detect pain; or caregiver bias about who really suffers pain, especially those with the mildest or most severe cases of dementia. Although the prevalence of pain in older adults is somewhere between 50% and 80%, pain in these individuals is both underidentified and undertreated, and a significant portion of demented older adults do not receive adequate interventions from caregivers to relieve their pain.

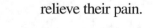

Pain Assessment

What makes pain assessment so challenging in older adults? "The indications of pain are frequently unclear in cognitively impaired people with limited communication abilities, and the only assessment possible is based on caregivers' perception through direct observations" (Cohen-Mansfield, & Lipson, 2002, p. 1039). Ability to truly assess pain and common perceptions of how older adults experience pain are flawed. Most nurses heard the following comment about pain among older adults: "every old person complains of pain." Ageist attitudes still thrive in practice. However, nurses must take older adults' complaints of pain seriously. Older adults expect to experience pain; they assume that it is a normal and inevitable part of the aging process. Patients do not want to be labeled as hypochondriacs or complaining patients and when they are identified as such, the ageist attitude is perpetuated (Fisher, Kutner, & Maier, 2002).

When evaluating the impact of pain on older individuals, remember that how pain is defined and its effects on the individual's activity influence the individual's response to that pain. Day-to-day pain can become second nature. Nurses must be able to assess and manage individual pain in order for the cycle of pain to be broken and to increase the quality of care for older adults.

The assessment of pain must be performed in a systematic way to successfully detect it and to effect early interventions. "Appropriate pain management can only be achieved through accurate pain assessment that is individualized, ongoing, and well documented" (Lane et al., 2003, p. 32). The Joint Commission on Accreditation of Healthcare Organizations (JCAHO) indicates that pain should now be considered the fifth vital sign and, as such, should be assessed each time blood pressure, pulse, and respirations are taken (JCAHO, 2003). The multiplicity of available assessment tools can be helpful, depending on individual communication capability. In the last 10 years, researchers have developed the following tools for assessing pain in noncommunicating older adults:

- Discomfort Scale-DAT (Hurley, Volicer, Hanrahan, Houde, & Volicer, 1992)
- NOPAIN (Snow, Hovanec, Passano, & Brandt, 2001)
- Checklist for Nonverbal Pain Behaviors (Feldt, Warne, & Ryden, 1998)
- Nonverbal Pain Assessment Tool (NVAT) (Fisher, Kutner, & Maier, 2003).

Vigilant surveillance by caregivers can help to determine the source of pain and strategies for its relief. Because of the communication difficulties and memory deficits present in patients with AD, the expression of pain differs each time for each person, even with subsequent assessments on the same day. Therefore, nurses can be more successful in assessment of pain by evaluating the present pain experience rather than asking the standard questions, such as "How long have you had this pain?" "When did your pain start?" or "How long does your pain last?" The assessment of pain is not always measured in terms of scales and ratings or verbal reports but rather in behavioral disturbances.

Look for cues that suggest the person with dementia is in pain. Staff observations are vital to assessment and interventions for pain. In long-term care facilities (LTCFs), nursing assistants spend the most time with patients and are, therefore, more sensitive to individual patient pain levels. Caregivers become surrogates for people with AD in reporting pain. Family members can be particularly helpful in this regard. They know how the patient or loved one normally responds to pain and may notice subtle changes in expression of pain as the disease progresses. As a result, they are reasonable assessors of pain for loved ones (Desbiens & Mueller-Rizner, 2000). Be sure to remember, however, that family caregiver reports alone are not always successful in determining pain in AD patients.

In 1992, Hurley et al., developed behavioral indicators for pain assessment of patients with progressive dementia. In 2003, most additional research agrees with these indicators (Briggs, 2003; Brummel-Smith et al., 2002; Cohen-Mansfield & Lipson, 2002). They are:

- noisy breathing   #54

- negative vocalisms or calling out

- absence of contented look

- sad appearance

- frightened appearance

- frowning or grimacing

- absence of a relaxed body posture

- tense appearance

- physical movements, such as fidgeting, rubbing, and guarding; agitation; and restlessness.

Other researchers include aggressive behavior as an indicator of pain, especially in demented older adults with two or more pain-related diagnoses

(Feldt, Warne, & Ryden, 1998; Horgas, 2003; Snow, Hovanec, Passano, & Brandt, 2001). Although these indicators have not been researched in great depth, they can be used as a basis of observational changes that require further investigation. Pain may be the cause. Assuming that these behavioral disturbances are the result of pain is problematic because these same behaviors can be expressions of cold, hunger, fatigue, fear, and other emotional and physiologic needs. Undoubtedly, there is a need to explain changes in behavior by attending to these disturbances and thus improving quality of life.

Whenever possible, pain should be treated immediately upon detection (see Table 6-1). Older adults are often responsive to nonpharmacological interventions for pain. Nonpharmacological pain treatment approaches fall into one of two categories: physical relief of pain or cognitive-behavioral practices. Physical relief strategies include the use of heat and cold therapies, massage, transcutaneous electrical nerve stimulation, and mild exercise. Cognitive-behavioral strategies are more difficult to implement in AD patients. They include guided imagery, relaxation, distraction, hypnosis, and biofeedback. Relaxation and distraction are most likely to be effective for patients with AD (Horgas, 2003).

TABLE 6-1: OUTCOMES OF UNTREATED PAIN
"Inappropriate pain management leaves both the elder and the nurse feeling unfulfilled and unhappy with the care" (Fulmer, Mion, & Bottrell, 1996, p. 225). Inappropriate measurement of pain can lead to: • Depression • Diminished function • Exacerbation of cognitive impairment • Sleep disturbances • Increased health care utilization costs.

It is essential that nurses review the nursing and medical literature in order to improve their practice and put in place the educational measures needed for continuous improvement of pain recognition and pain management (see Table 6-2).

TABLE 6-2: IMPLICATIONS FOR PRACTICE AND EDUCATION

- Pain assessment and identification inadequate
- As-needed analgesia inadequate
- Nonpharmacological strategies limited
- Observation assessment valid and reliable
- Cognitively impaired elders can self-report
- Improved pain management may maintain cognitive function
- Pain linked to depression
- Treatment of depression and improved physical function can reduce agitation
- Continuing education for nurses must focus on pain in cognitively impaired elders in relation to
  1) Observational assessment
  2) Self-reports
  3) Outcomes of poor pain management

Evaluation of Expected Outcomes

Evaluation of outcomes of interventions in the management of pain must include the person with AD, the nurse, and the institution. The outcomes should include:

1) Patient

   a) Absence of pain or level judged to be acceptable by staff or family caregivers

   b) Maintenance of functional ability

   c) No iatrogenic outcomes (falls, altered cognitive status, gastrointestinal [GI] upset or bleed)

2) Nurse

   a) Evidence of ongoing and comprehensive pain assessment

   b) Evidence of prompt interventional strategies

   c) Increased knowledge regarding pain management in AD patients

   d) Increased knowledge regarding medications

   e) Increased knowledge regarding assessment of pain

3) Institution

   a) Documentation of assessment of pain, plan, and effectiveness

      i) Documentation formalizes the pain assessment process, promotes communication between all caregivers, and has legal implications. Use the institution's normal charting process but remember to include the pain assessment document utilized. As the fifth vital sign, pain must be routinely assessed and charted with other vital signs. Pain behaviors and vocalizations of pain must be included in your charting because they are the only evidence of pain for those who cannot verbalize it.

   b) Possible increase in referrals to specialists

   c) Possible increase in referrals to outside providers

(Fulmer, Mion, & Bottrell, 1996)

Pharmacological Management of Pain

Research has demonstrated that older adults with dementia have lower rates of pain medication administration than those without dementia (Brummel-Smith et al., 2002). Standard medications for pain management can be worrisome and produce significant adverse effects. Age-related changes impact absorption, metabolism, distribution, and excretion of drugs. Caregivers are restricted in what pharmacologic interventions are available for pain.

When initiating pharmacologic management of pain, drugs with a short-half life are the initial considerations. Also keep in mind the guideline **start low and go slow!** The dose can be increased, so select the lowest dose available first, and slowly increase the dosage and frequency, as necessary. #56

Traditional nonsteroidal anti-inflammatory drugs (NSAIDs) such as ibuprofen and naproxen, although widely used, tend to increase confusion when used over a long period; they may also increase fluid retention and GI distress. Cyclooxygenase II (COX II) #57 inhibitors are often good alternatives to traditional NSAIDs for at-risk populations, especially those with known GI upset, renal impairment, or platelet dysfunction. At-risk patients include those with rheumatoid arthritis, osteoarthritis, hypertension, gastric ulcers, diabetes, or hepatic impairment.

Although opiates, such as morphine, are known to increase confusion in older adults, they are generally safe. Common adverse effects include sedation, respiratory depression, and constipation. Slow titration of the drug and frequent monitoring of patients taking opiates are very important. Studies have indicated that opioid analgesics hold particular promise in the treatment of pain in people with AD and should be used more frequently (Allen et al., 2003).

Some antidepressants and anticonvulsants are also helpful in treating pain, but these drugs can also increase confusion and cause weight loss. The adverse effects of these medications often leave caregivers with acetaminophen and mood stabilizers as the only choices for pain relief (Briggs, 2003; Cohen-Mansfield & Lipson, 2002; Lehne, 2004).

Caution must be used when administering any medication to older adults and is especially necessary in the use of pain medications. A conservative approach may help to control pain while limiting side effects.

HOSPITALIZATION

During the natural course of AD, individuals are likely to be hospitalized as a result of the disease itself, other diseases, or life events. The incidence of hospitalizations in persons with AD is significant. In a recent study, 24% of patients in the study, had experienced at least one acute hospitalization within the first 12 months of study follow-up (Andrieu et al., 2002).

Reasons for hospital admissions include sleep disorders, episodes of agitation, feeding issues, and pathological complications of the disease, such as gait disorders, falls, and anemia. Predictors of hospital admissions include behavioral problems, baseline educational level, and activities of daily living and bathing dependency. Andrieu et al. found that the severity of cognitive symptoms at baseline was not a predictor of admission (2002). Their findings also supported Neville, Boyle, and Baillon's findings (1999) that the number one cause of admissions to hospitals is behavioral problems. The leading behavioral problems included, in rank order, self-neglect #58 by community-dwelling persons with AD, general diagnostic treatment, wandering, and severe agitation. The second and third most frequent causes of hospital admissions were fractures and social factors such as family (Andrieu et al., 2002).

Hospitalizations, which can be frequent in some older adults with AD, can be stressful for the family and other caregivers and frightening for the patient. The Alzheimer's Association has produced a brochure for guiding family and nurses through the process of acute illnesses in persons with AD (Alzheimer's Association, n.d.).

Planning for Hospitalization

Planning for hospitalizations can enable a smooth transition from the home or LTCF into the acute care setting. Listed here are ideas for families and their caregivers to consider in those plans:

1) Be sure that people with AD are registered with the SAFE RETURN program through the local

Alzheimer's organization and that they wear their identification bracelets at all times.

2) Have a support system identified, with responsibilities clearly outlined. Be sure that these responsibilities have been reviewed with support team members prior to a trip to the hospital — for example, who the family member or caregiver can call to go with them to the hospital, who can take care of their home, who can assist with admission paperwork while someone is remaining with the AD patient, and so forth.

3) Family members must prepare an information folder for people with AD. This should include:

   a. Identification information: name, address, age, brief medical history

   b. Doctors names and contact numbers (this is especially helpful if the family is away from home)

   c. Insurance cards (company policy numbers and preauthorization telephone numbers)

   d. Medicare and Medicaid cards

   e. Current medication list

   f. Emergency contact numbers

   g. Important documents such as living will and durable power of attorney

   h. Card with the person's normal routine, personal habits, likes and dislikes, suspicions, falls, and other important personal information.

4) Family members should pack an emergency bag for the patient, including:

   a. Change of clothes

   b. Sanitary and personal item extras, such as adult diapers

   c. A reassuring object from home

      i. A recorder and tapes made of familiar voices or favorite music

      ii. Favorite pillow and pictures

      iii. Pain medication (acetaminophen or ibuprofen) for the caregiver. The family member is away from home and may need this.

      iv. A small amount of cash for food, magazines, and other small purchases

      v. A pen and notepad

      vi. Bottled water and a sealed snack, such as crackers, for the person with AD and the caregiver (emergency room visits and the process of being hospitalized can take a while)

4) Family members should not leave the emergency room without a plan for follow-up or, if the person with AD is being admitted, informing others of the AD patient's limitations, methods of communication, meaning of common behavioral problems, and so forth.

5) If the person with AD is admitted and if his or her insurance or finances allow, try to obtain a private room because this is quieter and less frightening.

6) Try to assure that the person with AD is never left alone in the hospital, even when tests are being conducted. This helps with reassurance and safety issues.

7) If behavioral disturbances do occur, insist that the staff avoid using restraints.

8) Make sure that the hospital staff knows when family members will be coming and leaving and what tasks they will perform for the person with AD, such as bathing, dressing, and eating.

SUMMARY

Quality of life is impacted dramatically by pain. Pain can develop as aging occurs and with various disease processes. The gold standard of assessing pain has always been the patient's self-report. This makes the ability to assess pain in individuals who are unable to communicate a challenge. Caregivers commonly become proxies for pain reporting but may miss some indications of pain. Caregivers must develop and refine observation skills in order to further evaluate pain in this vulnerable population (Fisher, Kutner, & Maier, 2002). Aggressive behaviors can often be attributed to two or more pain-related diagnoses, and attending to pain may significantly reduce behavioral disturbances.

Treatment of pain can include pharmacological and nonpharmacological strategies. Nonpharmacological treatments, such as behavior modification, distraction, and guided imagery are more difficult to implement for patients with AD because of already confounding behavior problems and inability to communicate. Researchers must continue to seek better methods of identifying pain and the most efficient means of treating pain in this at-risk population.

A large portion of the AD population will be hospitalized at some time for various disease-related problems. Nurses in the acute care setting must help the patient transition from the community or LTCF. Knowing what to anticipate in the care of persons with AD facilitates a much smoother course of hospital treatment.

EXAM QUESTIONS

CHAPTER 6
Questions 51-60

51. Quality of life in older adults with AD *focus on function*

    a. should focus on the impairment rather than the function of an individual.

    b. is rarely affected by the prevalence of pain.

    c. is easy to measure in people with terminal dementia.

    d. may be measured using a QUALID scale.

52. Pain influences quality of life. The best method of evaluating pain in people with AD is through

    a. caregiver and staff observations.

    b. observation of calm behavior.

    c. patient reports of pain.

    d. the knowledge that all older adults complain of pain.

53. The prevalence of pain in older adults with AD is difficult to measure because

    a. there are no tools for assessing pain in non-communicating older adults.

    b. the patient has a diminished ability to communicate.

    c. research shows patients with dementia tend to exaggerate their pain.

    d. research shows patients with dementia fabricate their pain.

54. When assessing the pain of a person with AD, the most appropriate action is to

    a. ask "How long have you had this pain?"

    b. assess the previous shift's nursing notes.

    c. look for cues, such as noisy breathing or tense appearance.

    d. assume that behavioral changes indicate pain.

55. A true statement regarding research and pain in older adults is

    answer sheet shows

    a. much research has focused on evaluating pain in noncommunicative older adults.

    b. historically, researchers have ignored people with dementia and severe communication restrictions.

    c. if no research exists on underidentification of pain in individuals with dementia, undertreatment of pain is likely.

    d. research has supported that those with advanced dementia receive almost identical treatment for pain as compared to those with higher levels of cognitive function.

56. When initiating pharmacologic management for pain in older adults with dementia

    a. start with drugs with a long half-life.

    b. start with the highest dose to bring on the effect and then titrate it down quickly.

    c. start with the lowest dose and slowly increase the dosage and frequency, as necessary.

    d. avoid Cox II inhibitors since they increase confusion.

57. Mrs. Payne, a 78-year-old woman with decreased renal function, has been restless, paces, appears sad, and grimaces. Your assessments reveal she is experiencing some form of discomfort and GI upset. When you review her medication administration record you find several drugs available for use. Your first choice of medication for Mrs. Payne would be

    a. naproxen.

    b. ibuprofen.

    c. a COX-2 inhibitor.

    d. morphine.

58. According to Neville, Boyle, and Baillon (1999), the leading cause of hospital admissions for people with AD in the community is

    a. self-neglect.

    b. fractures.

    c. falls.

    d. pneumonia.

59. Hospital admission can be traumatic for patients with AD and their families. A strategy for families to use to ease the transition into an acute hospital setting is

    a. encourage the staff to use restraints.

    b. present an information folder with personal information about the patient.

    c. avoid private rooms as they can be frightening and too quiet.

    d. avoid bringing personal items from home since they will think they are home.

60. A strategy that nurses in the acute care setting can use in managing patients with AD is

    a. use restraints for all behavioral disturbances.

    b. leave the patient alone at all times to reduce behavior problems.

    c. withhold pain medication to keep the patient alert.

    d. know what to anticipate in the care of people with AD.

CHAPTER 7

SPIRITUALITY, RELIGION, AND END-OF-LIFE ISSUES

CHAPTER OBJECTIVES

After completing this chapter, the reader will be able to recognize the need to incorporate holistic care into nursing practice and discuss the concepts of spirituality and religion as they relate to people with Alzheimer's disease (AD). The reader will also be able to acknowledge and provide for the special end-of-life needs of people with dementia.

LEARNING OBJECTIVES

After studying this chapter, the reader will be able to

1. discuss how to assess the spiritual and religious practices of people with dementia.

2. identify spiritual and religious interventions for people with dementia, including those with the potential to enhance quality of life.

3. identify the importance of a "good death" and its meaning to family members and caregivers.

4. discuss the grieving process experienced by people with AD and their caregivers.

5. identify the needs, including ethical and legal needs, of dying people with AD.

6. indicate the importance of monitoring and caring for the caregivers of dying AD patients.

7. discuss the care required for dying AD patients.

INTRODUCTION

Holistic nursing incorporates physical, psychosocial, and spiritual needs of human beings. All of these needs affect an individual's health status. Religion is a component of spirituality and comprises the formal beliefs and rituals a person uses to search for the meaning of his or her life. It is a bridge to spirituality and becomes a culture as it is shared with others. Life is a development concept that starts at conception and ends at death. A person may use his or her culture and various rituals and religious practices to help provide structure and meaning to daily life.

People who have AD or another related disorder are still capable of high levels of spiritual well-being. Just because they experience cognitive declines does not mean they cease to be relational and spiritual beings. Beliefs, rituals, and practices also influence people's perceptions of illness and their responses to it. People with AD continue, until the end of their lives, to need to be loved and wanted, to have hope, and to be valued as people.

It is understandable, even expected, that when faced with a diagnosis of AD, families may feel an overwhelming sense of loss. However, despite the physical and emotional damage that can occur with AD, certain people are able to transcend the hopelessness and find purpose and even peace amid the losses. Religion and spirituality play a role in this ability to cope (Stuckey, Post, Ollerton, FallCreek, &

Whitehouse, 2002). Even when faced with advanced dementia, people with AD have the ability to experience meaningful religious and spiritual events.

The largest portion of nursing literature that addresses the topic of spirituality does so mainly through theoretical and conceptual terms; it fails to provide functional guidance to support nursing actions (Dossey & Guzzetta, 2000; Mueller, Plevak, & Rummans, 2001). As caregivers, nurses must strive to remain sensitive to patient needs and must never fail to appreciate the importance of religion and spirituality to the well-being of patients and their families across the continuum of life. Patient care is much more than just managing disease; it must address all of the needs of the person. Spirituality is "a unifying force of a person's essence of being that permeates all of life and is manifested in one's being, knowing, and doing; the interconnectedness with self, others, nature, and God/Life/Force/Absolute/Transcendent" (Dossey & Guzzetta, 2000, p. 7).

SPIRITUAL AND RELIGIOUS NEEDS OF AD PATIENTS

Illnesses, such as AD, interrupt our routines and create situations of dependency. Throughout history, people have relied on religious beliefs and spirituality to cope with illness. More than 300 studies have demonstrated that individuals who rely on spiritual beliefs cope better and have better health outcomes than those who are without such beliefs (Mueller, Plevak, & Rummans, 2001). These studies have also shown that individuals who use spiritual and religious beliefs for coping have lower levels of depression during an illness (Mueller, Plevak, & Rummans, 2001). As previously discussed, depression is a common problem among patients with AD. Encouraging patients to rely on their established practices for coping can assist them in achieving better outcomes throughout the disease course. Religious and spiritual coping also appear to lessen the effects of stressful events on caregivers of the elderly population (Mueller, Plevak, & Rummans, 2001).

Body and soul are inseparable, so when nurses care for the body and mind, they are caring for the soul as well. Physical function and quality of life are definitely linked, but a potential chasm exists between them. This opening provides nurses the opportunity to enhance quality of life for older adults with dementia.

Many aspects of spirituality are intangible and not easily described. The concept of "soul" is mystifying. Johansson (2003) says that people know soul when they see it, in music, food, and paintings: "It is soul that gives depth to experience. It lives in the complexities and depths of our lives" (p. 228).

How does a nurse care for the soul? "Religion and spirituality, which are seen to have dominion over ways of connecting with the most essential features of the persons, i.e., the soul, offer potential pathways for maintaining meaningful connections between persons with AD and their families, friends, and other caregivers, even deep into the progression of the disease" (Stuckey, Post, Ollerton, FallCreek, & Whitehouse, 2002, p. 200). Nurses must provide care using their imaginations, honoring relationships, surrendering false impressions of control, and attending to the mystery that is part of each person (Johansson, 2003). They must realize that caring for patients involves much more than just managing disease. But, first of all, nurses must develop their own spiritual self-awareness as part of providing spiritual care to others.

Older adults with AD are whole beings with histories and relationships. Relationships with others contribute to psychosocial and physical well-being. For example, women with breast cancer who attend support groups report higher quality of life. Religion and spirituality can be at the center of an individual's responses to illness. Offering social support and relationships can be as simple as identifying resources available to people to meet their spiritual and religious needs. Simply placing a worn out comforter from home to which an older adult is attached in the room cares for the soul. It provides the comfort that quiets the soul and therefore the behavior (Johansson, 2003).

Spirituality plays a supportive role in the lives of certain people, especially older adults. It comprises important cultural factors and gives structure and meaning to values, behaviors, and experience.

Nurses may experience first hand the disregard of other care providers to the religious beliefs of people with AD. The reason for this disregard is a lack of training in religious awareness. Nurses should consider personal history when assessing patients' religious needs. It is important to remember that some people with AD have religious and spiritual pasts and may not be able to continue to participate in previous practices (Hilton, Ghaznavi, & Zuberi, 2002). For example, people of Jewish Orthodox, Muslim, and Hindu backgrounds are accustomed to food preparation that may include not mixing certain foods or not eating certain foods. Denying them such religious practices denies their heritage and their needs.

Meeting Spiritual and Religious Needs

Status of spiritual needs is assessed through informal, unstructured interviews. The nonverbal behavior of the interviewer helps to set up an open, friendly atmosphere in which the assessment can be conducted. The interviewer should determine what the patient's religious background is, what needs are met through the patient's spirituality, and how the spirituality is expressed, such as through community worship, music, nature, other people, or private prayer (Touhy, 2001).

Sensory aids (visual and auditory) are particularly helpful to cognitively impaired adults. Their life experiences are retained in the body. A simple cue may bring back childhood memories from a spiritual or religious past.

A number of books and journal articles focus on engaging people with dementia in worship or ministering to them. In one book, Everett (1996) remarks that traditional religious services use many cognitive-based expressions of faith, such as reciting scripture, listening to homilies or sermons, and responsive readings. She suggests that worship can and should be a multisensory experience. The use of touch, music, and even nature can serve as spiritual connections to people with AD. Similarly, Clayton (1991) argued for a "right-brain" approach to worship, that is, one that focuses less on intellectual skills and more on music, aroma, and touch.

Richards (1990) calls attention to the fact that early memories are often preserved in people with dementia and can be triggered using religious symbols that had important meaning in the past. Visual cues can include a picture of Mecca, a crucifix, prayer mats, prayer position of hands, a Bible, prayer bells, a skull cap, or a candle. Auditory cues can include hymns, the Lord's Prayer, davening, Shema and the Kaddish, or a call to prayer (see Table 7-1).

TABLE 7-1: SPIRITUAL AND RELIGIOUS TRIGGERS	
Visual Symbols	**Auditory Symbols**
• Mezuzahs	• Church bells
• Menorahs	• Shofar horn
• Yartzeit	• Organ
• Candles	• Hymns
• Crosses	• Scripture verses
• Rosaries	
• Bibles	
• Sculptures	
Other Sensory Symbols	
• Incense	
• Wine	
• Bread	

These cues can serve as bridges to the soul, a kind of mapping of how to reach the souls of individuals who have difficulty connecting with their spiritual or religious selves. Meeting these needs may require nurses to seek out help from others. Knowing when to call on professionals is important. Nurses' efforts are not enough to meet the spiritual and religious needs of their patients. Nurses can "create an environment of cues and religious encouragement and acceptance," but people need their spiritual and religious leaders and the practices only these people can provide (Buckwalter, 2003, p. 23).

Chaplains, who may be priests, rabbis, ministers, monks, or pastors, are important sources of spiritual care. Most facilities have chaplains on staff or have a referral list of different religious leaders. These individuals are able to provide support to patients and their families, provide spiritual counseling, and meet sacramental needs. Chaplains have a multitude of community resources that can assist patients and their families.

Many clinicians function using the biomedical model that fails to consider the relevance of spiritual matters. Interestingly, fewer physicians than patients fail to mention spirituality and religiosity as part of their personal characteristics (Loefler, 2003). These facts, as well as lack of time to address spiritual patient care, contribute to underrecognition and lack of consideration of patients' spirituality (Loefler, 2003). The ethical principles of beneficence and autonomy provide the opportunity for clinicians to respect and support patients' spirituality.

People with AD are not exempt from grieving, from suffering from life's losses. Times of grief or loss can be particularly difficult for patients with AD, not because they are grieving but because the disease may make it particularly hard to get to the core of the issue, causing the outward behaviors that are exemplified in the following case study.

Case Study

Martha was rifling through the phone book looking for her parents, who she claimed had "just died." Martha is 92. She cried, moaned, and even screamed that she lived in Oakbrook and she couldn't find her parents in the phone book. What would you do in this situation to help Martha?

1) A diversion may help in this situation.

2) Reality therapy may help, but many people question extensive application of reality orientation procedures. It may seem cruel and unnecessary to say to a confused patient, "Your mother has been dead for 20 years, and you are now living in Sunnybrook Nursing Home." Other more humane ways can be used to communicate with patients who have dementia. At times, reality orientation is a useful tool to orient a demented person to reality, especially during the early stages of the disease. Keep in mind that reality orientation should be used with discrimination. (See chapter 8 for further discussion on reality orientation.)

With continued and repeated conversations about the whereabouts of her parents, Martha finally said, "I know I don't live with my parents any longer. They are dead and are in heaven. I just still miss them so much." Martha was still grieving their death, but it took time, given the AD, to get to the core of Martha's problem.

Spiritual Assessment

One way of becoming sensitive to the spiritual needs of a patient is to simply conduct a spiritual history. A spiritual history taken at disease onset can prove to be helpful at a later time, when coping and behavioral interventions are required. Nurses know that before treating a wound, they must first verify the extent and characteristics of the wound and identify factors that may influence healing and outcomes of wound management. These same approaches apply to spiritual caregiving. Without these steps, nursing management is compromised.

A spiritual history informs the staff of the importance of spirituality in the life of the individual and the family, and it serves as a source of strength and coping. Some facilities have formal documents for spiritual assessment; if your facility does not, simply ask patients if they have religious or spiritual preferences and how they use these beliefs in their lives — for example, do they use them to get through rough times or deal with illness.

Incorporating spiritual care into nursing practice should include these steps:

- Include a spiritual history assessment for new patients.

- Learn about patient's religious denominations and their local religious or spiritual groups, with contact names and numbers.

- Prepare calendars for patients with special holidays so that they can participate, if appropriate.

- Become familiar with the skills necessary to attend to patients' spiritual and religious needs.

Assessment Tools

A number of spiritual assessment tools have been developed, three of which are included here. Fitchett (1993) developed a model for spiritual assessment that covers seven dimensions:

1. Beliefs and meaning (mission, purpose, religious and nonreligious meanings of life)

2. Authority and guidance (exploring where or with whom one places their trust and seeks guidance)

3. Experience (of divine or demonic) and emotion (tone emerging from one's spiritual experience)

4. Fellowship (involvement in an community that shares spiritual beliefs and practices)

5. Ritual and practice (activities that give meaning to life)

6. Courage and growth (ability to meet doubt and change oneself)

7. Vocation and consequences (what a person believes his or her calling is).

Maugans (1996) presented a mnemonic to assist nurses in remembering the components to cover during a spiritual assessment: **SPIRIT**.

Spiritual Belief: Religious affiliation and theology

Personal spirituality: Unique views on how life's experiences have shaped their spiritual transformation

Integration and **I**nvolvement: The individuals role and relationship with the larger spiritual community

Ritualized practices and **R**estrictions: Individual behaviors and activities that influence life (diets, rituals, holy days)

Implications: How do spiritual beliefs and practices influence the individual's health care?

Terminal events planning: End-of-life concerns; afterlife, cremation, meaning of death

In 1993, Highfield created the **PLAN** model for spiritual assessment and care. This model uses four tiers of increasing complexity:

Permission

Limited Information

Activating resources

Non-nursing referrals

The first level involves gaining permission by allowing and encouraging the individual to openly discuss his or her spirituality. The second level involves the nurse providing limited information to the individual's voiced concerns. The last tiers involve activating resources that are obtained from a more in-depth assessment, assisting the individual along the path to spiritual wellness, and making non-nursing referrals for spiritual concerns of the individual or concerns the nurse has for the individual.

Spiritual Needs Interventions

Albert Einstein (1879-1955) viewed religion and spirituality as follows: "My religion consists of a humble admiration of the illimitable superior spirit who reveals himself in the slight details we are able to perceive with our frail and feeble mind" (Calaprice, 2000).

Nurses often assume that a patient's spiritual needs are the same as religious preferences, affiliations, rites, and rituals. The word "religion" is from the Latin *religare*, which means "to bind together" (Mueller, Plevak, & Rummans, 2001). Religion can be defined as a system of beliefs and formal practices that are practiced individually or in a community group to provide focus and meaning to life, to understand death, and to maintain hope for the future (Mueller, Plevak, & Rummans, 2001; Sullivan, Smidt-Jernstrom, & Rader, 1995). However, religion is only one aspect of spirituality. The Latin word for spirituality is *spiritualitas*, which means "breath" (Mueller, Plevak, & Rummans, 2001). Spirituality is a much broader term that reflects the individuality of each person's beliefs about relationships, love and intimacy, forgiveness, hopes for the future, and methods of making peace with the past.

Spirituality is important to patients, caregivers, and practitioners. "It is not simply the application of technique. It requires both an internal and external attentiveness" (Johansson, 2003). Although some individuals regard themselves as spiritual, they do not always adopt a formal religion.

Nurses may try to avoid dealing with the spiritual needs of patients with AD because they think the needs are too personal or fear they could not recognize and communicate spiritual needs to patients with dementia. Listed here are possible indicators of unmet spiritual needs in elderly people:

- fear or anxiety
- anger or depression
- guilt
- grief
- regret
- loneliness
- separation or isolation

- lack of positive self-image
- need for reconciliation
- lack of self-identity
- alienation
- questions about the meaning of life
- sense of unfinished business.

(Mueller, Plevak, & Rummans, 2001; Sullivan, Smidt-Jernstrom, & Rader, 1995)

As illustrated in the case study involving Martha, living with AD means living in a world of fragments. Things do not seem connected. Patients may ask, "What am I doing here? What am I going to do next?" They may search for wholeness, their old identity, long-dead family members, control of familiar ground, or some kind of foundation to make sense of what is happening (Gwyther, 2001). Moving into a nursing home can intensify feelings of isolation and loss of identity and induce feelings about lack of privacy in a group setting. Nurses may recognize in people the indicators listed above in people with AD but may not be able to determine the needs associated with them. Nurses may find it useful to guess at the need that lies behind unexplained behaviors after exploring spiritual or religious background with the patient and the family.

Once needs have been recognized, several actions can be attempted to help patients with AD meet these needs:

1) Offer a supportive presence. Focus on one-to-one visits and involve clergy if possible and applicable. Help clergy or church visitors understand that being in the moment with a patient with dementia is more important than a religious discussion. Shared activities can be substituted for limited conversation.

2) Share in prayers, scripture readings, or other inspirational readings. Many patients can read words long after the meaning of the words is lost. Reading is a dignified activity that can be shared and is pleasurable. Prayer may be partic-

ularly helpful because it is thought that God listens and does not give advice. Patients with AD, as well as family caregivers, may gain a sense of peace from daily devotions.

3) Suggest attendance at religious services or worship, if possible. Give patients with AD opportunities to give as well as receive. Ask how situations were handled in the past in their community church. If appropriate, encourage clergy to include sacramental rites such as anointing or healing.

Interventions to meet spiritual needs should be comforting and reassuring to patients and help uphold their belief systems. Although many patients with dementia cannot express appreciation or even recognize what their spirituality meant to them in the past, they may be helped by the regular, calm presence of someone who cares about them.

The previous section discussed caring for patients with spiritual and religious needs. However, not all individuals are religious or spiritual people. Some people find meaning to life elsewhere. Furthermore, religion is not always the primary component of life satisfaction. The most important part of accepting the process of dying can be holding onto something that is personal and attaining a sense of contentment. Some people speak of a "simple" element of their life: memories. Memories can help keep these individual at ease despite conditions that many younger people would consider restrictions on quality of life (such as macular degeneration and inability to walk) (Endo, 2001).

END-OF-LIFE ISSUES

As much as 98% of older adults who have to be institutionalized in a long-term care facility (LTCF) or a hospital die there. Many of these individuals have dementia; estimates range from one-half to three-quarters. The incidence of dementia is especially high for the oldest old, who also have an increased likelihood of living in a LTCF. The number of people requiring care for dementia is expect-

ed to increase dramatically over the next 50 years (Moss, Braunschweig, & Rubinstein, 2002). These numbers have profound implications for how older patients will die or experience end of life. For example, when family members are questioned about the death of their loved one in a LTCF, 28% responded that their loved one did not experience a good death (Bosek, Lowry, Lindeman, Burck, & Gwyther, 2003). The reasons provided were as follows:

- did not want to die in a nursing home
- preferred to die a quick death (heart attack, die in sleep)
- physical or emotional circumstances impacted the death (difficulty breathing, scared, limited mobility)
- painful death for family members to watch.

In contrast, Bosek et al. (2003) listed the explanations given by family caregiver's belief that a good death did occur (reasons for a good death as perceived by family):

- family was present
- family was able to say goodbye
- death was sudden and quick
- death was expected.

In summary, a death was considered a good death if the death conformed to the person's preference regarding when and where to die and the death occurred without discomfort; the death was expected yet it was quick and painless. Families believed the reasons for a death without dignity may be linked to the fact that the person with AD suffered from a chronic debilitating disease that robbed the individual of a quick and peaceful death.

Many people in this country believe that a good death occurs when the dying person has made peace with God, family, and friends; completed unfinished tasks; fulfilled cultural death rituals; and said good-byes.

"If a good death is understood to be relinquishing of one's life with full awareness and acceptance...a 'good death' by this definition is not possible for those suffering from AD or a related dementia because that self-awareness has evanesced with the progress of the illness. Death can come only as a relief to the caregivers who usually have grieved long before this for the loss of their loved one's memories of self and family" (Margaret Borders, as cited by Bosek et al., 2003, p. 36).

Recently, terminal care for residents with dementia has gained some attention, but national data are light. In the majority of cases, dementia is not the primary diagnosis, nor is it usually listed as the cause of death. Nursing home residents with dementia who are terminally ill commonly suffer from multiple ailments; 91% have a major comorbid condition (Moss, Braunschweig, & Rubinstein, 2002).

Dying with AD

In the final stage of AD, a common path is traveled by people who have the disease. They gradually lose their motor skills to the point of loss of ambulation, no longer recognize family members, and lose the ability to understand and use language (see Table 7-2). Death usually results from a secondary cause, such as aspiration pneumonia, immobility, or infection. Moss, Braunschweig, and Rubinstein (2002) found that most of these people:

- have incontinence
- need complete assistance with eating and toileting
- no longer recognize loved ones
- have lost most or all verbal abilities.

Little is known about the way that nursing home personnel describe the care of terminally ill residents with dementia, specifically

- staff attitudes toward terminal care needs
- what constitutes a good death
- the actual care they provide to residents, family, and caregiving staff
- their attitudes toward hospice care

TABLE 7-2: CHARACTERISTICS OF PATIENTS IN THE LATE AND TERMINAL STAGES OF AD

- Dependence in activities of daily living, requiring the assistance of caregivers to survive
- Severe impairment of expressive and receptive communication, often limited to single words or nonphrases
- Loss of the ability to walk followed by inability to stand, or maintain sitting posture and a subsequent loss of head and neck control
- Development of contractures because of muscle rigidity and deconditioning
- Loss of ability to recognize food, self-feed, and swallow effectively
- Bowel and bladder incontinence
- Inability to recognize self and others

(Head, 2003)

- their perspectives on best practices.

Because of the lack of research into end-of-life issues for residents of nursing homes and how the nursing homes manage the needs of dying residents, their families, the caregiving staff, and surviving residents, recent research has looked closely at the care issues at end of life of persons with dementia (Blasi, Hurley, & Volicer, 2002; Moss, Braunschweig, & Rubinstein, 2002).

As a result of their research, Moss, Braunschweig, and Rubinstein (2002) suggest that

"Nursing homes should recognize the need to be proactive in leading residents, staff, and families to think in advance about the problems of pain, treatment, and comfort care. Building this stance into staff training and family outreach can potentially augment the scope and quality of terminal care for residents with dementia. We suggest that it is important to acknowledge the psychosocial impact of dying and death within the nursing home and to provide active support for residents, family, and staff. If end-of-life care were to become an agenda item for nursing home surveyors, that would be a major impetus in moving the facilities to maximize concern for residents, families, and staff around dying and death" (p. 245).

Other researchers recognize the barriers to adequate care of dying patients and have said

"Although many systemic barriers currently exist that impede the adequate provision of care for persons dying with dementia, the prospects for care improvement are positive. Some of these barriers can be addressed by legislation or policy changes, some by health care system changes, and some by educational interventions. Additional research is necessary to examine the barriers that cannot be clearly addressed by any of these changes. Armed with knowledge of these problems and their potential solutions, care providers, researchers, and policy makers will be able to enact changes that will result in improved care" (Blasi, Hurley, & Volicer, 2002, p. 64).

Therapies that were previously used to maintain function or cognition or improve communication may no longer be effective. Because of secondary illnesses that necessitate skilled medical care, hospitalization can often occur. These hospitalizations may actually increase functional deterioration and the risk of death.

Attitudes Toward Terminal Care for Residents with Dementia

In a study on terminal care of AD patients in nursing homes, Moss, Braunschweig, and Rubinstein (2002) found that a great majority of nurses and staff (93% of those who responded) believe that people with dementia who are dying have special needs. These special needs are primarily reflective of the limitations in their ability to communicate. Patients

with AD are unable to express discomfort and their feelings.

End-of-life care should focus on physical symptoms as well as psychosocial and spiritual concerns. Families do not always recognize the subtle changes that may signal the approach of death for their loved one. Part of nursing care is the ability to recognize signs and symptoms of the failing AD patient. Families may or may not have been counseled about the progression of the disease to death but are often shocked and not ready to accept the finality of this last phase of the disease when it occurs (Head, 2003).

Patients and their families, especially those of the Christian faith, have demonstrated religious justification for their insistence on aggressive medical care as the end of life approaches for their loved ones. The reasons cited are:

- hope for a miracle
- refusal to give up on the God of Faith
- a conviction that every moment of life is a gift from God and is worth reserving at any cost
- a belief that suffering can have redemptive value. (Brett & Jersild, 2003)

Although these reasons are commonly cited, some religious people do not desire aggressive medical care and cite other religious explanations. They believe in limiting medical interventions under certain circumstances. When medical interventions are demanded or refused on religious grounds, caregivers are not obligated to provide them. This is a time when chaplains or clergy should be present to discuss with family members the appropriate limits of life-sustaining interventions (Brett & Jersild, 2003).

Caregivers and Terminal Care

Research on the impact of end-of-life care on the family caregivers of people with AD and caregiver responses to their loved ones death is somewhat limited (Schulz, Mendelsohn, Haley, et al., 2003). Caregivers of people with AD report that they feel "on duty 24 hours a day." As a result of this level of attention to and care of the person with AD, they show evidence of depression while still providing the same level of care for their loved one. It is interesting to note that after the death of their loved one, they demonstrate astonishing resilience. Within approximately 3 months, these caregivers demonstrate substantial declines in the levels of their depression. A large portion of caregivers report that death of the loved one with AD is a relief to them as well as to their loved one. Staff in nursing homes have indicated that, "Usually by the time an end-stage dementia patient expires, we are all relieved, and the sadness is not there because we have watched this person deteriorate to where they are, and the death is like a relief" (Moss, Braunschweig, & Rubinstein, 2002).

End-of-life care can be particularly demanding on families of loved ones with AD. Because of this increased demand, families need to validate their effectiveness and especially their contributions to care of the loved one who is dying (Head, 2003). This finding suggests that nurses should allow family members to participate to the fullest extent possible in the care of their loved ones. Through their choice of activities, family members can derive much satisfaction from contributing to the care of their loved ones.

People with AD often withdraw and die gradually. This does not mean that interventions cease; in fact, it is often the case that nurses should become more aggressive in their assessment and treatment of people with AD as the disease progresses. Assessment of pain and other physical symptoms must be timely and aggressive in order to provide alleviation (Head, 2003). Hurley and Volicer identified that the dying process of AD patients can take between 5 and 38 days (2002) and that one in five deaths takes place in a nursing home.

Families often initially feel relief and then guilt as the end nears for their loved ones. Guilt may be the result of the family's inadequacy or impatience with the family member who is ill. It is a time when nursing support and assistance is vital to the well-being of the family members.

Care at the End of Life

Research in recent years has supported the belief that aggressive medical care for people with terminal dementia does not decrease progression of the disease, increase comfort, or extend survival. Despite these findings, aggressive medical interventions and inadequate pain management are commonly provided to dying persons with dementia in hospitals. Hospice and other community-based services are not appropriately accessed by this population (Blasi, Hurley, & Volicer, 2002).

Agreement on Treatments

Treatment decisions for people with terminal dementia must take into account previously expressed preferences for care and expectations for medical outcomes. Programs and services need to be made available as early as possible to all people with AD, and their family members, in order for them to make informed decisions. Advance directives and living wills should be discussed early in the disease process because these documents decrease the length of hospital stays and increase the likelihood of dying in a LTCF. Most health care professionals believe that advance care plans serve as mechanisms to improve end-of-life care. Nursing homes, LTCFs, and hospitals have a responsibility to provide information about advance care plans to all residents. Several authors have found that the presence of advance care plan documents is related to resident race, even after controlling for education and health status (Teno, Weitzen, Wetle, & Mor, 2001). Teno et al. (2001) found that African Americans are one-third as likely to have living wills and one-fifth as likely to have do-not-resuscitate (DNR) orders as Caucasians; Hispanics are about one-third as likely to have DNR orders as Caucasians. These findings help identify avenues for improving the quality of life of nursing home residents by increasing the attention nurses pay to patients' right to self-determination in end-of-life care.

Several medical specialty associations and societies, including the American Geriatrics Society, have identified core principles for care, such as advanced care plans, living wills, and DNR orders when caring for patients at the end of life. A review of these principles can be particularly helpful when improving quality of care or designing end-of-life services.

In their study, Moss, Braunschweig, and Rubinstein (2002) asked senior staff members from 391 nursing homes to reflect on the last resident with dementia who had died in their nursing home. The details of care for one resident from all the instititions is condensed in the following:

"There seemed to be substantial agreement between the resident's treatment wishes, the family's wishes, and the staff. Given the dementia and terminal illness of the resident, in general, it may be that prior statements or advance directives of the resident represented their wishes. In 79% of the cases, the family did not disagree at all with the resident's treatment wishes; in 84% of the cases, the staff did not disagree at all with the resident's wishes; in 76%, there was no disagreement between staff and the family's treatment wishes. When we combine these three areas of potential disagreement we find, however, that for 31% of the individual deaths reported, there was some disagreement in one or more of these pairs. In addition, we did not ask about disagreements within the staff or within the family. If the responding administrators were not closely involved in issues around terminal care in this case, they may have tended to underreport disagreements. Thus, this may be a conservative picture of disagreements. Nursing homes with special care units report fewer disagreements. The greater the

disagreement the more likely the nursing homes feel they have to make difficult decisions on care. In general, if staff does disagree with terminal care wishes of family or resident, staff may have to deal with conflicts in personal beliefs, cultural attitudes, and agency practices " (2002, p. 241).

Symptom Management

Satisfactory symptom management is a fundamental element of nursing care, especially care of terminally ill patients. Terminally ill persons with dementia have a unique set of needs because they are dying. Ineffective management of pain is all too common for dying people with dementia.

Evaluation of the quality of life of a dying person with AD is based on the following standards:

- Patients should be free from symptoms of pain, fear, skin breakdown, and shortness of breath.

- Death should occur in familiar surroundings (the person should not be moved within 3 days of death).

- Family members should be aware of the impending death and be at the bedside if they choose.

- Permission for autopsy should be sought when the cause of death is unknown.

As discussed in chapter 6, pain is a common problem for older people, and it is often improperly assessed or evaluated. It is more likely to be undertreated in LTCFs. Pain assessment is often difficult in residents with dementia, and physicians often find it easier to give analgesics to patients with cancer than to noncancer patients who have unrelieved pain. Research also suggests that nursing home residents with daily nonmalignant pain too frequently receive no analgesics (Brummel-Smith, London, Drew, et al., 2002; Sherder, 2000; Wynne, Ling, & Remsburg, 2000).

Harrold (1998) indicated that a lack of education and information are primary contributors to inadequate pain relief and management of other symptoms. Nursing staff and nursing assistants have been found to lack education or be misinformed about advance directives and palliative care. Nurses are not the only ones who lack information; physicians lack information about death as well. In fact, most physicians have little geriatric experience and approach care with the mind-set that they must cure the person who is ill; death is an enemy they must overcome. When physicians recognize that dementia is a terminal disease, it can be treated as such. With this lack of knowledge, it is obvious why people with AD who are in the terminal stage are not properly referred to hospice care. Education of caring professionals is necessary for the improvement of symptom management for persons with terminal dementia.

Symptom management is one area in which health care specialists can positively impact the quality of dying people with AD. Based on the various symptoms occurring near the time of death, such as pain, bowel and urinary elimination issues, shortness of breath, and feeding problems, nurses must remain alert to the problems and aware of proper interventions for their AD patients.

Caregiver burden, mood, and experience are variables that influence pain management. These factors can impact compliance with medication regimens and delivery of care; however, they are inappropriate determinants of symptom management. Researchers have found that lack of knowledge on the part of the caregiver can lead to low-quality care and inappropriate symptom management (Blasi, Hurley, & Volicer, 2002). One of the ways of overcoming caregiver variables and increasing quality of care is to offer educational opportunities, web-based information sessions, and educational handouts.

Palliative Care

The World Health Organization (WHO) defines palliative care as an approach that improves the quality of life of patients and their families facing the problem associated with life-threatening illness, through the prevention and relief of suffering by means of early identification and impeccable assessment and treatment of pain and other problems, physical, psychosocial and spiritual. Palliative care:

* provides relief from pain and other distressing symptoms;

* affirms life and regards dying as a normal process;

* intends neither to hasten or postpone death;

* integrates the psychological and spiritual aspects of patient care;

* offers a support system to help patients live as actively as possible until death;

* offers a support system to help the family cope during the patients illness and in their own bereavement;

* uses a team approach to address the needs of patients and their families, including bereavement counselling, if indicated;

* will enhance quality of life, and may also positively influence the course of illness;

* is applicable early in the course of illness, in conjunction with other therapies that are intended to prolong life, such as chemotherapy or radiation therapy, and includes those investigations needed to better understand and manage distressing clinical complications.

(WHO, n.d.)

Palliative care must focus on <u>providing comfort</u> vs. prolonging life. Those with the greatest knowledge about palliative care are people who work in the field of hospice care (Baer & Hanson, 2000; Shega et al., 2003). Hospice services provide skilled care to dying people and their loved ones. Hospice referrals should be made early in the disease process, and once again as death approaches. Hospice personnel, whether in a LTCF or a community dwelling, provide support for the staff and family. Baer and Hanson (2000) found that the quality of care increased significantly with the use of hospice in nursing homes (see Table 7-3).

TABLE 7-3: QUALITY OF CARE BEFORE AND AFTER HOSPICE					
Care of Pain and Other Symptoms			**Care for Emotional and Spiritual Needs**		
	% before hospice	*% after hospice*		*% before hospice*	*% after hospice*
Excellent	17	54	Excellent	21	48
Good	47	39	Good	43	43
Fair	29	6	Fair	23	9
Poor	7	1	Poor	14	1
(Baer & Hanson, 2000)					

In the Baer and Hanson study, it was found that family members rated the quality of care in all areas (physical, spiritual and emotional), with a higher rating after hospice services than before those services were initiated. Hospice personnel were chosen by 82% of respondents as the most important person for emotional and spiritual support, as compared with nursing home staff of 31%.

Once a terminal diagnosis is made, hospice Medicare benefits help to cover 24-hour on-call consultation, medications, and equipment related to the diagnosis. Some private insurance and state medical benefits also help to cover the expenses related to the terminal diagnosis (Head, 2003). The use of hospice services is growing at a rate of 10% to 20% per year. Of that growth, nursing home use of hospice care is expected to account for 17% of new enrollees (Baer & Hanson, 2000).

Nurses must follow primary care provider orders and implement nursing interventions that are appropriate for individuals in this final stage of life. A problem arises for nurses when they are given orders for interventions that are inappropriate for people with terminal dementia, including tube feeding, cardiopulmonary resuscitation, mechanical ventilation, and intensive care unit treatment. Inappropriate interventions are provided for different reasons: advance directive prepared by the person with AD about therapeutic options may not be made or honored, economic considerations, healthcare system factors, or health care provider factors may interfere with the restriction of inappropriate interventions (Blasi, Hurley, & Volicer, 2002).

Ethics committees can be helpful when decision-making becomes difficult. Fortunately, with increased education about AD, more primary care providers are urging people with AD to prepare advance directives in the early stages of dementia, which in turn should reduce conflicts over end-of-life care and the use of ethics committees to resolve inappropriate care.

Economic factors and health insurance issues make it particularly difficult for people with AD to gain access to hospice. Insurance companies put dollar limits on their reimbursement schedules and hospice benefits are not available in many insurance plans. Remember that the care of people with AD is a long-term option, but Medicare benefits are structured for short-term home care needs only. Blasi, Hurley, and Volicer (2002) indicate that the Medicare hospice benefit is not obtainable by many people because "hospice stays for persons with dementia tend to be quite short, and the benefit is essentially inaccessible for persons with dementia in its current form due to the difficulty in predicting 6 months of survival" (p. 62). It is interesting to note that advance planning and hospice care can reduce care costs for people with AD; hospice care can save between 10% and 17% in the last 6 months of life.

In community-dwelling people who are in the final stage of AD, burden and other specific characteristics of the caregiver have been linked to inappropriate interventions; in other words, caregivers were not aware of the services available to them. When caregivers became informed of their care options, more services were utilized (Blasi et al., 2002).

SUMMARY

Individuals who rely on spiritual beliefs actually cope better and have better health outcomes than those who are without such beliefs. Religious and spiritual coping also lessen the effects of stressful events on caregivers of the elderly population.

Nurses can enhance quality of life for older adults with dementia. The first step in that process is the use of a spiritual interview. The interview should determine what the patient's religious background is, what needs are met through the patient's spirituality, and how the spirituality is expressed. The spiritual history informs the staff of the importance of these matters in the life of the individual and his or her family and whether they can be used as a source of strength and coping. Nursing interventions to meet spiritual needs should be comforting and reassuring to patients and help uphold their belief systems.

End-of-life care should focus on physical symptoms as well as psychosocial and spiritual concerns. Death usually results from a secondary cause, such as aspiration pneumonia, immobility, or infection. A good death is one that conforms to the person's preference regarding when and where to die and dying without discomfort. Nursing interventions must address legal needs, such as living wills, advance directives, and powers of attorney, as well as all the physical needs of patients with AD and their family members.

EXAM QUESTIONS

CHAPTER 7
Questions 61-70

61. One of the better strategies to assist people with AD who are grieving is

    a. ignore the behavior.
    b. diversional activities.
    c. validation therapy.
    d. reminiscence therapy.

62. Assessment of spiritual and religious needs should include

    a. structured and formal questionnaires that the person with AD and the family complete.
    b. unstructured and informal interviews in which the nurse is able to assess the history and current needs of individual patients.
    c. referral to a chaplain who can perform a spiritual or religious assessment.
    d. simple observation of the religious practices of the person.

63. Sensory aids are particularly helpful to cognitively impaired adults. Visual cues can include:

    a. a crucifix or prayer mat.
    b. burning incense.
    c. scripture verse.
    d. church bells.

64. The statement that best reflects the difference between religion and spirituality is

    a. spiritual needs are easier to recognize in a person with AD than religious needs.
    b. religion is a system of beliefs and practices that give meaning to life; spirituality is more comprehensive.
    c. spiritual needs can be met by caregivers, but religious needs must be met by clergy.
    d. spirituality is one aspect of religious training.

65. According to Bosek et al. (2003), family members of dying patients with AD perceived a "good death" as when

    a. death was a slow and drawn out process.
    b. their loved one died in the LTCF but wanted to be home.
    c. family were present and able to say goodbye.
    d. their loved one died with pain and discomfort.

66. End-of-life care for persons with dementia should center around

    a. physical symptoms only.
    b. an aggressive medical cure.
    c. the physical, psychosocial, and spiritual being.
    d. the same as for any older adult without dementia.

113

67. Upon the death of a patient with AD, many caregivers feel

    a. rigidity and increasing depression.
    b. relief yet feelings of guilt.
    c. they must restrict their feelings of sadness.
    d. overwhelming grief and sadness.

68. When AD is first diagnosed, advance directives, living wills, and powers of attorney are needed. One of the far-reaching impacts of these early actions by families is

    a. these legal documents increase staff knowledge but decrease end-of-life care.
    b. the quality of life may be decreased but the length of stay in the LTCF is decreased.
    c. hospital stays are decreased and the likelihood of dying in a LTCF is increased.
    d. they are not related to end-of-life decisions and increase staff frustration.

69. Mrs. Terry is an 88-year-old woman who is nearing the end of her life. To assure quality care for Mrs. Terry, your care plan would include

    a. timely assessment, symptom management, and collaborative staff support.
    b. transfer her to an acute care facility once death is near.
    c. keep visitors to a minimum to assure privacy and dignity at the time of death.
    d. focus on prolonging life as long as possible.

70. Which of the following situations exemplifies palliative care?

    a. Hospice nurses and workers visit on a routine basis to provide comfort measures and family and staff support.
    b. At the fist sign of approaching death, the emergency medical services are called to transport a person with AD to an acute care facility.
    c. The physician orders various treatments to remove secondary disease signs and symptoms.
    d. Devices, such as feeding tubes and ventilators, are placed to maintain survival.

CHAPTER 8

NONPHARMACOLOGICAL TREATMENT

CHAPTER OBJECTIVE

After completing this chapter, the reader will be able to recognize common therapeutic approaches for managing the behavior of patients with Alzheimer's disease (AD) and incorporate these approaches into nursing practice.

LEARNING OBJECTIVES

After studying this chapter, the reader will be able to

1. identify problem behaviors of AD and the triggers that can initiate such behaviors.

2. describe a variety of therapeutic approaches for managing the behavior of patients with AD.

3. differentiate benefits of the therapeutic approaches of reality orientation, reminiscence, and validation therapy.

4. indicate techniques used in reality orientation, reminiscence, and validation therapy.

5. specify which therapeutic approaches are best for patients in early and late stages of AD.

6. identify specific factors for enhancing self-care of those with AD.

7. recognize environmental factors and psychosocial influences on the lives of those with AD and the nursing assessment for these factors.

8. identify the activities of daily living (ADLs) that are impacted by AD and the therapeutic activities intended to enhance ADLs in those with AD.

INTRODUCTION

A loving person lives in a loving world.
A hostile person lives in a hostile world.
Everyone you meet is your mirror.

—Ken Keyes, Jr.

Caring for someone with AD poses many challenges for both nurses and nonprofessional caregivers. Diseases of memory loss have a variety of symptoms that can baffle and overwhelm family members, cause injury of residents and staff within facilities, require physical or chemical restraint, and increase stress levels of caregivers and staff. Bizarre behaviors and memory problems make it difficult to understand and work with patients who have cognitive impairments. Patient behaviors can be the most distressing part of dementia or AD.

This chapter discusses therapeutic approaches to dealing with common problems. One way to approach irritating and bizarre behaviors is to attempt to understand what these behaviors mean. In other words, why do people act the way they do? It is known that dementia and AD damage the brain to the point that the patient cannot make sense out of what he or she sees and hears. Memory loss, anger, agitation, and other behaviors exhibited by the person with AD can cause embarrassment, frustration, and exhaustion to those providing care. Exploring what works best for each caregiver and what has worked for others helps alleviate these caregiver emotions and frustrations.

DEMENTIA-RELATED PROBLEM BEHAVIORS

AD can cause a person to exhibit unusual and unpredictable behaviors that challenge caregivers, including severe mood swings, verbal or physical aggression, combativeness, repetition of words, and wandering. Most behavioral problems do not occur early in the disease but rather occur when they are least expected. These behavioral changes can lead to frustration and tension for both people with AD and their caregivers. Nurses must remember that people with AD are not acting this way on purpose, and they must analyze probable causes and develop care adjustments. See Table 8-1 for common causes of behavior changes.

TABLE 8-1: COMMON CAUSES OF BEHAVIOR CHANGES

- Physical discomfort caused by an illness or medications
- Overstimulation from a loud or overactive environment
- Inability to recognize familiar places, faces, or things
- Difficulty completing simple tasks or activities
- Inability to communicate effectively

A range of verbal and physical behaviors are common and problematic in demented community-based populations. Researchers have found that having a dementia-related problem is associated with an increased risk of nursing home placement. In addition, these behaviors shorten the average survival time in the community by approximately 2 years (Phillips & Diwan, 2003).

Examples of Behavioral Problems

Nurses need to be able to identify behavioral problems. Examples include:

- accusing family members of stealing (usually, the person with AD has hidden these items)
- becoming irritated or belligerent late in the day
- telling untrue stories
- not recognizing familiar settings or family late in the afternoon
- threatening family members with violence
- refusing to bathe
- resisting directions or care.

Tips for Responding to Challenging Behaviors

Your response as a nurse can directly impact behaviors. The following are suggestions for responding to problem behaviors:

- Stay calm and be understanding.
- Be patient and flexible.
- Do not argue or try to convince the person.
- Acknowledge requests and respond to them.
- Try not to take behaviors personally.
- Accept the behavior as a reality of the disease and try to work through it.

Exploring Causes and Solutions

It is important to identify the cause of challenging behavior and consider possible solutions. Ask yourself these questions:

- What was the undesirable behavior? Is it harmful to the individual or others?
- What happened before the behavior occurred?
- Did something trigger the behavior?

Then explore potential solutions:

- Is there something the person needs or wants?

- Is the area noisy or crowded? Is the room well-lit? Can you change the surroundings?

- Are you responding in a calm, supportive way?

If these solutions are ineffective, try different responses in the future. Then ask yourself:

- Did your response help?

- Do you need to explore other potential causes and solutions? If so, what can you do differently?

Tips for Reducing Problem Behaviors

As a nurse, you must not only identify problem behaviors but also the therapeutics for reducing their risk. Here are some suggestions for doing this:

- Identify signs of frustration. Look for early signs of frustration during activities, such as bathing, dressing, or eating, and respond in a calm and reassuring tone.

- Do not take the behavior personally. The person is not necessarily angry with you. He or she may have misunderstood the situation or be frustrated with lost abilities caused by the disease.

- Avoid teaching or providing elaborate explanations and arguments. Be encouraging and do not expect the person to do more than he or she can.

- Use distractions. If the person is frustrated because he or she cannot perform a certain activity, such as unbutton a shirt, distract the person with another activity. After some time has passed, you can return to helping the person perform the original activity.

- Communicate directly with the person. Avoid expressing anger or impatience in your voice or physical actions. Instead, use positive, accepting expressions, such as "don't worry" and "thank you." Also use touch to reassure and comfort the person. For example, put your arm around the person or give him or her a kiss.

- Decrease the level of danger. Assess the level of danger for yourself and the person with AD. You can often avoid harm by simply stepping back and standing away from the person. If the person is headed out of the house and onto the street, be more assertive.

- Unless the situation is serious, avoid physically holding or restraining the person. He or she may become more frustrated and cause personal harm.

Behavior Triggers

In order to reduce the risk of some behaviors, it is essential to identify the triggers of the behavior. Common behavior triggers include illness, fatigue, change, and overwhelming stimuli.

Illness

Illness can induce a sudden onset of problem behaviors and confusion that do not go away with rest. Some of the common factors that contribute to sudden onset of problem behaviors include:

- Water intake: Pay attention to water intake because urinary tract infections are a leading cause of agitation.

- Arthritis: Look for signs that the patient is uncomfortable. Have activities such as excessive standing or walking contributed to stressing of the joints?

- Constipation: Provide adequate fiber and fluid; avoid laxatives and enemas.

- Alcohol: Advise the patient to avoid alcohol because it can worsen memory permanently. Changes in brain composition can also make AD patients overly sensitive to alcohol.

- Malnutrition: Malnutrition is a contributor to decreased mental status. When patients do not eat adequately, they lose weight. These individuals may simply need to take a multivitamin or ingest a higher amount of calories when they eat. Referral to a dietician can benefit people with AD.

Fatigue

Fatigue is most likely the biggest adversary of the person with memory loss because it causes them to tire easily. Fatigue is usually the result of the exacting toll of having to concentrate so hard most of the time. Table 8-2 lists suggestions for preventing fatigue.

TABLE 8-2: SUGGESTIONS FOR PREVENTING FATIGUE

- Give AD patients rest, such as quiet time and naps, both in the morning and in the evening.

- If patients get up during the night, do not keep them up all day. Forcing them to stay awake all day can make nighttime even worse.

- Get to know patients' "best time of day" and use that time to do activities, such as see friends and go to the doctor.

- Plan activities so that AD patients can get away for some rest.

- Make sure that activities are short in duration.

- Avoid offering caffeinated beverages.

- In the evening persons with AD may demonstrate increased agitation, activity, and negative behaviors. These characteristic behaviors of AD that occur late in the day have been referred to as "sundowning" and may be due more to being overly tired than the setting of the sun and night time. Be watchful in the evening hours for signs of sundowning, and then assess morning waking behaviors for improvement to provide clues to behavioral problems.

Change

People with AD need to have routines. The routine differs for each person but must remain fixed; keep the steps of the routine the same. If a well-meaning family member or friend suggests that it is time for a change in the routine, gently but firmly inform him or her that changing the routine is not in the patient's best interest.

The patient's environment needs to remain simple and stable. If families or facilities decorate for the holidays, these decorations must be kept to a minimum. The environment should also be kept relatively quiet — no big parties with lots of noise.

Although the person with AD is still able to attend family functions and social gatherings, it is best to consult with the host about keeping the festivity simple, including the number of guests, thus decreasing the opportunity for creating behavioral difficulties for the person with AD. Also advise the host that the person with AD may make demands at the party, may be rude to guests, or may wander off. These are all signals of fatigue or overwhelming stimuli.

Stimuli

Nurses must be mindful that people with memory deficits suffer from a host of problems, one of which is the inability to interpret properly what they see and hear. Noises and visual experiences can become distorted.

Here are some suggestions for diminishing overwhelming stimuli:

- Do not insist that people with AD remain in an environment that has created confusion or agitation. Remember that behavior is an outward sign of ability to tolerate a situation.

- If a person with AD states that he or she wants to leave a function, take the person away or get the person to an area of quiet and calmness and let the person rest.

- Misinterpretation of stimuli may cause an individual with AD to see figures that are not there. Find out what the stimulus for the behavior might be and remove it. For example, turn off the television, change the radio station to more soothing music, reduce the light in a room, cover the mirrors, and so forth.

- Do not argue or correct people with AD about what they think they are seeing or hearing. Remember that their brains are not functioning correctly and what they are experiencing is real to them. Reassure them that they are safe, that you understand their concern, and that you will take the problem away.

LOSS OF ACTIVITIES

Activities define who we are. When AD patients lose the ability to drive, work, do garden chores, cook, and perform other common activities, the resulting effects can be depression and anxiety. People with AD may say they are going crazy, deny the memory loss, or become angry when this occurs. Do not attempt to get them to admit that they are losing their memory. Rather, discuss with them the problem with their minds. Failure to have this discussion at an early point in the disease process can end in paranoia or suspicious ideas.

Exchange Activities

When the person with AD looses the ability to drive, work, garden, and perform other common activities, caregivers must change their activities. Exchange old familiar activities that a patient is angry about or grieving over with more simple tasks. Interventions at this time can include contacting an occupational therapist to help design substitute activities and taking advantage of adult day care. Remember that people with AD may be grieving and need time for this normal process. However, if grieving persists for more than 4 weeks or it affects appetite or sleep, seek treatment for depression.

The following recommendations can be used by caregivers to exchange lost activities for new ones:

- Have people with AD assist with chores around the house. The familiar tasks of sweeping, dusting, vacuuming, sorting laundry, and cooking help keep them focused and productive.

- Evaluate all activities for safety. Do not allow patients with AD to use sharp knives, power tools, or other dangerous objects.

- Minding pets, gardening, and listening to music can often result in positive behaviors and satisfaction.

- Physical exercise two to three times per week has been shown to assist in maintaining a positive mood and functional abilities.

- Being read to or listening to books on tape can be soothing.

- Show videotapes of favorite family gatherings, sports shows, and television programs. Be careful not to overstimulate the patient with violence on television or in movies.

When healthy individuals perceive a flaw in themselves or others they will test themselves or others and push to improve on the flaw. This behavior does not occur in patients with AD. It is not always best to exercise the minds of AD patients by testing and pushing them to achieve even simple tasks. Reminding them of their mistakes or pushing them to improve has a tendency to make AD patients uncomfortable. Although exercising a muscle in the body improves its function, this is not so with the brain; it is not a muscle. Accept the memory changes of people with AD and avoid quizzing them. When something is forgotten, such as how to perform a task, do not say "Think about it." They have lost the memory of it; rather help them with the task. Thinking about a forgotten task or activity only worsens the problem. Instead change the subject or distract them by introducing food or drink or calling a family member.

REALITY ORIENTATION

The basic format of reality orientation involves reminding patients with dementia or AD who they are and who is speaking to them, providing information about time and place, and giving a description about what is going on (Moffat, 1994). It is important for caregivers to speak clearly, keeping statements brief and specific. Demented patients are encouraged to rehearse the information given and to talk with staff members and with others, (if in a group). The original goal of reality orientation was to meet the sensory and emotional needs of patients who required long-term care. The needs would be met by: #73

- promoting <u>one-to-one</u> personal contacts in

which nursing assistants would spend more time with residents

- providing stimulating activities for residents

- encouraging positive attitudes in staff personnel.

The guidelines can be summarized as follows:

- New information is presented in a variety of formats, including routine communication and special learning groups.

- Staff correct incorrect or confused behavior or actions.

- Prompts, rehearsals, and reinforcement of adaptive behavior are used.

- Memory aids, such as reality orientation boards with date and time, are used to alleviate memory problems.

(Moffat, 1994; Spector & Orrell, 2001).

Historically, reality orientation was the mainstay of therapeutic activities in nursing homes, and it is a requirement in some states for long-term-care licensing (Ebersole & Hess, 2001). However, some people question extensive application of reality orientation procedures becaue they are so direct. It may seem cruel to say to a confused patient, "Your mother has been dead for 20 years, and you are now living in Sunnybrook Nursing Home." Other more humane and realistic methods can be used to communicate with patients who have dementia. At times, reality orientation is a useful tool for orienting a demented person to reality. It can be especially useful during the early stages of AD.

Over time, reality orientation has been modified to a more acceptable approach in which the aim is for staff members to respond to residents' initiatives rather than to initiate the interactions. An alternative to providing verbal information is to teach patients with dementia or AD to follow appropriately posted signs; this encourages them to find their own way around the facility environment or at home. Using such external memory aides as appointment books, alarm watches, and daily routine schedules may maintain memory in patients in the early stages of AD.

Reality orientation should be used with discrimination. Attitudes of staff members play an important part in the effectiveness of this intervention. Friendliness and a matter-of-fact approach are supportive and build self-esteem. The first steps in designing your care plan for a patient with dementia should consider whether it is better to orient the patient to the external world and surroundings or work within the patient's reality. In a clinical setting, an emphasis on reality orientation can lead to increased agitation and anxiety. However, the benefits of reality orientation have been confirmed by research, making this an intervention that can create a better social environment for little cost and brief training (Spector & Orrell, 2001). The beneficial returns depend on approaching demented individuals in a dignified and kind manner. Patients with dementia may become too impaired to benefit from such interventional activities as reality orientation.

REMINISCENCE

Reminiscing is considered a particularly adaptive function during the last stage of life. The concept of reminiscing has been used in many settings and for many purposes. Butler introduced life review in 1963 as a way to review the past in an attempt to examine conflicts and resolve and reconcile them or make order and meaning from them. Reminiscing is an enhancing and multifaceted experience that can have many purposes and functions when used with people AD. Patients with dementia or AD often retain remote memories long after their short-term memory is gone. The retention of remote memory can be used by nurses for maintaining patients' sense of self-esteem and identity (Ebersole & Hess, 2001). Because old memories are not judged for accuracy, they do not threaten the adequacy of the person who is reminiscing. Being able to have a conversation is an essential component of communication, but it declines in people with AD.

Group Reminiscence

During group reminiscence, triggers or aids can be used to access the memories. Such aids include photographs, foods, and smells that initiate recall and discussion of memories (Burns, Howard, & Pettit, 1995; Pittiglio, 2000; Remington, 2002). Group reminiscence is more effective when it is unstructured, and the value of group reminiscence lies in the enjoyment and satisfaction it gives to patients and to their families, if families are involved. Reminiscence therapy has been shown to have a significant effect on behavior and can be used as an alternative to chemical and physical restraints. It also has a positive effect on social behavior problems, improves social integration and cognitive function, and helps relieve depression (Finnema, de Lange, Droes, Ribbe, & van Tilburg, 2000; Moss, Polignano, White, Minichiello, & Sunderland, 2002; Pittiglio, 2000; Savell & Krinsky, 1998).

Reminiscence Therapy Guidelines for Nurses

Following these guidelines can help make reminiscence therapy a successful intervention:

- When beginning, discuss with patients the normal characteristics of a life review.

- Use open-ended questions.

- Show interest in what each person is sharing through nonverbal gestures and touch.

- Give each patient the chance to recap events in his or her life. Ask questions such as, "What do you remember about your first day of school?" or make requests such as, "Tell us about the first doll you had" or "Tell me what this picture means to you."

- Help patients put their lives in a broader or different perspective. For instance, ask them, "How did you manage?" or "Who helped you get through that?" or "How would you change that now?"

- Incorporate prompts that help to make connections between past hopes and dreams and the future, or make connections between members of the group to show common bonds.

- Focus on the individual as the central person in any story told. For example, ask, "What were you doing then?"

- Work toward the goal of increasing self-esteem of each person by recognizing the person's individuality.

- Share some of your own memories to help the demented person share his or her memories.

Benefits of Reminiscence Therapy

Reminiscence therapy has many therapeutic values. It can make memories more acceptable and can enrich the daily lives of people with AD, helping them experience life more fully. Sharing of memories by group members can stimulate other memories and talking about the loss of pets can help members recognize their coping styles for grief and loss. Other benefits of reminiscing include healing loneliness and isolation, giving a sense of continuity to life, and providing understanding from one generation to another (Moss, Polignano, et al., 2002; Pittiglio, 2000; Rader, 1995).

Studies have shown that reminiscing can also lead to positive changes in the attitudes of nursing assistants toward elderly people in nursing homes (Pietrukowicz & Johnson, 1991). In addition, reminiscence therapy requires little effort or time, so it does not intrude on the staff's work tasks. Another benefit of reminiscing is that nursing assistants may perceive elderly residents as more vital and unique, and this perception can increase the assistants' own self-esteem as health care workers whose work has often been undervalued or devalued.

Patients who reminisce most effectively are those who are highly functional. Reminiscence should be part of a comprehensive program to address the emotional, cognitive, and behavioral needs of patients who have dementia or AD. The loss of verbal ability and intact memory in the middle and later stages of AD makes reminiscence therapy less appropriate for patients in those stages.

VALIDATION THERAPY

Validation is based on accepting the reality and personal truth of another's experiences. Validation accepts the old person who mentally returns to the past. Often, his/her retreat is not a form of mental illness or disease, it is a survival technique; they must return to the past in order to survive today's personal mental and physical losses. It assists those with AD to reduce stress and enhance dignity and happiness.

The validation therapy approach was established for people with AD between 1963 and 1980 by Naomi Feil (Neal & Briggs, 2003). It tunes into the patients' inner worlds and helps them restore the past by reliving good times and resolving past conflicts. Based on respect and empathy, validation helps reduce stress, enhance dignity, and increase happiness (Feil, 1982). It assists in restoring self-worth, minimizes the degree of withdrawal from the outside world, promotes communication, reduces problem behaviors such as agitation and anxiety, and facilitates independent living (Neal & Briggs, 2003). See Table 8-3 for components of validation therapy.

Validation therapy can be useful in restoring a sense of well being in nursing home populations that include residents with AD. It is based on a developmental theory of aging. As controls relax in old age, disoriented, elderly individuals need to express long hidden or buried emotions in order to die in peace (Feil, 2001). This theory is truly about life's final struggles. The changes at the end of older adults' lives occur because of physical decline and as a result of their individual desire to return to their past; a past that can be filled with long hidden or

TABLE 8-3: VALIDATION THERAPY COMPONENTS

1. Older adults struggle to resolve unfinished life issues before life ends. Their behavior is age-specific. Their behavior demonstrates human needs.

2. Validation therapy classify older adult behaviors into four evolutionary stages:

   a. Malorientation — A means of expressing past conflicts in masked forms.

   b. Time confusion — Older adults retreat inward, no longer holding onto reality.

   c. Repetitive motion — Words do not hold the means of working through the unresolved discords and now physical movement replace those lost words.

   d. Vegetation — The older adult shuts out the entire world and gives up trying to figure out living.

3. Validation therapy includes psychosocial, physical, and social characteristics, as well as helping techniques for older adults in each of the four stages.

4. Validation therapy can be used with individuals or within groups. When using group therapy, the interventions must be decidedly structured and the group must contain between five and ten individuals. This therapy is designed to encourage energy, social interaction, and social roles.

(Feil, 2001; Neal & Briggs, 2002)

buried emotions that have never been resolved. Now, at the end of their life, there is an urgency to wrap up the loose ends of life, such as these buried emotions. These individuals need someone to listen to them during this time, and if no one is there to do so, the very old and especially those with dementia withdraw. Older people who are trying to tie up loose ends by retreating into fantasy or confusion are often brought closer to reality and security by validation therapy.

The foundation of validation therapy lies in the examination of the meaning of apparently senseless or bizarre behavior. Focus shifts away from the reality of the situation. For example, if an elderly woman in a nursing home says there was a man under her bed last night, it does not help to argue with her. But caregivers cannot agree with her either, because on some level, she knows the man was not there even though she saw him clearly in her mind's eye. What they can do is rephrase what she said: "You saw a man in here? Who was he? When did you see him? What did he look like?" If a caregiver can get the woman to talk about her feelings and validate that they are real, they lose their strength. If they are ignored, they only become stronger.

Validating a patient's particular need or feeling can restore self-esteem and promote a deeper understanding of the patient by staff members. Validation therapy involves following the patient's lead and responding to the issues that are important to the patient rather than interrupting to supply factual data, as in reality orientation. Even the most strange or fantastic words or actions carry a message if caregivers are willing to listen. Validation therapy does not mean that the patient's inappropriate words or actions are reinforced. Nurses should respond sensitively and reorient the patient only when they have a legitimate reason for doing so. Using validation therapy both individually and in groups, validation workers tune into the world of the elderly. Traveling back in time with them, the caregiver can begin to understand the underlying life themes that are being expressed. Through careful listening, eye contact, and touch, the trained person can build a sense of mutual respect and trust with the elder. Most important, feelings can be understood and interpreted. See Table 8-4 for principles of validation.

Consider this example: Mrs. Smythe continually stuffs paper tissues in her purse. The nurse asks if the paper is important. When Mrs. Smythe nods "Yes," the nurse suggests that being organized and putting things where they belong is important. The nurse asks if stuffing the tissues away makes Mrs. Smythe feel better. When Mrs. Smythe responds affirmatively, the nurse has validated the action and its meaning to Mrs. Smythe. Making sense of the activity is helped by the nurse's knowledge that Mrs. Smythe was a bookkeeper and often put important papers in envelopes and file cabinets. Pointing out that Mrs. Smythe no longer has a job and lives in a

TABLE 8-4: PRINCIPLES OF VALIDATION

1. All older adults are valuable and accepted without judgment no matter how disoriented they become.

2. All older adults are one of a kind and must be treated as individuals.

3. There is a reason for the behavior being displayed by the disoriented person.

4. As a function of aging, the anatomy of the brain changes and changes in behavior can take place. These changes exhibit the physical, psychosocial, and social changes that have and are taking place during the individual's life.

5. As memory fails, older adults have a need to restore balance to their lives by recapturing memories from their past.

6. As health care providers, nurses cannot change the behaviors of older adults unless these individuals want to change those behaviors.

7. Each of life's stages has a task that must be completed and if not resolved may lead to psychological troubles.

8. Empathy for older adults who are disoriented builds trust, restores dignity, and lessens anxiety.

9. Health care providers must become trusted listeners in order to allow older adults to express painful feelings. They must acknowledge and validate those feelings because, if these feelings are disregarded, they will gain strength.

(Feil, 2001; Neal & Briggs, 2002)

nursing home now would serve no useful purpose. However, another approach in this instance could be to occupy Mrs. Smythe in stuffing envelopes as a purposeful and useful activity.

Validation Therapy Techniques

Listed here are techniques that can be used by health care providers during validation therapy:

- Use nonthreatening and factual words to build trust.

- Ask questions such as who, what, when, where, and how, but not why.

- Validate feelings only after they are expressed.

- Rephrase the statement, but be somewhat vague. Repeat in your own words what was said; use the same pitch, tempo, and even facial expression, as those used by the patient.

- Use polarity. Ask the patient to describe the extreme form of his or her experience. Try to help the patient imagine the opposite. Was there a time when the behavior did not occur?

- Reminisce. Explore the past to establish trust and find familiar coping methods to use again.

- For patients who are less verbal, use touch, voice, and eye contact. Music can also be helpful.

Validation therapy can restore a sense of well being, increase trust, improve speech, increase clearness of thinking, and provide more social interaction. Although some medical practitioners are skeptical about the scientific rationale for its use, those who have seen the beneficial results of validation therapy continue to advocate for its use and further studies (American Psychiatric Association [APA], 2000; Neal & Briggs, 2003).

ENHANCING SELF-CARE

Research indicates that people with AD can assume normal ADLs and that with proper guidance and interventions these individuals experience functional gains in ADLs. The earlier self-care

begins, the greater the success in maintaining ADLs or slowing functional decline.

When problem behaviors occur during the early stages of AD, the patient can prepare a list of self-care items. AD patients may find familiar tasks such as ADLs difficult and staff members need to find ways to help them overcome problem areas.

Dealing with Memory Changes

Dealing with memory changes can be made easier by:

- posting a schedule of the things to do every day, such as meal times, regular exercise, medication schedules, and bedtime

- having someone call to remind about meal times, appointments, or medication schedules

- preparing a calendar with events for the week and month

- labeling photos in albums

- labeling cupboards and drawers

- organizing closets

- posting reminders to turn things off.

One of the most difficult tasks of caring for people with AD is taking away responsibility and restricting activities. However, nurses commonly see bills go unpaid or poor judgment in the spending of money, hundreds or thousands of dollars spent on strange items. Early in the disease, making things simpler and less confusing can help individuals with AD. Recommendations include:

- making arrangements for direct deposit of checks and other income

- making arrangements for help paying bills

- having meals delivered at home

- having someone check on smoke alarms and house safety

- having someone call or visit daily.

Doing difficult tasks can become frustrating. Some suggestions to assist in reducing the frustration include:

- doing difficult tasks during the best times of the day

- allowing time to accomplish a task

- taking a break if something is too difficult

- arranging for others to help with tasks that become too difficult.

Difficulty communicating with others can signal a milestone in decreasing function. When people with AD begin to experience difficulty understanding what others are saying or finding the right words to express themselves, they may find the following recommendations helpful:

- Take time to say what is being said.

- Ask the other person to repeat a statement, speak slowly, or write down words they do not understand.

- Find a quiet place if there is too much distracting noise.

Driving

Nurses must recognize that, at some point, it may no longer be safe for patients with AD to drive. Discuss with the family and primary care provider how and when decisions about driving will be made. If this is not accomplished early, family may not recognize driving limitations until a calamity occurs. For example, a father tells his daughter that he and his wife will be safe taking a drive. Many hours later, he calls from 300 miles away and has no idea how he got so lost in areas he traveled in for 50 years. Now the daughter must go find him.

The decision concerning the issue of driving is not always made by the person with AD. Primary care providers or family members may make it. The decision to "take away the keys" can be devastating for the person with AD. It may be the person's last bastion of maintaining control; the loss of driving takes away freedom. Individuals go to great lengths to keep driving, and taking away the keys may not be enough; the car may need to be disabled or sold. This issue raises ethical and legal concerns of decision-making for the person with AD.

When family members or caregivers make decision to discontinue their loved one's driving, they need to make plans for other transportation options, such as family members, friends, and community services. They can contact the local chapter of the Alzheimer's Association to learn what transportation services are available in their area.

DECISION-MAKING AND AD

As AD progresses, the decision-making capacity of the individual is harder to evaluate. Care providers tend to overestimate and underestimate the decision-making capacity of individuals with AD. If an individual's decision-making capacity is underestimated, his or her right to autonomous choice is denied (Volicer & Ganzini, 2003). When decision-making capacity is overestimated, these same individuals may make choices that are not in their best interest. Overestimation generally occurs in the early stages of the disease, when the individual is able to keep up the appearance of being able to operate in the social world. Overestimation generally occurs while the person with AD is still in the home and family, friends, and primary care providers overlook cognitive impairment. Underestimation generally occurs in long-term care facilities (LTCFs) when individuals have AD or schizophrenia (Volicer & Ganzini, 2003).

How do we identify when overestimation or underestimation has occurred? A few inquiries posed to the person with AD can be beneficial in determining their decision-making capacity:

- Can they understand the information relevant to making a choice?

- Can they express a choice?

- Can they provide subjective rationale for a choice?

- Can they make reasonable treatment choices when an alternative treatment choice is unreasonable?

- Can they appreciate the consequences of the decision for themselves?

Please keep in mind that "although making an unusual choice might be a warning flag that decision-making capacity requires further assessment, it is the ethical concept that individuals have the right to make idiosyncratic choices that lies at the core of decision-making capacity" (Volicer & Ganzini, 2003, p. 1272).

DIFFICULT BEHAVIORS

As AD progresses, behavior problems become much more evident and harder to manage. Listed here are specific behavior problems and some of the suggested interventions for those behaviors.

Agitation

The term agitation is used to describe a behavior that is multidimensional and complex. The complexity lies in the behavior as well as in the management of the behavior. As AD progresses, most people experience agitation in addition to memory loss and other symptoms. Sloane, Mitchell, Preisser, Phillips, Commander and Burker (1998) indicate that agitation is inappropriate verbal, vocal, or motor activity that cannot be explained by individual needs or confusion. Table 8-5 provides examples of behaviors that suggest agitation.

Agitation is reported in more than half of community-dwelling patients with dementia and affects up to 70% of nursing home residents. According to some researchers, agitated and aggressive behaviors become more common with increasing severity of dementia; others have found no such correlation. Nevertheless, understanding these behaviors and the factors that precipitate

TABLE 8-5: EXAMPLES OF AGITATION
• Repetitive mannerisms and nonloud verbal repetition and questions (most common)
• Wandering
• Demanding to leave during an activity or event the individual was looking forward to
• Waking up in the middle of the night to get dressed and start the day
• Not recognizing familiar settings, home, or family late in the afternoon
• Becoming belligerent and irritated late in the day
(Hall, 2003b)

them, as well as ways to manage them, are critically important to all caregivers in determining the need for nursing home placement, regardless of the severity of cognitive impairment. Dementia patients with uncontrolled agitation or wandering are institutionalized sooner than subjects without behavioral disruptions because they are more difficult to care for (Poole & Mott, 2003).

Do not simply dismiss changes in behavior. When agitation is sudden, it requires medical attention; there is most likely a cause other than the AD. Medical causes of behavior problems in people with AD include malnutrition, medications, infection, dehydration, or blood glucose abnormality. Changes in appetite or sleep may also be attributed to other factors. Nonmedical causes include loud noises, loss of recognition or surroundings, crowds, new places, and difficulty with accomplishing a task.

In the early stages of AD, people may experience personality changes such as irritability, anxiety, and depression. As the disease progresses, other symptoms may occur, including sleep disturbances, delusions (firmly held beliefs in things that are not real), hallucinations (seeing, hearing, or feeling things that are not there), pacing, constant movement or restlessness, checking and rechecking door locks or appliances, tearing tissues, general emotional distress, and uncharacteristic cursing or threatening language.

Possible causes of agitation

Agitation may be caused by a number of different medical conditions and drug interactions or by any circumstances that worsen the person's ability to think. Situations that can lead to agitated behavior include moving to a new residence or nursing home, other changes in the environment or caregiver arrangements, misperceived threats, or fear and fatigue resulting from trying to make sense out of a confusing world. Table 8-6 lists examples of behaviors that suggest agitation.

TABLE 8-6: CONTRIBUTORS TO AGITATION
• Anger and personality changes
• Aggression
• Suspicious thoughts
• Loss of recognition
• Anxiety

Identifying Agitation Triggers

Correctly identifying what has triggered agitated behavior can often help in selecting the best behavioral intervention. In many cases, the trigger is some sort of change in the person's environment:

- change in caregiver
- change in living arrangements
- travel
- hospitalization
- presence of houseguests
- bathing
- being asked to change clothing.

Treating Agitation

A person exhibiting agitated behavior should receive a thorough medical evaluation, especially when agitation comes on suddenly. Treatment of agitation depends on a careful diagnosis, determination of the possible causes, and the types of agitated

behavior the person is experiencing. With proper treatment and intervention, significant reduction or stabilization of the symptoms can often be achieved.

There are two distinct types of treatments for agitation: behavioral interventions and prescription medications. Behavioral treatments should be attempted first. In general, steps in managing agitation include:

1) identifying the behavior
2) understanding its cause
3) adapting the caregiving environment to remedy the situation.

Managing Agitation

Historically, changing the environment has been reported to reduce agitation. Environmental factors that can be manipulated to reduce agitation include room size, layout, and room configuration. Included in manipulation of the environment are specific protections for wanderers, such as incorporating means of controlling exits to decrease the opportunities for unauthorized leaves from a facility. Noise reductions in the environment will also assist in lessening agitation. Staff and caregiver factors that can affect agitation include the ratio of caregivers to AD patients, consistency of staff members or caregivers, organized activities, and the level one-on-one care.

Nursing responsibilities include the management of agitation in older adults, yet research indicates that nurses do not understand or manage agitation well (Poole & Mott, 2003). If they do not understand or manage agitation well, how do they care for an older adult who is agitated? This question is not easily answered because there are so many extenuating circumstances.

Consider the nurse's attitude toward an agitated person with AD. Caring for a person with AD who is agitated increases a nurse's risk of injury, increases the demand on her time, and demands quick response time. Now consider that this nurse has four other patients to care for, the staffing level is insufficient, and it is this nurse's third day of working under these conditions. Would you think that the nurse's attitude might be negative? Why would this nurse want to take care of a high acuity patient load, knowing that there aren't enough staff to provide the best possible care to these patients?

Poole and Mott (2003) investigated the feelings and actions of nurses caring for agitated older adults. They discovered that, although some nurses had adequate training and understanding of all the complexities of managing agitated patients, others were ill equipped for the same responsibility. Because of disparities such as this, nursing actions did not meet best practice standards.

Understanding the medical problems leading to agitation of people with AD was problematic for nurses in Poole and Mott's (2003) research. The following are excerpts of nursing comments demonstrating both positive and negative understanding:

Positive

- It was not the patient's fault, he or she was really sick.

- You've got to actually diagnose what's wrong.

- Get someone else to sit with the patient, or hire a special duty nurse.

Negative

- You think you've calmed them down and they seem sweet or whatever, but people can just change.

During an episode of agitation

- **Do:** Redirect the person's attention, back off and ask permission, use calm positive statements, reassure, slow down, use visual and verbal cues, add light, offer guided choices between two options, focus on pleasant events, offer simple exercise options, and limit stimulation.

- **Do not:** raise voice, take offense, corner, crowd, restrain, rush, criticize, ignore, confront, argue, reason, shame, demand, condescend, force, explain, teach, show alarm, or make sudden

movements out of the person's view.

- **Say:** May I help you? Do you have time to help me? You are safe here. Everything is under control. I apologize. I am sorry that you are upset. I know it is hard. I will stay until you feel better.

Interventions for Agitation

Managing agitation can include medications and restraints. The lack of understanding of medication dosing and the injurious nature of mechanical restraints are serious concerns. Training is imperative for ensuring that staff use best practices (see Table 8-7). Nurses in Poole and Mott's (2003) study demonstrated lack of knowledge in this area as well.

TABLE 8-7: GENERAL STRATEGIES TO PREVENT OR REDUCE AGITATED BEHAVIORS
• Create a calm environment: remove stressors, triggers, or danger; move the person to a safer or quieter place; change expectations; offer a security object, rest, or privacy; and limit caffeine use.
• Provide an opportunity for exercise, develop soothing rituals, and use gentle reminders.
• Avoid environmental triggers, such as noise, glare, insecure space, and too much background distraction, including television.
• Monitor personal comfort: check for pain, hunger, thirst, constipation, full bladder, fatigue, infections, and skin irritation; ensure a comfortable temperature; and be sensitive to fears, misperceived threats, and frustration with expressing what is wanted.
• Simplify tasks and routines.
• Allow adequate rest between stimulating events.
• Use lighting to reduce confusion and restlessness at night.

The following are statements made by nurses regarding medication dosing:

- "The dose of medication ordered didn't touch her."

- "....won't even numb a little finger."

- "The restrained patient has more rights than I do."

The following are statements made by nurses regarding mechanical restraints:

- "....better than chemical restraint because you just release it after a couple of hours."

- "Sometime the restraints make them more agitated but you'd rather that so you can get out and get some of the other work done and come back to them later and calm them down."

An important factor in nurses attitudes about agitation is perceived lack of support from the medical staff. Many of the nurses in Poole and Mott's (2003) research also demonstrated a lack of understanding of recommended medication practices. Nurses requested larger doses of psychotropic drugs, which were denied by the physician, and this was perceived as lack of support rather than an understanding of low dosing of medications.

These findings demonstrate inadequacies in education of nurses, system inadequacies in the staffing required for best practices, and pervasive negative attitudes that increase the problems surrounding caring for agitated older adults (Poole & Mott, 2003; Hurley & Volicer, 2002).

Interventions for Agitation and Aggression in Dementia

Interventions to reduce agitation in people with AD have included a myriad of approaches. These categories include modification of the environment, interpersonal strategies, and use of physical or chemical restraints. Physical restraints should be avoided as much as possible. Anxiety and agitation that cannot be remedied through nonpharmacological interventions may require treatment with short-acting anxiolytics, such as alprazolam and lorazepam. The largest body of research on non-

pharmacological interventions for agitation was performed in the 1990s. These studies focused on the use of communication, music therapy, massage, amelioration of sleep-wake cycles, room redesign, animal therapy, mirror usage, and bathing as ways of reducing agitation.

In more recent years, studies have focused on balancing behavioral, environmental, and pharmacological interventions (Zeisel, Silverstein, Hyde, et al., 2003); developing conceptual frameworks from which to develop educational programs on behavioral interventions (Volicer & Hurley, 2003); formulating methods of describing and measuring the success of specific interventions for specific behaviors to achieve desired outcomes (Czaja, Schulz, Lee, & Belle, 2003); and developing special resources for enhancing caregiver health (Mahoney, Jones, Coon, et al., 2003).

Caregiver education delays nursing home placements of AD patients. It is important to teach the three R's: Repeat, Reassure, and Redirect. Repeat questions or directions as needed. Reassure the AD patient when they are troubled or confused. Redirect their focus to something about which they are confident. Redirection is the same practice some people use on children when their behavior is inappropriate. These measures can assist caregivers in reducing problematic behaviors, which can then reduce the use of pharmacologic interventions.

Interventions For Problem Behaviors

- Nurses need to determine when it is necessary to consult with a geriatric psychiatrist, who can be most beneficial in addressing the agitation of a person with AD.

- Restraints should be used only as a last resort to control behaviors. Although some research indicates a correlation between low physical restraint use and reduced agitation, it is more important to evaluate the cause of the behavior. The best rule of thumb is don't use physical restraints. Remember, prevention is a better solution, if possible. Look for signs of frustration and intervene early.

- Reduce the size of the unit. Research suggests that the larger the unit size, the greater the agitation of the population because it increases patient's stimulation.

- Medical evaluation should be performed to rule out physical and medical problems, side effects of medication, and the need for medication.

- Separate the patient from stressful situations, people, and places.

- Alternate rest and activity times; do not over-stimulate. Research has shown that having patients in bed for some time during the day was associated with reduced agitation. Daytime rest periods, directed at reducing overstimulation, also help to decrease agitation.

- Distract versus confront. Distract with food, activity, or conversation.

- Back off, if necessary; decrease your level of danger; and seek help as needed.

- Use gentle touch; respond calmly and slowly.

- Do not respond with anger or confrontation.

- Reassure the person.

- Utilize good communication techniques.

- Be conservative in the use of force or restraint.

- Reduce environmental stressors (such as noise, crowding, caffeine, and television).

- Find creative outlets, such as repetitive activity, music, exercise, and dance.

- Experiment with objects that have a soothing effect (dolls, stuffed animals).

- Use reminiscence and validation.

- Respond to feelings; for example, say "I know you are upset; let me see if I can help" or "This is really making you frustrated, isn't it? Why don't we do something else."

- Avoid taking comments or outbursts personally.

- Give adequate time to complete tasks.

- Learn from experience; keep a log to see if a pattern exists.

- Recognize that anger and agitation may be symptoms of dementia and frustration over losses, not deliberate responses.

(Sloane, Mitchell, Preisser, et al., 1998; Alzheimer's Disease and Related Disorders Association, Inc., 2002; Volicer, 2001; Cummings & Cole, 2002; Volicer & Hurley, 2003).

Resistive Behavior

Caregivers, whether professional or family, often help patients with dementia eat, bathe, use the toilet, dress, and take medications. Providing this assistance can be a source of stress for the caregiver, especially when the patient resists the efforts. Coltharp, Richie, and Kaas (1996) defined resisting care as behavior by the individual in any form that may prevent or hinder the nurse or caregiver in performing or assisting with ADLs. These ADLs can include bathing, eating, toileting, dressing, and grooming. Patients with AD or dementia may angrily object to the assistance, become verbally or physically abusive, hit, slap, bite, scream, run away, argue, or become agitated. As the behavior escalates, mental, emotional, or physical abuse of the patient by the caregiver may occur.

The first principle of nursing management of patients who resist help with ADLs is to determine the cause of the problem (assessment). If a physical problem such as pain or constipation is discovered, it should be dealt with first. Ask, what is the behavior, who is involved, and where, when, and how does the behavior occur? It is also important to consider for whom the behavior is a problem. Is it simply annoying to the staff?

Nurses should examine their own or other staff members' feelings and responses to the situations that occur (Coltharp et al., 1996). The activity the patient resists should be carried out in a calm, friendly, gentle manner without rush or hurry (Mace

& Rabins, 2001). For example, the environment for the bath can be altered. Possible changes include covering mirrors; installing grab bars; using a shower or tub seat; avoiding bath oils or bubble bath; and, in general, making the bathroom a gentler, softer, quieter place. In some rare instances, low doses of lorazepam (Ativan) are effective and well tolerated and have minimal side effects when other interventions to decrease resistance have been unsuccessful (Stewart, 1995, 2000).

Goals should be realistic. When a patient resists help with dressing, expectations can be modified. Wearing the same clothing for 2 days in a row is all right. Removing a patient's soiled clothing from the room at night avoids arguments. If choices are confusing, they should be eliminated. Dressing can be simplified to sturdy, washable clothing with Velcro fastenings.

Resistance to toileting can be met by determining underlying causes, such as burning or pain associated with a urinary tract infection. Also, easily pulled on and off pants and slacks can be substituted for ones with complex zippers and buttons. The bathroom and toilet can be marked with signs that cue patients to the use and location of these facilities. The key to management of resistance to care is to be flexible and imaginative. The trial-and-error method is useful for finding what works. Keep in mind, however, that what works today may not work tomorrow. This notion cannot be stressed enough to caregivers of patients with AD or dementia.

Catastrophic Reactions

Becoming overwhelmed and overreacting to a situation leads to what is called a catastrophic reaction. In patients with dementia, catastrophic reactions are characterized by sudden emotional outbursts and feelings of terror related to being overwhelmed, distressed, or confused by situations (Mace & Rabins, 2001). During a catastrophic reaction, people display behaviors such as:

- stubbornness

- overcriticism
- rapidly changing moods
- worry and fear
- anger and suspiciousness
- excessive crying
- increased restlessness, pacing, and wandering
- striking out (combativeness).

These reactions appear to be set off by inconsequential situations, many times related to the inability to perform a simple task, such as hair brushing; inability to find something (glasses or teeth); or washing dishes. A sudden increase in catastrophic reactions may be an early indicator of a developing medical problem such as an infection (Rader, 1995). Catastrophic reactions most commonly occur in the morning hours in a health care facility, when daily care activities are greatest. At this time, staff members are under pressure to follow a schedule and place more demands on patients to complete bathing and grooming tasks.

Managing Catastrophic Reactions

Catastrophic reactions are disturbing and cause stress to caregivers and nursing staff. The best management technique is to try to understand the cause of the behavior and head off the reaction before it occurs. Adverse drug reactions should be considered first and ruled out by the clinician. Then, the communication techniques discussed in chapters 3 and 4 and the strategies listed here may be helpful:

- Create a no-fail, low-demand environment with a consistent, predictable schedule. One preventive activity found to be useful for residents who like to rock is a glider swing (Snyder et al., 2001). The intervention was found to produce pleasure, comfort, and relief of anxiety and is safe and practical for nursing home residents.

- Give directions one step at a time, in simple language. Break tasks down into easy steps and limit choices.

- Help patients accept their inability to perform

certain tasks by staying calm and not becoming irritated or angry at failure to perform these tasks.

When a catastrophic reaction is occurring, these strategies may be more helpful:

- Let the person with the best relationship with the patient respond.

- Do not ask questions, argue, restrain, or try to reason with an agitated person.

- Give verbal reassurance that you understand the patient's fear and embarrassment. Use touch if the patient is responsive to it; pat the patient's arm or shoulder and use soothing music.

- Guide the patient to a quiet place or offer distraction with a conversation or activity.

- Get other staff members to assist and, if necessary, get out of range or leave the room. If attempts to divert the reaction are unsuccessful, do not take the outcome personally.

If catastrophic reactions occur frequently, caregivers and nurses can keep a log of what happens, when it happens, who was around, and what helps. They can use the data to look for patterns of events or times that may trigger the reaction. After the reaction is over, they should reassure the patient that they recognize that this reaction can be upsetting to the patient as well as to staff members and that they will continue to care for the patient.

Delusions and Hallucinations

Delusions and hallucinations are the prominent signs of psychosis in people with AD. Wilson, Gilley, Bennett, Beckett, and Evans (2000) found that more than 40% of people with AD experience hallucinations, and these hallucinations are associated with a lower baseline cognitive score and more rapid decline on all cognitive measures when compared with people without hallucinations. Delusions were found to be present in 30% to 55% of AD patients, but the delusions were not significantly related to cognitive decline. Effective interventions

for delusions and hallucinations include decreasing environmental stress (discussed earlier in this chapter) and simplifying the environment.

A hallucination is a false perception of objects or events involving the senses. When a person with AD has a hallucination, he or she sees, hears, smells, tastes, or feels something that is not there. The person may see the face of a former friend in a curtain or may hear people talking

If the hallucination does not cause problems for caregivers, the patient, or family members, it may be best to ignore it. However, if hallucinations occur continuously, consult a physician to determine if there is an underlying physical cause. Also, have the person's eyesight and hearing checked, and make sure the person wears his or her glasses and hearing aid on a regular basis, if applicable.

Managing Hallucinations

Here are some tips for managing patients with hallucinations:

Offer reassurance

- Respond in a calm, supportive manner.

- A gentle tap on the shoulder may turn the person's attention toward you.

- Look for the feelings behind the hallucinations. You might want to say, "It sounds as if you're worried" or "I know this is frightening for you."

- Avoid arguing with the person about what he or she sees.

Use distractions

- Suggest that the patient take a walk or sit in another room. Frightening hallucinations often subside in well-lit areas where other people are present.

- Try to turn the person's attention to music, conversation, or activities.

Modify the environment

- Check for noises that might be misinterpreted, such as noise from a television or an air conditioner. Look for lighting that casts shadows, reflections, or distortions on the surfaces of floors, walls, and furniture.

- Cover mirrors with a cloth or remove them if the person thinks that he or she is looking at a stranger.

Depression

Depression is covered thoroughly in chapters 2 and 3 but deserves a mention here. The significance of depressed mood and depressive syndromes in patients with AD remains a controversial issue. Studies of depression in patients with AD conducted in the last 10 years have created discrepancies in estimation of prevalence, main clinical correlates, and response to treatment (Chemerinski, Petracca, Sabe, Kremer, & Starkstein, 2001). According to the research, "Depressed patients with Alzheimer's disease rated their depression (on the Hamilton Depression Scale) as less severe than did their respective caregivers, suggesting that depressed patients with Alzheimer's disease may not be fully aware of the severity of their depressive symptoms" (Chemerinski et al., 2001, p. 71).

Most research indicates that depression occurs in nearly 4 million of the 31 million older adults in the United States. Depression is associated with disability and a diminished quality of life. It is very important to differentiate dementia of AD from depression. Primary care providers recognize less frequently than is desirable, the fact that dementia is known to occur more frequently in older persons with AD than those without AD (Kroenke, 2002).

Currently, some researchers support using antidepressants for treatment of depression. Selective serotonin reuptake inhibitors (SSRIs) may be the drugs of choice, based on the clinical presentation of the individual with AD (Lehne, 2004; Serby & Yu, 2003).

Nurses must be able to distinguish between apathy and depression. Apathy is loss of motivation; it is commonly mistaken for depression but is actually a form of executive cognitive dysfunction. When peo-

ple with AD are in a state of apathy, they rely more on others to care for them daily. This, in turn, places even more stress on family members and caregivers. Difficult as it may be, assessing apathy means that the practitioner must be able to distinguish loss of motivation from loss of abilities resulting from cognitive decline. Differentiating apathy from depression or other syndromes is important because treatments differ for each condition (Landes, Sperry, Strauss, & Geldmacher, 2001). However, this difference is just being recognized, and instruments that assist in differentiating between syndromes need research to support their efficacy.

A depressed mood in AD has been associated with a range of depressive symptoms — guilt, suicide, insomnia, loss of interest, retardation, agitation, worry, anxiety, loss of energy, loss of libido, loss of weight, and hypochondriasis — suggesting that both affective and autonomic symptoms of depression are frequent among patients with AD. Researchers find a similar prevalence of depressive symptoms among depressed patients with AD and patients with primary depression without dementia, except for loss of appetite, loss of weight, suicide, and anxiety, which were more severe in the latter group (Chemerinski et al., 2001; Serby & Yu, 2003).

Managing Depression

A wide variety of interventions are available to treat depression and improve levels of functioning:

- *Counseling:* Although many older adults with AD can be treated by their primary care provider, a referral to a geriatric psychiatrist may be of assistance, especially when the symptoms of depression are atypical.

- *Day-care activities:* Involving the individual in social activities can be beneficial.

- *Medications:* The choice of an antidepressant depends on a number of factors. Many of the drugs for people with AD lessen behavior disturbances and improve ADLs but do not improve cognition. Always ask if the drug has

demonstrated efficacy and safety. SSRIs are preferred.
(Serby & Yu, 2003)

Sleep Disorders

Sleep disorders are common among people with AD. Sleep patterns change with aging. Older adults sleep lighter and awaken more easily because of degenerative changes in the central nervous system. Nocturia, muscle cramps, and noise interrupt sleep for older people, and older people may require more time to return to sleep (Eliopoulos, 1995).

Normal sleep is divided into two types: rapid-eye-movement (REM) and non-REM. Each night, sleep begins with non-REM sleep, which is followed in about 2 hours by REM sleep that recurs three to four times each night at regular intervals. With age, people have less deep sleep (stage 4 non-REM sleep) and less REM sleep. Patients with AD have even less non-REM and REM sleep (Eliopoulos, 1995). Patients with AD may not be able to connect the meaning of sleep cues in the environment (such as darkness and quiet) to the sleep cycle.

Nurses must evaluate changes in sleep patterns in order to rule out other causes. Contributors to loss of sleep can include pain, fear, depression, and adverse effects of medications. An analysis of the contributing factors to loss of sleep helps facilitate a decrease in early pharmacologic interventions.

Sleep hygiene interventions are practical in community settings and natural in institutional settings (McCurry, Gibbons, Logsdon, Vitiello, & Teri, 2003). With training, all caregivers can assist in the changing of sleep hygiene practices for people with AD. However, research has established that simply educating caregivers is not always enough. Caregivers need active assistance in establishing individualized sleep hygiene programs.

Effective Interventions for Enhancing Sleep

Establishing a routine in the daily schedule not only benefits overall behaviors but it also improves sleeping habits. Some suggestions for effective sleeping patterns are listed here:

- Keep the sleeping area free from distractions.
- Use a nightlight, if helpful.
- Keep the individual dressed during the daytime hours.
- Decrease caffeine consumption.
- Decrease fluid intake after 5 p.m.
- Administer diuretics no later than 5 p.m.
- Increase daytime activity levels or the daily exercise regime.
- Individualize sleeping habits.
- Avoid confrontations about bathing and putting on pajamas at bedtime.
- Warm milk and tryptophan may be successful sleep aids.
- Recommend a warm bath just before bed.
- Offer a light snack high in carbohydrates before bed.
- Refer the patient to a geriatric psychiatrist.
- Offer respite care services for people with AD and their family members.
- Address the fatigue but do not interrupt nighttime sleep.
- In the early stages of AD, 15- to 30-minute rest periods are usually sufficient; longer rest periods can interfere with nighttime sleep.

Pharmacological treatment for sleeping disorders depends on the reasons for the disorder. Once the evaluation process rules out other causes, such as pain, fear, and side effects of other medications, it may be prudent to provide short-term pharmacological treatment for a sleep disorder. Only when nonpharmacological treatments have failed should drugs such as benzodiazepines be used. Terminate their use at the earliest possible time.

When putting patients with dementia to bed at night, caregivers should use a nightlight and follow an established regular bathroom and bedtime ritual. Put a commode at the bedside for use during the night, if necessary. No attempts should be made to keep patients in bed by using bed rails or, at home, placing a chair next to the bed. Keep in mind that nighttime wandering can be dangerous and puts an added burden on the caregiver, whether at home or in a health care facility.

If the patient awakens because of pain, pain medication can be provided at bedtime. Massages or back rubs at bedtime can be calming and relaxing as well. One study looked at the effects of upper back, slow-stroke massage to manage agitated behaviors (Rowe & Alfred, 1999). The results revealed an added beneficial effect of uninterrupted sleep for demented individuals.

The most important strategy used to manage sleep disorders is to allow patients who wake up to get out of bed if they wish. For example, Mr. Foster went to bed early every evening. He had been a railroad engineer and had always been an early riser. He would wake up at 2:00 or 2:30 a.m. and want to get up. Staff members would take him to a safe, quiet place near where they worked, give him a snack, and turn on the television or read to him. If necessary, they let him sleep in a recliner chair either in his room or near them. The key is supervision and responding to the individual patient's needs.

Caregivers can make the home as safe as possible by lighting the bathroom, keeping the area around the patient's bed clear, and using nonskid strips by the side of the bed to prevent the patient from falling or slipping when getting up. Caregivers should also block stairs, lock doors and windows, and lock up dangerous items, such as knives and scissors, any time people with AD are present, but especially at night when they might be up alone. A room monitor may be helpful if the caregiver sleeps in another part of the house. Caregivers at home may need to consider respite or in-home care if sleeping problems persist.

Use of sleeping medications is not particularly effective in patients with dementia. Common side effects of these drugs are unsteady gait, which increases the risk of falling, and incontinence. Antihistamines such as diphenhydramine (Benadryl), which are commonly present in over-the-counter sleep medications, can increase confusion and cause anticholinergic effects (dry mouth, constipation, urinary retention or hesitancy). The use of sedatives, such as zolpidem (Ambien) and trazadone (Desyrel), at home may help the caregiver get much needed sleep (APA, 2000). However, sedatives should be avoided in a health care facility, because staff members are available at night to meet the individualized needs of patients with AD (Mace & Rabins, 2001) and undesirable side effects may be intensified. Minor tranquilizers or benzodiazepines may be adequate only on a short-term basis for sleep disorders.

Communications Disorders

Communication difficulties increase frustrations for both the caregiver and the individual with AD. Communication difficulties arise from the loss of memory. Communication is covered in depth in chapter 3.

Repeated Questions

One of the contributors to caregiver frustration is the repeated questions that usually come from people with AD. For people with AD, repeated questions are usually the result of several factors: they don't remember having asked the question; they have lost all sense of time; the question is really not what they want to know. Usually they are trying to discover when something will happen. A problem arises when their questions become obsessive and intrusive. Repeated questions are discussed in more detail in chapter 3.

THERAPEUTIC ACTIVITY

Nursing research has identified therapeutic activities for AD patients. A host of interventions have been recognized to enhance well-being. Well-being can simply be defined as a resolution of the problem behavior. Quality of life can be enhanced by promoting a feeling of well-being. Self-reported mood and observations of affect are often used as indicators of emotional well-being; however, because people with AD are unable to vocalize their emotions, behavioral manifestations are substituted as expressions of personal emotions.

Interventions to enhance well-being may include:

- stimulating cognition
- creating an emotional response
- encouraging movement
- calming agitation
- enhancing sleep
- creating pleasure
- assisting in maintaining or reestablishing dignity
- providing meaningful tasks
- impeding mental decline
- facilitating friendships.

Nursing literature details an expansive array of activities for AD patients. Probably the most frequently used intervention is music. Music can be used alone or in combination with other interventions to relax and stimulate individuals. It has been used to increase or maintain the physical, mental, and social functioning of older adults (Humphrey, 2002). In a study by Cohen-Mansfield (2001), verbally disruptive behavior was reduced by 31% during music groups. Music therapy has also been found to increase socialization and decrease agitated behaviors (Aldridge, 2000; Gerdner, 2000; Poole & Mott, 2003; Remington, 2002; Sandbandham & Sphirm, 1995; Zeisel & Raia, 2000; Zeisel et al., 2003).

Music has been found to positively affect almost all behaviors and improves active involvement of individuals as well as their social, emotional, and cognitive skills. Researchers have hypothesized that music forms a bridge between the cognitive and creative sides of the brain. A nursing home in Michigan started a music therapy program for individuals with dementia based, in part, on the "Mozart Effect" discovered in 1993 by University of California researchers. These researchers found that listening to Mozart before an IQ test boosted scores and suggested that listening to the music helped organize the firing patterns of neurons in the central cortex. For patients with AD, listening to Mozart may improve concentration and enhance remaining abilities. No particular type of music or patient background increases these benefits.

One goal of the Omnibus Budget Reconciliation Act (OBRA) of 1987 was to maintain quality of life and pleasurable activity for patients with dementia. Individualized recreational therapy, as an intervention for disturbing behaviors, should be unique for each person based on three factors: the individual's needs, current functioning level, and past interests. Research shows that 91% of non-pharmacological interventions produce a benefit in treating the disturbing behaviors of dementia (Cohen-Mansfield, 2001). Achievable outcomes include increased strength, endurance, and flexibility; maintained or improved self-capability with ADLs; fall prevention; decreased sleep difficulties; increased nutritional intake; increased socialization; increased verbalization; and decreased disturbing behaviors, anxiety, apathy, passivity, and depression. These goals were reached by gaining insight into the special emotional needs of each patient with AD, by exploring the patient's strengths, and by attempting to understand which activities provide satisfaction and meaning to that patient.

A distinction should be made between diversional activities and therapeutic activities. Bringing in a barbershop quartet or someone to sing

Christmas carols or hymns or play the accordion is not a therapeutic activity unless the event has a measurable outcome specific to each patient present. Nurses must have an awareness of each patient and his or her unique needs.

To meet the needs of individual patients, therapeutic activity programs may include the following types of activities (Gibb, Morris & Gleisberg, 1997; Turnbull & Turnbull, 1998):

- *Mental stimulation:* Reading, talking, reminiscing
- *Socialization:* Discussions during mealtimes or other group gatherings
- *Creative activity:* Crafts, needlework, storytelling
- *Productive activity:* Building something, providing a service to another
- *Emotionally supportive activity:* Support group, one-to-one attention
- *Physical activity:* Walking, exercise, movement to music
- *Personal care:* Bathing, dressing, eating

A nursing home in Ohio developed programming for a dementia unit based on Montessori methods (Bruek, 2001). Maria Montessori designed an educational setting in which children engage in a series of individualized activities to foster independence and make meaningful choices. The concept is founded on rehabilitation concepts; it breaks down tasks into simple steps and guides individuals through one step at a time. Activities are anything the resident does during the course of a day; they focus on recognizing strengths and interests and enabling residents to demonstrate their remaining abilities. Intensive in-service training was conducted with staff, volunteers, and families. The results of the study interventions were enhanced resident engagement with others and positive emotional states. Cognitive capabilities are maintained when patients with AD are challenged and stimulated (Bruek, 2001).

Observant nurses notice when a patient is becoming anxious and can respond with an appropriate therapeutic activity. Many traditional nursing interventions encompass the benefits and characteristics of therapeutic activity. These therapeutic activities can be provided by nurses or can be taught to other staff members or caregivers in settings that do not have specific people to handle therapeutic activities.

In today's world of care for people with dementia, nurses and other staff provide recreation therapy and activities with measurable goals and outcomes (see Table 8-8). The environment of therapeutic activity for patients with AD should be failure-free, have limited goals, and provide structure. Some interventions have been directed specifically at overcoming obstacles or difficult behavior. The key is that the activity must have meaning for the individual patient and provide feelings of increased success and self-esteem.

TABLE 8-8: THERAPEUTIC ACTIVITIES
- Art
- Games, such as table games or dominoes
- Musical instruments
- Physical activities to improve conditional and overall health and provide distraction in times of wandering or troubled behavior
- Activities to enhance level of alertness
- Reading (can assist in maintaining language skills, comprehension, and expression)
- Movies (can serve as distractions and reality orientation)
- Reminiscence
- Music tapes

ENVIRONMENTAL INFLUENCES ON BEHAVIOR

The environment threatens many people with AD because the objects in it become unrecognizable. A frightened or disoriented person with AD may wander or develop disruptive behavior such as agitation. Dysfunctional behavior may indicate a progressive lowering of the threshold for stress, which hinders the individual's functioning in the environment. As signs of anxiety and anxious behavior appear, the environment can be modified and simplified to assist in decreasing anxiety.

Staff personnel and administrators of nursing facilities must look closely at the amount and kinds of stimuli and demands the nursing home environment creates for patients who have AD. The environment may need to be modified or at the very least have clutter cleared away (Schultz, Ellingrod, Turvey, Moser, & Arndt, 2003).

The OBRA outlines guidelines for the physical environment in nursing homes. The emphasis is on providing care in a manner and in an environment to promote the maintenance or enhancement of the quality of life of each resident. The physical environment should support and expand the experience of daily living through contact with food preparation (sounds and smells), a homelike setting for watching television or people, and group settings to encourage socializing (Young, 2001; Kolanowski & Whall, 2000; Sloane et al., 1998).

Modifying the Environment

Nurses should look at the areas in a nursing facility, hospital, or home that make up the physical environment. They should assess and personalize the immediate patient area, the noise level, and the lighting (the average 80-year-old patient requires three times more light than does a 20-year-old).

When asked, elderly people say that what makes any environment positive is being treated with dignity, respect, and kindness. Therefore, creating a positive psychosocial environment is essential. The psychosocial environment involves staff members' attitudes, communication skills, behavioral approaches, and willingness to nurture healthy interpersonal relationships with patients with dementia; the structure of activities; an atmosphere of friendliness and caring; family support; and educational services. Staff members' attitudes reflect how they view their jobs and how they value residents and families. How the staff responds to difficult behaviors is key for patients with dementia. The staff members at a nursing home should recognize the equality of patients with dementia and enable patients to do as much as possible for themselves.

A less obvious component of the organizational environment is the structure of the day. For patients with dementia, the predictability of the daily schedule makes them feel secure and less fearful. Nurses have the opportunity to affect the organizational environment for patients with AD and other dementias. It is critical for nurses to examine each aspect of the environment (physical, psychosocial, and organizational) for clues to patients' unmet needs that may precipitate inappropriate behaviors. Nurses must be involved in all aspects of planning and analyzing the environment of patients with AD.

Nurses can use a patient's anxiety as a barometer to determine what the patient can handle at any particular time. As anxious behaviors occur, activities can be modified and environmental stimuli simplified until the anxiety disappears. This may mean moving objects around, lowering the level of noise or decreasing the amount of glare or light in a room, or making the necessary safety and security evaluations and changes. Nurses should not move furniture around in patients' houses or in LTCFs because this can interfere with patients' memory of where objects are in their surroundings. Uncomplicated designs in the layout of furniture or even the patterns in fabrics on furniture and drapes help decrease disorientation. Grouping favorite items together assists in signaling familiarity and decreases discomfort. Mirrors and bright daytime glare can be particularly distracting to people with AD. The use of translucent sheers or shades and removal of mirrors can help reduce distraction and disorientation and can create a soothing environment (Young, 2001). All of these factors play a role in minimizing anxiety related to the physical environment in patients with AD.

When people with AD have an unsteady gait, thorough evaluation of the environment for safety hazards and the need for safety appliances is usually necessary. Handrails, ramps, raised toilet seats, and shower bars may be necessary. When installing handrails, doors, or other safety items, it is important that they be noticeably different than the color on the walls or floors. Remember that people with AD can develop gait disturbances and such items as throw rugs, extension cords, and decorative items located low on the floor can be safety hazards and should be removed. Because of the tendency of people with AD to hide things in strange places, such as toilets and cupboards, and because these people cannot distinguish hazardous materials, it may become necessary to place locks on dangerous items.

To avoid confusion and encourage independence, provide cues to the environment. For example, hang a picture of a toilet on the bathroom door. Memory boxes have shown great success in helping patients identify "home." Memory boxes are recessed holders or frames that contain pictures of the individual, a favorite belonging, and items the person can relate to and remember.

One activity commonly associated with behavioral problems is bathing. An author once wrote that no one with AD ever dies from not bathing. But it can sure be a struggle to get them to bathe. Patients try telling you they have already bathed and do not need to or just simply refuse to bathe. This can certainly be considered resistive behavior.

BATHING

Case Study

Mrs. Nelson, a 75-year-old woman with dementia, wears glasses and usually wears a favorite yellow sweater with her blouse and slacks. She walks around the nursing unit and is often found in the television room on the far side of the residence. She smiles, is friendly, eats well, and enjoys small-group activities. Her caregiver reported that Mrs. Nelson appears to get along just fine, until shower time. At this time, she becomes aggressive, loudly objects to being showered, and has hit and slapped some staff members. During a conversation about the shower incidents, the caregiver stated there was only one nursing assistant that Mrs. Nelson liked. This assistant was a woman who worked nights. The assistant never had any trouble with Mrs. Nelson. Staff members recognized, with the help of the patient's family, that Mrs. Nelson was a morning person and had always been shy, particularly around men. Letting the staff person who had the best relationship with her care for her and honoring her preference for female caregivers were the first steps in managing the behavior.

Assisting with Bathing

Here are some suggestions that may decrease resistive patient behavior regarding bathing:

- Let the person choose the time of day to bathe.

- Set consequences for not bathing, such as the patient cannot go to the park if he or she does not bathe today.

- Reinforce positive behavior of bathing with rewards the person enjoys.

- Make bath time enjoyable: color the water, play favorite music, or use floating animals.

- Allow patients to keep their underwear on if that is the reason for resistance.

- Instead of asking if the individual wants to bathe, change the way the question is stated and change the context. For example, say, "Let's get freshened up."

- Have the room ready. Keep it warm with low lighting.

- Use equipment that assists in providing dignity, privacy, reduction in anxiety, or comfort for the person, such as
  - a shower head
  - a blanket for covering the body
  - a wash basin and chair
  - no-rinse soap and shampoos.

- Begin the bathing process in the least sensitive area first. Try legs and feet first with the face last.

- Wash the hair last or at a separate time.

When a patient refuses to take a bath or shower, the reason may be that the whole process has become confusing and perplexing. The ability to process incoming stimuli decreases as dementia increases, and the environment outside becomes the only way for the patient to interpret what is happening. The patient perspective might be as follows: A person comes in to see you, removes you from your bed, and takes your clothes off. If you object, you are given a smile and a pat on the arm. Your calls for help are often ignored. Often, in a nursing facility, you are taken down a cold, public hallway, with a thin sheet or blanket covering your most private parts, and then taken into a cold, noisy, strange room where all covering is removed (Brawley, 2002).

Bathing and showering are extremely private activities. Many people have never had anyone see them bathe or shower. The bathing process should be individualized to the needs and routines of the patient involved (Dougherty & Long, 2003; Rader, 1995). It is not necessary to bathe every day or to shower or bathe on particular days or at prearranged times. If Mrs. Nelson accepted a shower early in the morning from her favorite staff member, she had her shower then. If she refused, staff members altered plans to meet her needs.

SAFETY

Early in the disease process, people with AD lose their sense of danger. This can easily result in injury. As caregivers, nurses are responsible for decreasing the potential for any harm coming to those in their care. Initiating some simple safety practices can help:

- Safety-proof the house or facility. Treat the environment as though you have a toddler to be concerned about. Get down to their eye level and survey the environment for all possible safety hazards. Put covers over unused electrical outlets.

- Be sure the facility contains smoke detectors and fire extinguishers.

- Remove all guns and hunting knives from the premises.

- Remove all power tools from the premises.

- Put safety locks on the drawers that contain knives. Put all kitchen equipment that could cause harm (food processors, choppers, scissors, irons) away.

- Turn the hot water heater temperature down to less than 120 degrees.

- If the individual smokes, set up "smoking areas" that do not include upholstered furniture.

- When the stove is not being used, remove the knobs.

- Hire out lawn care to reduce the danger from lawn mowers and weeding and edging equipment.

- Taste the person's food before serving it so they do not burn their mouths or skin (if spilled).

- Serve food on unbreakable dishes.

- Put safety gates at the tops and bottoms of stairs.

- Remove throw rugs and clutter from floors.

- Store all medications in tamper-proof or locked containers.

- Install assistive devices, such as grab bars in bathrooms.

- Try to eliminate furniture with sharp corners or pad them.

DRESSING

Some people with AD want to wear the same clothes day in and day out. This generally signals difficulty handling change, which is normal for these individuals with AD. So what can you do? When you shop for clothes, buy two or three of the same articles of clothing. Then when the person takes off the dirty article, switch it with a clean article. Try to get pictures of the individual in their favorite pieces of clothing so that if they should wander off you have an easy reference for the police.

Keep clothes simple. Clothes that fasten with Velcro are a great idea because they are easier to get on and off. (Though at times you may wish they were not so easy to get off.)

HIDING ITEMS

Hiding and losing personal items can become frustrating for caregivers and patients. Sometimes people with AD hide items because they are suspicious that someone may try to steal them. It is important to remember that items such as keys get hidden and go unfound. Duplicate these items and keep them in a safe place. If a person with AD does not drive, let the keys stay "lost" by actually removing them from the premises.

Some ideas to assist with minimizing the loss of valuable items are listed here:

- Remove valuables and use safety deposit boxes for money and jewelry.

- Put clappers on house and car keys so they beep when lost.

- When items are lost, check common hiding places, such as:

  - under the mattress
  - in the pages of a book
  - under pillows
  - in the freezer
  - in food containers
  - behind bricks in the basement
  - in the trash
  - in the toilet
  - in the hems of curtains
  - in the backs of picture frames
  - in tissue containers or toilet paper cylinders.

WANDERING

Consider these actual incidents that occurred in 2001:

A 70-year-old man with dementia wandered into a retaining pond not far from his home, where he was mauled by an alligator and bled to death.

An 88-year-old woman with dementia died of exposure after she wandered from her home into a small area of thick brush. After an intense 5-day search, her body was found within half a mile of her home, only 20 feet from a well-searched road.

Another man with dementia, 77 years old, wandered from his front porch, where his wife had left him, and was hit and killed by a firetruck that was sent to help find him.

These actual incidents had terrible outcomes. Unfortunately, stories such as these about people with dementia who have been found walking aimlessly in their communities, often suffering from exposure to the elements, wearing no clothing, or otherwise endangered, occur all too often. The Alzheimer's Association estimates that 60% of people with AD will wander and become lost in the community at some point (Rowe, 2003).

Research on Wandering

Family and other caregivers indicate that wandering is one of the most difficult behaviors to manage in patients with AD (Hope, Keene, McShane, et al., 2001). Despite this, there have been very few research articles published on the subject in the last 15 to 20 years. Lai and Arthur (2003) have summarized the findings of the literature in their description of the attributes of a wanderer:

- relatively young member of the older population
- more cognitively impaired
- more likely to be a man
- might have experienced sleep problems
- had a more active premorbid lifestyle
- used more psychotropic medications.

An increased risk of becoming lost, even in familiar environments, results from deficits in the areas of memory, abstract thinking, and judgment. A person with dementia may forget his address, his name, or the names of those with whom he lives. He may not recognize his own home or neighborhood. Poor judgment may lead him into unsafe, potentially fatal, situations. Dementia may also render him unable to interpret sensations of heat, cold, thirst, or hunger. Impairments in abstract thinking may cause the person to leave home in search of a caregiver who is in the next room. Once a person with dementia becomes lost outside the home, he may either fail to recognize that he needs help or may be unable to seek it.

Physical frailty, loss of balance, and increased risk of injury often accompany dementia (Rowe, 2003). Wandering can result in serious injury to the patient or placement in a nursing home.

It's a common mistake to treat wandering and becoming lost as the same problem. However, people who wander may never become lost and those who never wander may become lost. Therefore, the literature on wandering is not particularly useful in understanding this problem.

In a study conducted by Rowe (2003), the reasons for people becoming lost during a 1-year time period were analyzed. Listed here are the findings:

- The various circumstances in which people

with dementia were reported missing sometimes included wandering, but not always. The most common reasons cited for those lost while being looked after by an informal caregiver were that the caregiver was distracted or asleep, the person with dementia was left at home alone, or the person with dementia became agitated and left the house by himself in anger. Because many people with dementia who live at home retain some ability to function independently, some became lost when they were on normal outings, either walking or driving.

- Some who were living or being cared for in professional settings became lost, even though such settings often have electronic monitoring systems to prevent unattended exits. Medical transportation services also accounted for some of the incidents; for example, a driver would leave a person with dementia outside the home and drive away before he or she was inside.

- Almost 90% of the people who were lost were found within five miles of home, and 37% of those were found within one mile of home. It is important to note that they were found in a variety of indoor and outdoor locations, including (in order of decreasing frequency) residential yards, streets, health care facilities, libraries, shopping centers, highways, convenience stores, and restaurants.

- There were few indications in the Safe Return data that people with dementia who became lost sought help; rather, lost people were found only when someone recognized that they needed help and offered assistance. (The education of police officers, community groups, and caregivers is therefore essential.) The kind of person who made the discovery of the lost person was reported in 468 cases; 36% (167) of the lost people were found by police officers and 34% (159) by Good Samaritans.

Thomas (1995) indicated that wandering is behavior that is unchanging and attempts to meet some particular need defined by the wanderer. This impaired behavior is typified by excessive motion and walking, and it often leads to safety or irritation-related predicaments. Wandering has also been defined as aimless movement (Colombo et al., 2001).

In 2001, Hope et al. conceptualized wandering as a motor dysfunction that implicated a disruption in the ability of people with dementia to self-monitor their behavior. Some researchers have described wandering as aimless movement (Colombo et al., 2001), but others have made a distinction between aimless and purposeful movement in AD, such as someone who is hungry and searching for food (Kiely, Simon, Jones, & Morris, 2000). No matter how wandering is defined by researchers, nurses will tell you that the behavior exists and it is a complex behavior.

Triggers

Triggers for wandering include sleeplessness with normal aging, sundown syndrome, and inactivity during the day, including too many daytime naps. Sundown syndrome occurs as a result of changing light; the person with AD may not be able to tell if it is day or night. At dusk, the lighting can induce disorientation in people with AD. This is a good time to keep the individual busy with household tasks that are quiet in nature (Young, 2001).

Types of wandering include day and night wandering. People with AD may wander in the evening simply due to inactivity during the day. Caregivers may be exhausted, but inactivity or napping during the day leaves people who have AD with unspent energy. This is why it is so important to maintain the daily activities of people with AD (Geldmacher, Heck, & O'Toole, 2001).

Hussain (1985, 1987) identified four types of institutionalized wanderers based on their intent rather than their pattern of movement. These classifications have been quoted frequently in the literature by clinicians and researchers (Lai & Arthur, 2003). They are:

1) *Exit seekers:* Whether looking for someone or something, the person wants to leave the building.

2) *Akathisiacs:* The person is restless, pacing, and agitated. The wandering may be due to prolonged use of psychotropic drugs (neuroleptic-induced pacing and restlessness).

3) *Self-stimulators:* The person wants to stimulate himself or herself by touching walls or doors or turning doorknobs.

4) *Modelers:* The person follows others around and copies what they do by going where they go.

Researchers since Hussain have specified that because different features of wandering can occur in the same individual; therefore, compartmentalizing people who wander according to intent is not acceptable (Hope et al., 2001).

More recent researchers (Hope et al., 2001; Kiely et al., 2000) have used research rigor to investigate wandering, attempting to identify characteristics of institutionalized residents or those living at home who wander. The characteristics discovered include discomfort or unsettled states, cognitive impairment, medication use, clinical factors such as pain, stress, boredom, feeling lost, need to act out past work roles, or need to urinate.

Managing Wandering

By creating an outline of when (especially time of day) and under what circumstances wandering occurs, nurses can develop a plan for dealing with the behavior (see Table 8-9). Managing the environment is one method of dealing with wandering. Visual barriers across doorways, on the floor in front of doors, or over doorknobs are effective interventions. Another intervention found to decrease wandering is the use of a wanderer's cart. This mobile cart helps individuals who do not stay seated at mealtimes by making finger foods available from the cart as they wander. The wandering cart prevents agitated wandering into other patients' rooms and into housekeeping areas. Providing a tabletop activity near an exit was most helpful for individuals who

TABLE 8-9: GUIDELINES FOR NURSING MANAGEMENT OF WANDERING

1. Look for the basis of the behavior.

2. Restructure the environment using visual barriers, electronic alerting systems, and visual cuing. Decrease noise and confusion.

3. Encourage interaction with others in areas set aside for socialization.

4. Use activities that promote self-esteem, such as a collage of pictures supplied by the patient's family or an audiotape or videotape.

5. Go out with the patient through one door and back in another, or take him or her for a walk.

6. Provide regular exercise and diversion.

7. Use simple language and simple signs to provide cues.

8. Monitor often for physiological needs and meet the patient's need to feel secure and safe.

9. Have patients with dementia wear some type of identification, and alert all staff (or neighbors if at home) to patients who wander.

(Coltharp, Richie, & Kaas, 1996)

were attempting to exit because it served as an active diversion for them (Buettner, 1999).

Wanderers generally do not respond well to drug therapy. Some psychotropic medications make wandering worse by stimulating akathisia. Alprazolam was investigated as a pharmacotherapeutic intervention for wandering, because it was believed to be less toxic and potentially more effective than other pharmacological interventions (Szwabo & Tideiksaar, 1991); staff reports were that wandering decreased with use of the drug.

All people with AD should be registered with the Alzheimer's Association Safe Return Program, which helps to identify, locate, and return lost people with AD. AD patients should wear identification at all times in order to maintain their safety. For people with AD who have a tendency to wander, it is important to provide unrestricted areas to wander. These areas can include enclosed backyards or supervised walking paths. For continued safety, gates, alarms, and chimes can all be used to prevent unsupervised wandering.

Informal caregivers and health care professionals must learn to differentiate becoming lost from the wandering that is often associated with dementia. Although it is true that some wanderers become lost, people with dementia become lost for many reasons other than wandering. All people with dementia, whether they live alone, with an informal caregiver, or in an institution, should be considered capable of becoming lost (Rowe, 2003).

Another implication for practice is that successful searches must begin immediately (see Table 8-10). The best way to prevent death is to find those who are lost before they enter areas where it will be more difficult to find them, such as fields, junk yards, or unpopulated areas. Resources such as police departments and search-and-rescue teams should be employed as early as possible in the search. If the missing person has not been found in 6 to 12 hours, the search should be refocused on undeveloped areas or areas of thick vegetation near the place where the person was last seen (Rowe, 2003).

Doll Therapy

Many adults still love to cuddle their children and grandchildren's teddy bears or some other stuffed toy. Giving someone with AD a doll as therapy can make a lot of sense, especially if it makes them happy, less anxious, more occupied, and appears to be a creative way of caring. Since pets have been used to assist in reduction of anxiety and disruptive behaviors, a doll might also serve the same purpose when pets are not practicable. Doll therapy, which seems to have begun in the mid 1990's, is a way of using dolls to awaken memories or a previous role in life, especially if it assists in focusing for reminiscence and conversation.

TABLE 8-10: AD WANDERING AND GETTING LOST: A PLAN FOR SEARCHING

To prevent the person with dementia from becoming lost, a caregiver should:

1) Use all available resources to avoid leaving a person with dementia alone in the home.

2) Secure the home environment so that a person with dementia cannot leave alone while the caregiver is asleep or distracted.

3) Ensure that all outside doors are locked or, if the person with dementia can work the door lock, place a lock out of reach or change the type of lock used. People with dementia often cannot learn to work locks they have not seen before, because the disease prevents them from learning new information.

4) Consider using motion detectors on doors. Such devices sound a tone when motion is sensed, alerting the caregiver to potential danger.

5) Consider a home security system that would alert residents when someone is moving through the house or opening a door to the outside.

6) Register the person with dementia in the Safe Return Program of the Alzheimer's Association and keep contact information updated. Ensure that the person with dementia wears the Safe Return jewelry or clothing tags at all times.

7) Let neighbors know that a person with dementia lives in the neighborhood, and ask them to escort him home if they see him out alone.

8) Prepare a search plan in case the person with dementia becomes lost.

9) Keep copies of up-to-date photographs ready for distribution to searchers, police officers, hospitals, and media.

10) Do not rely on past behavior in predicting current behavior; becoming lost in the community is an unpredictable event.

When a person with dementia is discovered missing, a caregiver should:

1) Conduct a search immediately. A person with dementia is unlikely to find his way home independently; it is essential to find him while he is still in a populated area.

2) Call the local law enforcement agency and the Safe Return Program to report the missing person.

3) Enact the prepared search plan:

    a. Get help searching and assign a section of the neighborhood to each searcher.

    b. Ensure that someone remains at home in case the missing person returns or is found; the caregiver should be reachable by phone.

    c. Search all areas that might be accessible to the lost person, including front yards and backyards, public buildings, stores, streets, and highways.

    d. Begin the search in the area immediately surrounding the location where the person with dementia was last seen. Judgments about when to expand the area to be searched depend on the number of searchers available, the kind of terrain to be searched, and the physical capability of the missing person.

    e. If the person with dementia is not found within 6 to 12 hours (or sooner, if weather conditions are extremely hot, cold, or inclement), search wooded areas or fields near where the person was last seen. Areas of thick vegetation must be searched in an organized manner by as many searchers as are available, working very close to one another. People with dementia are unlikely to seek help or respond to calls and frequently try to hide from searchers; it is often necessary for searchers to come directly upon a lost person in order to find him in such an environment.

Note. From "People with Dementia Who Become Lost: Preventing Injuries and Death" by M.A. Rowe, 2003. *American Journal of Nursing, 103*(7), 32-39.

Because people with dementia have childlike behavior it can seem natural to believe that a doll is an appropriate means of establishing a rapport with them, providing comfort through cuddling or simply companionship (Bailey, Gilbert, & Herweyer, 1992).

This therapy may work better for women, as they have played with dolls as children and may have had the role of mother and held babies. Perhaps dolls may not work for men if they did not play with dolls as a child or were not fathers. But remember that there are no perfect treatments for people with AD. Try something new and if it works then you have a successful intervention.

A successful intervention in using doll therapy is demonstrated in its incorporation into an award-winning nursing home unit with reduction in wandering and reduced anxiety during hospitalizations and out-of-facility physician visits (Optima, 2000).

THE NEED-DRIVEN DEMENTIA-COMPROMISED BEHAVIOR MODEL

Another innovative framework, The Need-Driven Dementia-Compromised Behavior Model, looks at disruptive behaviors of demented people as "potentially understandable needs" (Kolanowski, 1999; Kolanowski & Whall, 2000). In this model, dementia-compromised behaviors, such as wandering and calling out, are viewed as reflective of quite stable background factors and somewhat changing proximal factors (see Table 8-11). The interaction of background and proximal issues produce the need-driven behaviors. This model focuses on interventions that respond to the underlying problems of the demented individual. The background factors are long-standing, less changeable, and often strengths of the individual, while the proximal factors are more easily manipulated to produce changes in behavior in a manner preferred by the individual. The implication is that all behavior has meaning and is driven by need (Colling & Buettner,

2002; Ebersole & Hess, 2001). More research is needed to identify how the model can enhance the quality of life for individuals with dementia.

SUMMARY

Managing the care of patients with AD and other dementias is an enormous challenge for health care providers. As much as 80% of all people who live in nursing homes behave in ways that cause problems for professional and family caregivers at some time. Effective coping with behavior problems requires that staff members be understanding, flexible, and creative and listen with the "third ear" — that intuitive listening that nurses do so well. Vollen (1996) offers a framework, using the mnemonic **TIME**, for dealing with disruptive behaviors:

Together: Work together and plan together to get the best results.

Investigate: Explore the causes of the behavior.

Measure: Quantify the occurrences of specific behaviors to picture behavioral patterns.

Empathize: Try to see the behavior from the point of view of the person with dementia.

A basic premise for dealing with these problems is that all behavior has meaning. Caregivers and nurses may not understand or recognize the meaning, but it is there.

The focus on caring for patients with AD and other dementias has often been on the tasks involved rather than on the patients. A number of therapeutic approaches can be used to deal with patients' behaviors. Behavioral problems encountered when caring for patients with AD and other dementias include wandering, resisting care, sleep disturbances, and catastrophic reactions.

The research discussed in this chapter tries to understand what this behavior means and how to deal with it. Nurses who think that behavior has meaning act differently toward patients than nurses who think things just happen. Therapeutic

TABLE 8-11: NEED-DRIVEN DEMENTIA-COMPROMISED BEHAVIOR MODEL

BACKGROUND FACTORS

Dementia-compromised functions
    Circadian rhythm
    Motor ability
    Memory
    Language

General health state
Demographic variables
    Gender
    Race and ethnicity
    Marital status
    Education
    Occupation

Psychosocial variables
    Personality
    Individual response to stress

PROXIMAL FACTORS

Physiological need state
    Hunger or thirst
    Elimination
    Pain
    Disturbance of sleep

Psychosocial need state
    Affect

Physical and social environment
    Light, sound, and heat level
    Staff mix and stability
    Ambience of environment
    Companionship or isolation

BEHAVIOR
Aggression
Wandering
Crying out

Note. From "An Overview of the Need-Driven Dementia-Compromised Behavior Model." by A.M. Kolanowski, 1999, *Journal of Gerontological Nursing, 25*(9), 7-9.

approaches give nurses a framework for dealing with the erratic behaviors of patients with dementia. Nurses can encourage behavioral changes by teaching and modeling methods of coping for staff and family caregivers. Continuing to learn and expand the repertoire of management strategies is essential in caring for patients with AD.

EXAM QUESTIONS

CHAPTER 8
Questions 71-80

71. Fatigue is a common trigger of problem behavior in patients with AD. A strategy for preventing fatigue is to

    a. offer caffeinated beverages.

    b. plan for periods of rest and quiet time.

    c. provide excess stimulation to keep them awake.

    d. ensure the activities are long so they have ample time to complete them.

72. During a crowded and loud holiday party, your patient with AD is starting to get agitated and becomes verbally inappropriate. The factor that may contribute to this behavior change is most likely due to

    a. illness.

    b. fatigue.

    c. stimuli.

    d. change.

73. The therapeutic approach used to orient a demented person to reality in the early stages of AD is

    a. reality orientation.

    b. validation therapy.

    c. life review.

    d. individualized care.

74. Patients with AD benefit most from reminiscence when they

    a. do not need to understand the guidelines.

    b. are not part of a group.

    c. have not lost their verbal ability.

    d. have not lost a good sense of humor.

75. People with AD often retain remote memories long after their short-term memory is gone. The process of thinking or telling about ones past experience to enrich ones life is known as

    a. reality orientation.

    b. self- care.

    c. reminiscence.

    d. validation therapy.

76. A nurse's first response to agitation in a person with AD should be to

    a. simply to dismiss changes in behavior as normal and move on.

    b. remain calm and reassuring to the person with AD and identify the trigger of the agitation.

    c. remove the person with AD from the present environment and restrain them immediately.

    d. administer an antianxiety medication to relieve agitation.

77. Catastrophic reactions are

    a. the result of becoming overwhelmed and overreacting.

    b. continuous emotional feelings of fear.

    c. a late indicator of a developing medical problem.

    d. always best resolved through chemical restraint.

78. Delusions and hallucinations are prominent signs of psychosis in people with AD. John is a patient who is hallucinating on your unit. An appropriate therapeutic approach to him is to

    a. say, "John, that is not a spider on the wall and you must go sit down."

    b. say, "John, I think you should go to a nice dark room to relax by yourself."

    c. say, "John, you seem upset. Why don't you join Jim in the sun room to listen to music."

    d. cover the mirror in John's room, turn down his lights, and restrain him so he doesn't harm himself.

79. Melinda is an 85-year-old lady with AD who seems to have lost her appetite, sits around ringing her hands, has a slower than normal gait, and may be sleeping less at night than usual. You believe she is depressed. Which nursing intervention should you attempt?

    a. Question the administration of an SSRI as ordered.

    b. Consult with the activities director to try to get Melinda involved in more social activities.

    c. Let Melinda rest and sleep during the day time because she is failing to sleep enough during the night.

    d. Administer a benzodiazepine as ordered.

80. The Need-Driven Dementia-Compromised Behavior Model's primary focal point is that

    a. not all behavior has meaning, so interventions cannot be designed to respond to the underlying problems of the demented individual.

    b. dysfunctional behavior may indicate a progressive lowering of the threshold for stress and thus interventions cannot be specific.

    c. behavior such as wandering causes the person with AD to want to change contributing factors such as sound, heat, or problems with memory or language.

    d. all behavior has meaning and interventions must address the underlying problems of the demented individual.

CHAPTER 9

PHARMACOLOGICAL TREATMENT

CHAPTER OBJECTIVE

After completing this chapter, the reader will be able to identify and implement the pharmacological principles that guide the care of older adults with Alzheimer's disease (AD).

LEARNING OBJECTIVES:

After studying this chapter, the reader will be able to

1. summarize the basic principles of pharmacology for older adults.

2. describe pharmacological, nonpharmacological, or combination treatments for AD and recognize when they may be indicated.

3. recognize drug classifications used for treatment of AD and their pharmacokinetic and pharmacodynamic properties.

4. recognize adverse effects of medications used for treating AD.

5. differentiate between drugs used to improve cognition and those used to treat behavioral problems.

6. recognize the indications and considerations for discontinuation of medications.

7. discuss the relevance of new research in medication regimes for people with AD.

INTRODUCTION

The management of AD includes pharmacological and nonpharmacological interventions. People with AD and their families should participate in the decision process for all therapies. They should have a clear understanding of the risks and benefits of any treatment, and treatments should be based on individual preferences.

Medications to reverse or cure AD have not been shown to be successful. However, medications can slow the progression of AD by addressing the chemical messengers of the nerve cells (neurotransmitters); cholinesterase inhibitors have shown to improve symptoms. Medications that are currently used to treat psychiatric conditions can successfully be used for secondary symptoms of AD. Other drugs may also be used in an attempt to alter the course of AD. These include ginkgo biloba, anti-inflammatory drugs, hormones, and many others.

Nurses must be competent in understanding the medications administered to patients. They must also be able to educate individuals and families about the intended use, adverse effects, and effectiveness evaluation of these medications.

PHARMACOLOGY AND OLDER ADULTS

Four out of five individuals over age 65 have at least one chronic disorder. This fact helps us understand why the older population consumes more drugs than any other age-group in the United States. Drug therapy can help prolong and improve the quality of elderly people's lives. Yet, there is an inherent danger in medication usage and the concurrent use of multiple drugs to manage multiple disorders.

Nurses are instrumental in managing the many tasks involved in care of older people, one of which may be medication administration. Another task may be assisting with activities of daily living. No matter the level of care you provide, you will expand your knowledge and enhance care of older individuals by understanding how drugs work, adverse reactions to medications commonly used by older persons, costs issues related to medication usage, and how to enhance individual compliance with medications (Chisholm & DiPiro, 2002).

Demographics of Medication Usage in Older Adults

- 50% of older adults consume multiple drugs. Polypharmacy is defined as the use of more than one agent to affect a therapeutic endpoint.

- Older adults consume 25% to 30% of all prescription medications and 40% of all nonprescription medications.

- Older adults comprise 12% of the U.S. population, yet they receive 32% of all prescriptions dispensed.

- Older adults spend an estimated $3 billion annually on medications.

- Ambulatory older adults use two to four prescription drugs regularly.

- Long-term care residents use two to ten prescription drugs regularly.

- Misuse of drugs is the fifth leading cause of death in elderly persons.

(Allen, 2003; Alzheimer's Organization, 2004)

UNDERSTANDING THE NURSE'S ROLE

Remember that *you* are the patient's last line of defense against errors. The nurse's role in medication administration include:

- *Preadministration assessment:* Collect baseline data for future comparisons.

- *Dosage and administration:* Deliver the correct dose and administer it safely.

- *Evaluate the drug response:* Observe the patient's reaction. Did the drug do what it was supposed to do, or did it have a negative impact on the patient?

- *Minimize adverse effects:* When do adverse effects occur? What are early signs? What actions are needed for those adverse effects?

- *Minimize interactions:* What other medications and substances are being used?

- *Make as-needed decisions:* Does the patient need acetaminophen versus a narcotic?

- *Manage toxicity:* Assess for physical and mental signs and symptoms that indicate medication toxicity.

(Allen, 2003; Lehne, 2004)

Nursing Management of Drug Therapy

When managing drugs for any patient, you need to have a core knowledge.

- Drug knowledge
  - Pharmacotherapeutics: Why the drug is prescribed
  - Pharmacokinetics: What the body does with the drug
  - Pharmacodynamics: What the drug does with the body
  - Contraindications: Reasons for not administering a particular drug
  - Precautions: Closely monitoring drug therapy
  - Adverse effects: The unwanted effects of drugs

– Drug interactions: What effects may occur when drugs are administered with other drugs, foods, or other substances

• Patient variables
   – Current or past illness
   – Gender
   – Age
   – Diet
   – Health habits

It is also important to understand the basics of drug properties:

• Effectiveness: The drug should elicit the response for which it was administered.

• Safety: The drug should not produce harmful effects even if given at high doses and for a long period.

• Selectivity: The drug should elicit only the response for which it is given. Other responses are called adverse effects or side effects.

• Reversibility: Certain drug actions should be reversible — for example, general anesthesia and birth control pills.

• Predictability: The patients response to the drug should be somewhat predictable. Remember, however, that everyone is an individual and not everyone will respond to a drug in the same way. Drug therapy must be tailored to the individual.

• Ease of administration: Drugs need to be easily administered.

The goal of drug therapy is to provide the maximum benefit with minimum harm (the effects should do more good than harm).

The usual benefit of using a drug is the drug's therapeutic effect. Defining benefits more broadly can include what the patient or the patient's family sees as the benefit of a particular medication. The discussion of benefits should include a look at all drugs being taken, including over-the-counter and social drugs, such as alcohol and nicotine. For example, benefits from the use of psychoactive drugs can include increased appetite, weight gain, decreased agitation, increased function, and increased ability to socialize.

CLINICAL PHARMACOLOGY AND GERIATRIC CONSIDERATIONS

Pharmacokinetic Changes

Absorption

Physiologic changes that occur with age, such as changes in gastrointestinal (GI) motility and pH changes, can alter drug absorption. However, there has been little evidence to suggest that this has major consequences. Reduced absorption in the elderly has been observed for some compounds that are actively absorbed (such as galactose, calcium, thiamine, and iron). The absorption of most drugs by passive processes generally is not affected.

Distribution

Major changes in body composition occur as people age. Body fat increases from 15% to 30% and lean body weight decreases in proportion to total body weight .

Although total plasma protein concentrations remain relatively constant, albumin concentrations are lower in the aged. Drug interactions based on protein binding, and other factors, can be more pronounced in the elderly because these patients tend to be taking more drugs.

Cardiac output is also reduced in the elderly, thus drug distribution to the kidneys and liver are reduced. This can alter the overall elimination of some drugs.

Metabolism

The liver is the main organ involved in metabolism. Liver blood flow and liver mass tend to decrease with age. Protein binding is also reduced, especially to albumin. For some drugs that undergo metabolism (oxidation and reduction), metabolism decreases with increasing age. Examples are lidocaine, phenytoin, propranolol, and theophylline. For drugs that undergo metabolism through conjugation, metabolism does not change greatly with age. Some example drugs are isoniazid and temazepam.

Elimination

With increasing age, glomerular filtration rate deceases due to a reduction in kidney size (20%), reduction in the number of nephrons (35%), reduction in the number of functioning glomeruli (30%), and a decrease in renal blood flow (40% to 50%). Serum creatinine also decreases with age because of reduced muscle mass. Creatinine clearance, as a function of age, should be computed in order to make dosage regimen adjustments. Drugs that are excreted renally, and therefore require dosage adjustments in elderly patients, include aminoglycosides, digoxin, lithium, methotrexate, quinidine, and tetracyclines (except doxycycline).

Dosing Recommendations

The effects of age on drug disposition depend on the particular compound in question and the characteristics of the population. When evaluating geriatric studies, it is important to distinguish between long-term care patients who are not considered to be healthy and the active elderly (age > 65 years) living in the community. Some changes attributed to the elderly may be due to immobility or underlying diseases. Furthermore, because of differences in body composition between males and females, it is often important to distinguish between these groups (Allen, 2003; Lehne, 2004).

CASE STUDY

Sarah Miller, a 67-year-old woman, has been brought to her physician's office by her husband because she has begun to get lost in familiar surroundings and is currently fearful of going out alone because she feels she will not find her way home. After further questioning, her physician, determines that she has experienced a slow decline in short-term memory over the past 18 to 24 months. Sarah's father and his brother both had AD.

The physician conducts a Mini-Mental Status Exam (MMSE), on which Sarah scores a 23. He also administers the Clock Face Test, and Sarah cannot draw a clock set for 10:20. The physician decides to begin Sarah on a low-dose cholinesterase inhibitor (CEI). He asks to see her again in 2 weeks for follow-up. At that time, Sarah is tolerating the medication. At a 6-week visit, Sarah exhibits no change in her test performances, so her physician increases the drug dosage and has Sarah return in 1 month. At this follow-up visit, Sarah still scores 23 on the MMSE but can correctly draw the clock face. Her next visit is scheduled for 1 month later.

At her next visit, Sarah's MMSE has increased to 26 and her husband reports that she is less fearful and seems to have more energy. Her next appointment is set for 6 months later. At this time, Sarah is maintaining a 26 on her MMSE, she is reading novels again, and she has begun to participate in volunteer activities. She does not venture out unaccompanied because she is still somewhat fearful of getting lost.

Sarah's physician continues to see her every 6 weeks for medication surveillance. After a total of 18 months of treatment with a CEI, Sarah's MMSE score is 23, she is reading less, and she has stopped her volunteer work but still tries to complete her normal household tasks and work on different word puzzles. Her energy level seems to be diminishing slightly. Her medication regime is maintained for another 20 months. At this time, Sarah seems to no longer benefit from the medication, so it is gradually withdrawn.

PHARMACOLOGICAL TREATMENT OPTIONS

Treatment options and a wide variety of clinical trials focus on three main aspects of AD:

1) improving memory and enhancing cognition

2) delaying the onset or slowing the progression of AD

3) treatment of medical and behavioral symptoms.

Pharmacological treatments for improving memory, enhancing cognition, and delaying the onset or slowing the progression of AD include many different preparations, some of which are approved by the U.S. Food and Drug Administration (FDA) and others that have not demonstrated efficacy or safety in drug trials. These latter preparations are still used in treatment by physicians and family members. These include cholinesterase inhibitors (CEIs), antioxidants, monoamine oxidase inhibitors (MAOIs), nonsteroidal anti-inflammatory drugs (NSAIDs), gingko biloba, metrifonate (ProMed), hormones, antiglutamatergic therapy, acetyl-L-carnitine HCL (ACL) (Alcar).

Cholinesterase Inhibitors

Pharmacological treatments for AD are limited to approximately four prescription drugs approved by the FDA (at the time of this printing). The classification of medications to delay the progression of the disease are known as CEIs. They include donepezil (Aricept), rivastigmine (Exelon), galantamine (Reminyl), and tacrine hydrochloride (Cognex). CEIs inhibit acetylcholinesterase (AChE) and butyrylcholinesterase (BuChE).

Acetylcholinesterase breaks down acetylcholine; people with AD have decreased levels of acetylcholine in the brain. The physiological role of butyrylcholinesterase is unknown, but levels of this enzyme have been shown to increase as AD progresses, whereas acetylcholinesterase decreases. Both of these enzymes are found in neuritic plaques, and their inhibition by CEIs may modify the deposition of beta-amyloid, which has been found to be a key component of the pathology of AD (see chapter 2) (Gauthier, 2002).

Acetylcholine is important to the brain cells that control memory, thought, and judgment. For people with mild to moderate AD, these medications have produced modest improvements in memory, as evidenced by performance on tests (such as the MMSE), when compared with a placebo. CEIs have the potential to delay the memory loss progress of the disease by 1 year or longer (Clark & Karlawish, 2003; Kawas, 2003; Long & Dougherty, 2003).

Donepezil has been studied in multiple controlled trials (Rogers & Friedhoff, 1996; Rogers, Doody, Mohs, & Friedhoff, 1998; Feldman, Gauthier, Hecker, Vellas, Subbiah, & Whalen, 2001; Lehne, 2004). One such study on donezepil indicates that it is the most effective, simplest to use, and the best tolerated of all CEIs (Jones, 2003).

Tacrine and donepezil are classified as short-acting, or reversible, agents because they are hydrolyzed within minutes of binding to acetylcholinesterase (AChE). Rivastigmine is classified as an intermediate-acting or pseudoirreversible agent due to its long inhibition on AChE of up to 10 hours. Galantamine is also classified as an AChE inhibitor. It appears to act on nicotine receptors in the brain. Both acetylcholine and nicotine receptors have been suggested as areas related to cognitive impairment (Hines, 2001).

Mechanism of Action

These drugs do not slow the disease process which involves senile plaques and neurofibrillary tangles; rather they attempt to increase the available amount of acetylcholine by blocking the enzyme AChE, which breaks down acetylcholine. By inhibiting AChE, these drugs make more acetylcholine available at cholinergic synapses. For AD patients, this can mean increased transmission by cholinergic neurons that have not been destroyed by AD.

Therapeutic Effect:

These drugs have a low percentage, probably less than 30%, of patient response. The response is very modest and is only short term for mild to moderate AD. Remember, however, that AD is irreversible and so any increase in function that can be gained for these patients is very helpful. An unexpected benefit of some CEIs is their ability to reduce some of the neuropsycological symptoms associated with AD, such as apathy and visual hallucinations (Clark & Karlawish, 2003; Lehne, 2004).

Pharmacokinetics

- Tacrine (Cognex): administered orally; if administered with food, absorption is decreased. First pass effect impacts bioavailability. Peak is 2 hours and half-life is 3 hours. It crosses the blood-brain barrier and is retained in the central nervous system (CNS) (Lehne, 2004).

- Donepezil (Aricept): basically the same as tacrine (Lehne, 2004).

- Galantamine (Reminyl): rapidly absorbed from the GI tract with peak concentration occurring in about 1 hour; absorption is not affected by food; half-life is 7 hours; protein binding is 18%; metabolized in the liver; excreted in the urine; plasma concentration increases in patients with moderate to severe liver impairment (Scott & Goa, 2000; Janssen, 2003).

- Rivastigmine (Exelon): is rapidly absorbed with bioavailability of about 40%. Drug half-life is about 1.5 hours; excreted in the urine. Peak plasma concentrations occur approximately 1 hour after administration. Administration with food delays absorption by 90 minutes. Rivastigmine penetrates the blood-brain barrier, reaching peak cerebrospinal fluid concentrations in 1.4 to 2.6 hours. Rivastigmine is about 40% bound to plasma proteins (Novartis, 2003).

Adverse Effects

The adverse effects of CEIs are directly related to the rate of dose increase. When starting individuals on these medications, dose intervals should be gradually increased until the optimal therapeutic dosage has been reached. The interval between dose increases may be extended or the dose step size may be reduced accordingly if adverse effects occur. Adverse effects can be worrisome and lead to discontinuation of the medication. "Treatment with CEIs results in a modest but significant therapeutic effect and modestly but significantly higher rates of adverse events and discontinuation of treatment" (Lanctot et al., 2003, p. 557).

- The major adverse effect of tacrine (Cognex) is liver toxicity. Other side effects include nausea and vomiting, diarrhea, dyspepsia, and ataxia. Levels of alanine aminotranferase (ALT) must be monitored approximately every other week. These levels are usually elevated in those taking more than three times the normal level of tacrine. When these levels are reached, the medication dosage must be reduced or the medication stopped. Upon discontinuation of the drug, liver damage is reversed. Watch for clinical jaundice (bilirubin of 3 mg/ml) or signs and symptoms of hypersensitivity (such as a rash and fever) in association with elevated ALT. If seen, the drug must be discontinued.

- Donepezil (Aricept) side effects include nausea and vomiting and bradycardia.

- Galantamine (Reminyl) side effects include nausea and vomiting, diarrhea, and anorexia.

- Rivastigmine (Exelon) side effects include nausea and vomiting, diarrhea, and anorexia.

Drug Interactions

- Tacrine, donepezil, rivastigmine, and galantamine have different pharmacological properties that can potentially increase patient risks for several different types of drug interactions:

- Tacrine can interact with drugs metabolized by the cytochrome P450 (CYP)1 A2 enzyme, as well as interact with donepezil and antipsychotics. These last interactions produce parkinsonian symptoms.

- Bioavailability of galantamine is increased by coadministration with paroxetine, ketoconazole, and erythromycin.

- Rivastigmine is metabolized by esterases other than the CYP enzymes; it is unlikely to be involved in pharmacokinetic drug-drug interactions.

- CEIs can introduce central or peripheral hypercholinergic effects through drug interactions with antipsychotics or antiarrhythmics.

  • Central effects: excitation or agitation

  • Peripheral effects: bradycardia, loss of consciousness, digestive disorders.

(Bentue-Ferrer, Tribut, Polard, & Allain, 2003; Clark & Karlawish, 2003; Long & Dougherty, 2003; Mohs et al., 2001).

CEIs Notes

Tacrine, donepezil, galantamine, and rivastigmine have no effect on senile plaques or neurofibrillary tangles. Their effects include:

• delay progression of disease symptoms by exerting a modest, temporary effect on cognition

• influence attention, concentration, mental acuity, and speed of information processing

• "after effectiveness" (the rate of decline continues at the rate prior to administration; discontinuation may lead to regression).

Treatment with CEIs should be started at the time of diagnosis of AD. Treatment must never be delayed. Delays reduce the maximum possible response to CEIs; do not wait thinking that CEIs will be more effective on more severe deterioration. People with AD should be expected to be treated with CEIs for 3 to 5 years, or until the therapeutic benefit is not effective for the deficits of AD.

When it has been determined that the drugs are of no further benefit to the individual, they should be discontinued, but *do not withdraw these drugs all at once.* They should be tapered off by reducing the dose by approximately 50% every 2 weeks. Individuals should be closely monitored as the drugs are discontinued. If deterioration of cognitive status, behavior, or function occurs, the optimal dosage of the drug should be reinstated because these changes suggest that the individual is still deriving benefit from the treatment.

People with AD who stop taking CEIs do not derive any additional benefit if they resume taking them at a future time. In fact, they may not regain the full initial benefit of the drugs.

The costs of treatment of AD can be high, especially with the cost of acquiring medications such as CEIs. One is left to wonder about the long-term cost effectiveness of such treatments. People with AD who suffer from more severe effects of the disease realize higher total costs of care. Those with less severe disease are cared for by informal caregivers and their formal costs are much less. People with AD who take and tolerate CEIs are able to be cared for by informal caregivers (family) for longer periods, thus reducing the formal costs of AD. It seems reasonable to assume that savings in formal care can offset the increased drug costs incurred by the use of CEIs. Although some studies support this notion, it may be too early to affirm. Long-term studies to demonstrate this benefit are still underway (Jonsson, 2003; Kawas, 2003; Neumann et al., 1999)

Nonsteroidal Anti-Inflammatory Drugs

Although controversial, some evidence suggests a connection between inflammation and AD, indicating that regular use of nonaspirin NSAIDs may reduce the risk of AD; the longer the use, the lower the risk. "In a study of elderly twins, the risk of AD was 10 times lower in the twin who used NSAIDs" (Lehne, 2004). Aspirin and acetaminophen do not seem to protect against AD. Some of the drugs suggested that do provide benefit include nonspecific cyclo-oxygenase (COX) inhibitors (such as indomethacin). The adverse GI effects can be significant, however, thus reducing the adherence to the drug regime (Clark & Karlawish, 2003; Lehne, 2004). Two herbs, flaxseed and evening primrose, may also have a role in preventing or treating AD because they exhibit anti-inflammatory properties (Miller, 2001).

Other trials using COX-2 inhibitors have been disappointing. Dr. Paul Aisen of Georgetown University Medical Center conducted a study that compared three treatments: Vioxx, the recently recalled anti-inflammatory drug formerly made by Merck & Co., which is generically known as rofecoxib; naproxen, an over-the-counter medication sold under several trade names, including Aleve; and a placebo. The two drugs showed no better results than the placebo (Clark & Karlawish, 2003; Lehne, 2004; Rubin & Rubin, n.d.).

The National Institute on Aging (NIA) also conducted a recent study of anti-inflammatory drugs. The results of the study failed to show that these drugs slowed the progression of AD. The National Institutes of Health are also conducting a 7-year study to determine if NSAIDs can help prevent AD (Rubin & Rubin, n.d.). Despite these failures, the promise of anti-inflammatory drugs leaves much research to be conducted on this topic.

Antioxidants

Some researchers hypothesize that the pathogenesis of AD is due to oxidative injury. The inflammatory response results in production of free radicals that injure the brain. Since 1997, vitamin E (alpha-tocopherol) and selegiline (Eldepryl) (a selective MAOI) have been suggested to be beneficial for patients with moderately severe AD by delaying institutionalization and losses in ADLs (Kawas, 2003; Lehne, 2004). However, even when combined, these drugs do not improve or retard

cognitive decline, the hallmark of AD, thus leaving researchers questioning their true efficacy.

Here is how antioxidants are believed to work for AD:

1) Vitamin E
   a. Prevents cell damage by scavenging free radicals in cell membranes
   b. Preferred over selegiline
   c. Only high-doses have shown any effect on progression of AD

2) MAOI-B blockers such as selegiline increase the brain levels of certain neurotransmitters and have the potential to lead to cognitive improvement

3) Vitamin C
   a. New information released in the media (CNN, 2004) has indicated that research shows decreased risk of AD when vitamin C and vitamin E are taken together prior to AD onset (see Table 9-1). As of this publication, no research is available to support these claims.

Hormones

AD is more common in women than in men by a ratio of two-to-one. This implies an association between gonadal hormone levels and AD. Serum concentrations of gonadotropins, luteinizing hormone, and follicle-stimulating hormone are sensitive to changes in estrogen; gonadotropins are the primary regulators of estrogen production. In postmenopausal women, estrogen loss increases gonadotropin circulation. In women taking estrogen replacement therapy (ERT), the concentration in circulation falls due to estrogen's suppressive influence on the hypothalamic-pituitary-gonadal axis. Thus, the effects of ERT may be due more to hormones other than estrogen. In the early postmenopausal period, gonadotropins are highly elevated, but they fall over ensuing years. ERT might be more beneficial during this period of high

TABLE 9-1: REDUCED RISK OF AD IN USERS OF ANTIOXIDANT VITAMIN SUPPLEMENTS

The Cache County Study

Background: Antioxidants may protect the aging brain against oxidative damage associated with pathological changes of AD.

Objective: To examine the relationship between antioxidant supplement use and risk of AD.

Design: Cross-sectional and prospective study of dementia. Elderly (65 years or older) county residents were assessed from 1995 to 1997 for prevalent dementia and AD, and again from 1998 to 2000 for incident illness. Supplement use was ascertained at the first contact.

Setting: Cache County, Utah.

Participants: Among 4,740 respondents (93%) with data sufficient to determine cognitive status at the initial assessment, researchers identified 200 prevalent cases of AD. Among 3,227 survivors at risk, researchers identified 104 incident AD cases at follow-up.

Main Outcome Measure: Diagnosis of AD by means of multistage assessment procedures.

Results: Analyses of prevalent and incident AD yielded similar results. Use of vitamins E and C (ascorbic acid) supplements in combination was associated with reduced AD prevalence (adjusted odds ratio, 0.22; 95% confidence interval, 0.05-0.60) and incidence (adjusted hazard ratio, 0.36; 95% confidence interval, 0.09-0.99). A trend toward lower AD risk was also evident in users of vitamin E and multivitamins containing vitamin C, but researchers saw no evidence of a protective effect with use of vitamin E or vitamin C supplements alone, with multivitamins alone, or with vitamin B-complex supplements.

Conclusions: Use of vitamin E and vitamin C supplements in combination is associated with reduced prevalence and incidence of AD. Antioxidant supplements merit further study as agents for the primary prevention of AD.

Note. From P.P. Zandi, et al., Cache County Study Group, 2004. *Archives of Neurology, 61*(1), 82-88. Reprinted with permission from the American Medical Association.

levels of gonadotropins (Smith, Perry, Atwood, & Bowen, 2003).

Estrogen plays a role in some brain regions involved in learning and memory and in the protection and regulation of cholinergic neurons. The increased incidence of AD in women has not been observed in women who have a history of ERT replacement of more than 10 years. This suggests that ERT is ineffective during the latent preclinical stage of AD, which can be as much as a decade or more before the onset of diagnosable dementia (Resnick & Henderson, 2002).

A decline in estrogen occurs after menopause. Low estrogen levels may be linked to cognitive function regression associated with AD. Previously, some argued that ERT had beneficial effects on memory and learning in postmenopausal women, and that estrogen protected the brain against neurotoxic

events through cholinergic regulation. The benefits of estrogen on the health of elderly women have been a controversial subject for many years, but interest in its effects on health outcomes may have never been higher. It had been suggested that estrogen enhances cholinergic activity by improving memory and cognition in women, thus reducing the risk of AD (Fillit, 2002; Resnick & Henderson, 2002; Smith & Levin-Allerhand, 2003; Waring, Rocca, Petersen, O'Brien, Tangalos, & Kokmen, 1999).

Because of controversy over the use and benefits of ERT, it is helpful to review the basics of these studies. Several cohort studies have addressed the association between ERT in postmenopausal women and AD. Research suggested that postmenopausal women who used ERT had a reduced risk of AD; other studies have not confirmed this (Waring et al., 1999). Some studies differentiate between women's risk of acquiring AD based on length of medicating with estrogen prior to diagnosis of AD (Breitner & Zandi, 2003). Other studies report reduced mortality among women with AD who were on long-term ERT (Lehne, 2004; Waring et al., 1999).

Current evidence does not support the use of estrogen in the treatment of AD patients. The Women's Health Initiative (WHI) randomized clinical trial of postmenopausal hormone therapy terminated the combined estrogen-progestin portion (but not the estrogen-only portion) of the trial early, after only 5 of the planned 8.5 year trial duration (Shumaker, Legault, Rapp, Thal, Wallace, Ockene et al., 2003). "Women who received estrogen plus progestin experienced a small but significant increase in the primary outcome, coronary heart disease; a nonsignificant trend toward an increase in the primary adverse outcome, invasive breast cancer; an significant increase in a global index (which included stroke, pulmonary embolism, endometrial cancer, colorectal cancer, hip fracture, and death due to other causes) summarizing risk and benefit... the WHI did focus on risk of dementia and cognitive decline, but these outcomes are not considered in the WHI risk-benefit profile" (Resnick & Henderson, 2002, p. 2170).

A recent study of the effects of estrogen-progestin treatment in women over age 65 found deleterious effects, meaning an increased incidence of dementia occurred. It is believed that the combined hormones may have been responsible for this increase, but the researchers did not rule out the late age at which therapy was begun (Breitner & Zandi, 2003).

The most recent research indicates that not only does ERT have no significant effect on the clinical course of AD in elderly women, but a higher frequency of breast cancer occurs in women taking ERT. Furthermore, dementia increased with combined estrogen-progestin therapy. This may, however, suggest that ERT may be beneficial as a primary, rather than secondary, means of preventing AD.

Hormone use involving estrogen unopposed by a progestin may offer the greatest potential for neuroprotection (Fillit, 2002; Resnick & Henderson, 2002). However, ERT should not be started in old age in the hopes of preventing or treating AD (Breitner & Zandi, 2003).

Antiglutamate Therapy

Antiglutamate drugs were identified in Europe in the 1990s as useful in the treatment of AD because they may limit the neuronal damage that can occur as a result of excessive glutamate stimulation. Glutamate, an amino acid, is the predominant excitatory neurotransmitter in the brain. Lundbeck, a Danish pharmaceutical company, and the German pharmaceutical company Merz, indicated their clinical studies of the drug memantine (Namenda) does slow the progression of AD. It has been marketed in Germany since 1989 for treatment of moderate to severe AD "dementia syndrome." An improvement in functional independence and a reduction in the required level of care in advanced AD was found. The FDA's Peripheral and Central Nervous System Drugs Advisory in September, 2003 unanimously agreed that memantine is effective and safe for the treatment of moderate to severe Alzheimer's Disease.

Memantine's mechanism of action is different from that of the cholinesterase inhibitors currently available for treating AD. Glutamate binding stimulates the N-methyl-D-aspartate (NMDA) receptor, and long-term overstimulation has been linked to neurological disease. Memantine is an NMDA receptor antagonist which prevents the binding of glutamate. It has been approved for treatment of moderate to severe AD, and is being evaluated for use against additional forms of dementia. Adverse effects associated with memantine include both cardiovascular events (hypertension, heart failure and fainting) and CNS effects (dizziness, confusion and headache). The drug should be used with caution in patients with seizure disorders, or liver or kidney impairment.

In a recent study, memantine was combined with Aricept, the most commonly prescribed AD drug in the United States. Individuals who took the drug combination experienced a sustained improvement in cognition and ADLs. Keep in mind that neither of these drugs have cured, halted, or reversed the process of cell damage that eventually leads to AD (Rubin & Rubin, n.d.). The impact is that patients enter long-term care facilities later in the disease process, thus reducing overall costs (Winblad & Jelic, 2003).

Cholesterol-Lowering Drugs

Researchers have wondered if cholesterol-lowering drugs might help prevent or treat AD. Two retrospective studies indicated there was a 60% to 73% lower risk of AD in patients who had been taking statin drugs as compared to those with untreated hyperlipidemia. Atorvastatin is currently under investigation and is in phase II clinical trials (Dougherty & Long , 2003).

ACL (Alcar)

ACL is similar to CEIs and may, therefore, interact with cholinergic receptors. It may also undergo conversion to acetylcholine in the CNS, thereby increasing acetylcholine levels. The manufacturer of the drug believes that it may provide a protective effect against neuritic tangles and, therefore, improve communication between cells. In clinical trials, the drug has improved cognition in those with AD. It also has the potential to slow the progression of the disease (Lehne, 2004; Rubin & Rubin, n.d.).

Other Treatments

One of the most interesting advances in the search for treatment of and a cure for AD has been in the field of immunization. In July of 1999, the Cable News Network posted a story about an experimental vaccine that showed promise in reducing brain deposits linked to AD in mice. The vaccine was designed to attack the plaques deposited in the brains of people with AD. Scientists think of the plaques as foreign invaders in the body, similar to viruses and bacteria (Cable News Network, 1999).

In one experiment, conducted by Elan Pharmaceuticals, mice that were genetically engineered to acquire AD were later vaccinated with active and passive A beta serum against it and, 13 months later, showed no signs of the disease. In subsequent experiments to help determine the effectiveness of the vaccine on mice already showing signs of AD, the mice showed no signs of improvement after 7 months of treatment. In phase I of the clinical trial, which has already taken place, humans were vaccinated with A beta immunization. No adverse effects were reported in phase I. Approximately 5% of the patients in phase II developed meningoencephalitis, ending the trial in March 2002. These adverse effects will be further studied and may assist in developing newer and safer vaccines for use in future human trials (Lemere, Spooner, Leverone, et al, 2003; Cable News Network, 1999).

Although the AD found in mice only partially resembles the AD of humans, research in this area could yield important information. The research also poses questions about who should receive vaccinations and when. This may require developing better ways for determining who is at risk for the disease (Cable News Network, 1999).

Alternative Medical Treatments

Ginkgo Biloba

Ginkgo biloba is a popular Chinese herb or dietary supplement that is derived from maidenhair tree leaves. This herb is used widely in countries outside the United States to prevent and treat AD (Miller, 2001). Studies on the use of ginkgo biloba are limited and have used small sample sizes. In most studies, the benefits demonstrated have been about the same as those for tacrine. Although ginkgo biloba may enhance cognitive function, dietary supplements are not regulated and the purity and potency of the preparations can vary from manufacturer to manufacturer and pill to pill (Kawas, 2003: Lehne, 2004).

Ginkgo preparations exhibit antioxidant, antiplatelet, and anti-inflammatory actions, which have been linked to such adverse reactions as bleeding. Therefore, drug-to-drug interactions run high with such medications as antiplatelet drugs (aspirin) and anticoagulants (such as warfarin [Coumadin]), and these combinations must be used cautiously (Kawas, 2003; Lehne, 2004).

Huperzine A

In Chinese medicine, an extract from moss has been shown to have similar properties to a number of FDA-approved drugs, such as acetylcholinesterace inhibitors, in the United States. One of these is huperzine A, an unregulated dietary supplement. Studies that have been conducted question the use due to unregulated dosing and administration. (Long & Dougherty, 2003; Mahi, 1999; Pepping, 2000).

Melatonin

Melatonin is a naturally occurring hormone that is used as an over-the-counter medication to treat insomnia (regulation of sleep-wake cycles). Researchers have indicated that this may be a helpful antioxidant that can reduce lipid levels. Melatonin levels decrease in older adults, and this drug has been suggested to assist in circadian rhythms. No current clinical trials are underway (Long & Dougherty, 2003).

The future of AD therapy seems to be focused on several testable hypotheses, which are listed in Table 9-2.

Remember from Chapter 2 that mild cognitive impairment (MCI) can carry with it a risk of conversion to AD, possibly at a rate of 12% to 15% a year. Recent studies look at giving individuals with MCI a CEI, vitamin E, or COX-2 inhibitors for 3 years. These agents may protect or slow the progression of AD. When this type of information is released in the media, people flock to their physi-

TABLE 9-2: POTENTIAL THERAPIES BASED ON HYPOTHESES

Potential Therapy	Hypothesis	Mechanism of Action
1. Gamma-secretase inhibitors	Excessive deposition of beta-amyloid fibrils	1. Increased amyloid metabolism by alpha-secretase and shift to nontoxic pathway
2. Immunotherapy (amyloid vaccine)		2. Breakdown of amyloid-containing plaques by antibodies to beta-amyloid
3. Cholinesterase inhibitors		3. Inhibition of acetylcholinesterase and butyrylcholinesterase in neuritic plaque
4. Alzhemed		4. Prevention of fibrillinogenesis plaque formation
NSAIDs	Excessive brain inflammation	Suppression of microglial and complement activation
1. Statins	Insufficient brain plasticity due to mutation of apolipoprotein E	1. Induction of apolipoprotein E to compensate for lower cholesterol levels
2. Neotrophin		2. Enhanced activity of nerve growth factor
Vitamin E	Premature cell death	Antioxidant protection
Calcium channel blockers	Systolic hypertension in middle age, causing leuko-araiosis and stroke	Control of blood pressure

(Gauthier, 2002)

cian's office seeking the "new" medication. Problems arise, however, because there are no guidelines in place for such treatment. In 2003, the Consortium of Canadian Centers for Clinical Cognitive Research held a research conference on MCI to formulate such guidelines. The United States should not be far behind (Gauthier, 2002).

Miscellaneous Agents

Additional drugs for AD include those that are used in treatment of behavioral problems, such as antipsychotics, antidepressants, anticonvulsants, and other psychotropic medications.

Research is now taking place on the use of nerve growth factor (NGF) to prevent cholinergic neuron atrophy and improve functional capacity. The Ciba Foundation held a symposium in 1996 on NGF to explore the use of this drug for neurological and sensory disorders. They reported that when nerve growth factor was used "...the results were that the postsynaptic cholinergic system was almost completely spared from degeneration" (CIBA Foundation Symposium, April 1996). These results suggest that NGF may play a role during central cholinergic development.

Gangliosides have also been shown to slow the progress of AD by exerting an effect on the synthesis of membrane phospholipids.

Nootropic drugs exert a regulatory effect on neuronal metabolism and influence synaptic plasticity and learning behavior. Preliminary data from a worldwide study indicate that these drugs show promise in providing symptomatic relief for patients in early to intermediate stages of AD. These drugs are not metabolized or eliminated by the liver, which holds promise for those with liver disease.

Hundreds of drugs are currently undergoing trials in the United States and Europe. It is interesting to follow the clinical trials to see where researchers are focusing their energies in the treatment regarding AD.

Listed here are several sites where you can review such development.

- Clinical Trial Web Sites
  www.clinicaltrials.gov

- AD Clinical Trials Database, a joint project of the FDS and NIA. Provides directories of clinical trials by state, with detailed information on experimental drugs.
  www.alzheimers.org/trials/

- Center Watch Clinical Trials Listing Service
  www.therubins.com

- Alzheimer's Association
  www.alz.org

- National Institutes of Health
  www.nih.gov

TREATMENT OF SECONDARY SYMPTOMS OF AD

Remember that practically all people with AD have symptoms other than cognitive losses. These symptoms may include depression, paranoia, delusions, hallucinations, agitation, aggression, and wandering (see chapter 8 for further discussion of these behaviors). These behaviors can require medication in order to improve quality of life for individuals with AD and their family members and caregivers.

At the same time, nurses must keep in mind that the response to pharmacological treatment of secondary symptoms of AD is never predictable, and choosing a dose and duration of treatment can come down to clinical judgment of the prescriber. Behavior-controlling medications must be used cautiously and used for specific clinical symptoms. The old adage of prescribing medication for older adults, especially those with dementia, is so true: **start low and go slow!!!**

Antipsychotic Medications

Psychotropic medications have been shown to be effective in the treatment of secondary symptoms of AD. Caution is always required, however, because demented patients are particularly susceptible to adverse effects of these medications. Antipsychotics are not appropriate for the treatment of wandering, restlessness, or dementia. They are useful for the treatment of behaviors caused by psychosis-related conditions, those that become a threat to the patient and a danger to others, including staff members, or interfere with the staff's ability to care for the patient. In these instances, behaviors must be documented and quantified. The American Society of Consultant Pharmacists has made the following recommendations for the appropriate use of antipsychotics in long-term care settings (Wachter, 1996):

1) Use one-time-only dosing of antipsychotics for acute situations and avoid as-needed orders.

2) Set specific criteria for periodic reevaluation of the need for antipsychotic medication. Titrate the dose down to the minimum dose and use only for the shortest time span.

3) Encourage the patient's family and others affected by the patient's behavior to become more informed and to improve their communication and knowledge.

Through education and clinical practice, nurses are equipped to detect and assess changes in physical and mental functioning. Knowledge of the risks versus the benefits of psychoactive drugs and of pharmacokinetic changes can enable nurses to recognize actual and potential problems and intervene quickly and effectively. The reality is that other forms of management for behavioral problems should be tried before any physical or chemical restraints are considered.

All drug therapies have an adverse side. Side effects, toxic effects, idiosyncratic reactions, and allergies are some of the risks to consider. Because elderly patients have higher fat-to-lean ratios, lower concentrations of serum albumin, less total body water, and slower liver metabolism and renal clearance, they need far lower doses of drugs than do younger people. Antipsychotic drugs are stored in fat, so both therapeutic and adverse effects last much longer. Another rationale for using smaller doses of antipsychotics is that lower concentrations of albumin mean that less of the drug is protein-bound, meaning more drug is free to circulate (Lehne, 2004). Most elderly patients need only one-tenth to one-third of the usual adult dose to start.

Adverse effects

Adverse effects of antipsychotic agents include anticholinergic effects, such as urinary retention, constipation, blurred vision, dry mouth, and confusion, which is more likely to occur in elderly patients with dementia. Other possible adverse effects are sedation, orthostatic hypotension, dizziness, anxiety, irregular or rapid heartbeat, photosensitivity, impaired temperature regulation, and depression. Abnormal, involuntary movements, such as lip smacking and lateral movements of the tongue, characterize tardive dyskinesia, a side effect that occurs after long-term use of antipsychotics. Neuroleptic malignant syndrome is a rare but potentially fatal side effect. This medical emergency is characterized by muscle rigidity, high fever, elevated levels of creatine phosphokinase, unstable blood pressure, and confusion. Management involves treating the signs while stopping the medication.

Extrapyramidal side effects of antipsychotics include pseudoparkinsonism (in 20% to 30% of patients), dystonia (25%), tardive dyskinesia (32% after 5 years, 68% after 25 years), and akathisia (20% to 40%) (Carvey, 1998). In akathisia, restless movements often mimic agitation. The ultimate adverse effects can be falls that result in fractures; loss of connection with the environment by decreasing cognition, communication, and loss of function; and eventually a poorer quality of life (see chapter 5).

Adverse drug reactions are the fourth leading cause of death in hospitalized patients (Delafuente, 2000). Only heart disease, cancer, and stroke are more prevalent. In fact, some geriatric advocates stress that any symptom in an elderly patient should be considered a drug side effect until proven otherwise. (This refers to adverse drug reactions in all classes of drugs, not just psychotropic drugs.)

Summary of Pharmacological Treatment of Secondary Symptoms of AD

1) Use only those classes of medications that have been shown to be efficacious in managing secondary symptoms of AD.

   a. Antidepressants for depression and irritability: The medications most useful for treating depression resulting from AD are those with minimal anticholinergic adverse effects. Selective serotonin reuptake inhibitors appear to be the most effective. Remember that the major adverse effect of these drugs is sedation (Bronstein & Pulst, 2003; Lehne, 2004).

   b. Anxiolytics for anxiety, restlessness, verbally disruptive behavior, and resistance: Remember, do not use restraints. When gentle reassurance does not work, short-acting anxiolytics such as alprazolam or lorazepam may be beneficial. The major adverse effects of these drugs is sedation. It is best to avoid using benzodiazepines due to their adverse effects. Nonbenzodiazepine anxiolytics such as buspirone may also be used (Bronstein & Pulst, 2003; Clark & Karlawish, 2003; Lehne, 2004).

   c. Antipsychotics for hallucinations, delusions, and agitation: The major problem with these drugs is that parkinsonism symptoms can develop or be exacerbated (Clark & Karlawish, 2003; Lehne, 2004).

   d. Anticonvulsant mood stabilizers, antipsychotics, trazadone, anxiolytics, and beta blockers for hostility, agitation, and unco-operativeness: Antipsychotics, trazadone, and anticonvulsant mood stabilizers have the highest efficacy. Atypical antipsychotics such as clozapine and risperidone have low adverse effect profiles and probably are safer than other antipsychotics (Bronstein & Pulst, 2003; Lehne, 2004).

   e. Sleep disorders may be adverse effects of other medications. Conditions such as pain and depression may also cause insomnia. When administering medications for insomnia, use extreme caution because reactions such as incontinence, instability, falls, and agitation commonly occur (Lehne, 2004). Minor tranquilizers or benzodiazepines may work but only in short-term dosing. These drugs should be avoided if possible and terminated as soon as possible if used. Melatonin or a short-acting sedative (such as zolpidem) may help insomnia. When stronger sedation is required, a very low dose of an atipsychotic is preferable to longer-acting benzodiazepines because the latter generally have lasting effects. Diphenhydramine hydrochloride, an over-the-counter medication, may be effective but it also has anticholinergic adverse effects that may increase confusion (Bronstein & Pulst, 2003; Clark & Karlawish, 2003; Lehne, 2004; Wallace & Buckwalter, 2003).

2) Prior to initiating any medication regime, consider the behavior and determine if this behavior is being caused by or exacerbated by a current medication.

3) Delirium and acute medical conditions (such as urinary tract infection, constipation, and pneumonia) must be ruled out prior to prescribing a medication for managing secondary symptoms.

4) Single agents should be tried prior to starting multiple drug regimes for secondary symptoms.

5) Start with a low dose and gradually increase

either the dose or the frequency until a therapeutic effect is realized.

DEVELOPMENT OF NEW DRUGS

Just a few years ago, people with AD and their families had very few options for treatment. Today, research progress instills hope of more treatment options becoming available in the future.

Research and development of new drugs can be an expensive and lengthy process, commonly taking, on the average, 17 years for development. However, reading about drugs for AD can make development appear to move at a rapid pace. One can read about new drugs for AD weekly, as evidenced by the following excerpts from recent headlines:

08/05/04 *Merck Signs Deals in Oncology and Alzheimer's*
Merck and Celera Diagnostics have begun to collaborate to find drug targets and biomarkers for Alzheimer's disease (Marx, 2004).

07/29/04 *Celera, Merck to Tackle Alzheimer's*
Celera Genomics has signed its third big research partnership this month. The company says Merck will help fund research into potential treatments for Alzheimer's disease based on Celera's gene discoveries (Clabaugh, 2004).

07/23/04 *Two Alzheimer's Drugs Show Potential – U.S. Studies*
Two experimental Alzheimer's drugs have the potential to prevent or halt the progress of the brain-wasting disease, doctors said on Wednesday, July 21, 2004 (Hurdle, 2004).

07/22/04 *Study Examines Seroquel for the Treatment of Agitation in Elderly Patients with Dementia*
Study results suggest Seroquel may reduce symptoms of agitation associated with dementia in long-term care patients; analysis shows no evidence of an increased risk of cerebrovascular adverse events (Astra Zeneca, 2004).

04/29/04 *Ceregene Confirms Plans to Further Develop Alzheimer's Disease Gene Therapy*
Ceregene, Inc., today announced that based on preliminary findings in a study conducted at the University of California, San Diego, it will advance its gene therapy for Alzheimer's disease into further clinical development.

04/28/04 *Large New Study Supports Statins For Alzheimer's Disease*
A large new study has found strong further evidence that statin drugs have therapeutic benefit for Alzheimer's Disease (AD).

04/08/04 *Alzheimer's Drugs Frustrate Doctors*
The drugs now available to treat the memory and thinking problems of Alzheimer's patients have failed to live up to the public's high expectations and offer such modest benefits that many doctors have doubts about prescribing them (Grady, 2004).

Full articles mentioned above may be found at ProHealth's Alzheimer's Support.Com http://www.alzheimersupport.com/articles/pastdrugnews.cfm

Managing medication regimes for patients with dementia, especially AD, is a challenging task. So far, therapies intended to change the underlying course of the disease have for the most part been unsuccessful. Because the drugs currently available for AD have side effects that vary from person to person, it is adventitious to have many drugs available to primary providers.

Many researchers have difficulty supporting their claims about drugs they have developed for AD; the FDA does not approve these drugs. However, researchers such as Shumaker, Legault, Rapp, et al. (2003) have recently substantiated claims about the use of old drugs, such as estrogen, in the treatment of AD. Nurses and other health care providers must remain current about new drugs intended for the treatment of AD. Nurses must be knowledgeable about these drugs in order to provide comprehensive education to patients and their families.

SUMMARY OF OBRA INTERPRETIVE GUIDELINES

The Health Care Financing Administration (HCFA), now the Centers for Medicare and Medicaid Services (CMS), an agency responsible for regulating nursing homes participating in the Medicare and Medicaid programs, developed interpretive guidelines for fulfilling OBRA requirements, including use of medications. These guidelines were implemented nationally in 1990 (see Figure 9-1). Updated guidelines were implemented in July 1999 and again in 2002. The Program Memorandum from the Department of Health & Human Services (DHHS) sets out the 2002 revisions (see Table 9-3).

Fick, Cooper, Wade, Waller, Maclean, and Beers (2003), in their article entitled "Updating the Beers Criteria for Potentially Inappropriate Medication Use in Older Adults: Results of a U.S. Consensus Panel of Experts," have set out tables similar to those originally developed by Beers in 1997 (see Tables 9-4 to 9-6). For nurses working with older adults, especially those with dementia, it is particularly helpful to be able to review these quidelines when considering medication care plans for older adults.

All psychotropic drugs (antidepressants, anxiolytics, sedative-hypnotics, and antipsychotics) are subject to the "unnecessary drug" regulation of OBRA. According to HCFA guidelines, "residents must be free of unnecessary drugs," which are defined as those that are duplicative, excessive in dose or duration, or used in the presence of adverse effects or without adequate monitoring or indication. The remaining regulations apply to anxiolytic, sedative-hypnotic, and antipsychotic drugs only (see Tables 9-7 through 9-11).

SUMMARY

Research and development of new drugs moves at a rapid pace, making managing medication regimes for patients with dementia, especially AD, a challenging task. So far, therapies intended to change the underlying course of the disease have for the most part been unsuccessful. The disease has no cure, and no magic bullet can stop the progression of the disease. AD remains a relentless and devastating disease, and researchers desperately continue to search for a cure. Monies are being dedicated by hundreds of organizations to aid in the fight against this disease. With this escalation of interest and investment in stopping the disease, several new drugs have been developed and are somewhat successful in slowing the progression of AD or improving its symptoms. The hope is that as researchers discover more about the disease and its biological markers, they will be able to initiate disease-modifying treatments and, eventually, find a cure for AD.

Most patients with AD have symptoms secondary to their cognitive losses. These symptoms may include depression, paranoia, delusions, hallucinations, agitation, aggression, and wandering. The goal of nurses is to improve the quality of life for people with AD; sometimes that means treating these behaviors with medications. Nurses must be knowledgeable about these medications and remember to use only those classes of medications that have been shown to be efficacious in managing secondary symptoms of AD. This is important because the risk of adverse reactions and ultimate harm to the person is high. Inappropriate use of prescription drugs is a serious health risk for the general older adult population and a more serious risk for those with dementia.

FIGURE 9-1: SUMMARY OF THE HEALTH CARE FINANCING ADMINISTRATION (HCFA) GUIDELINES

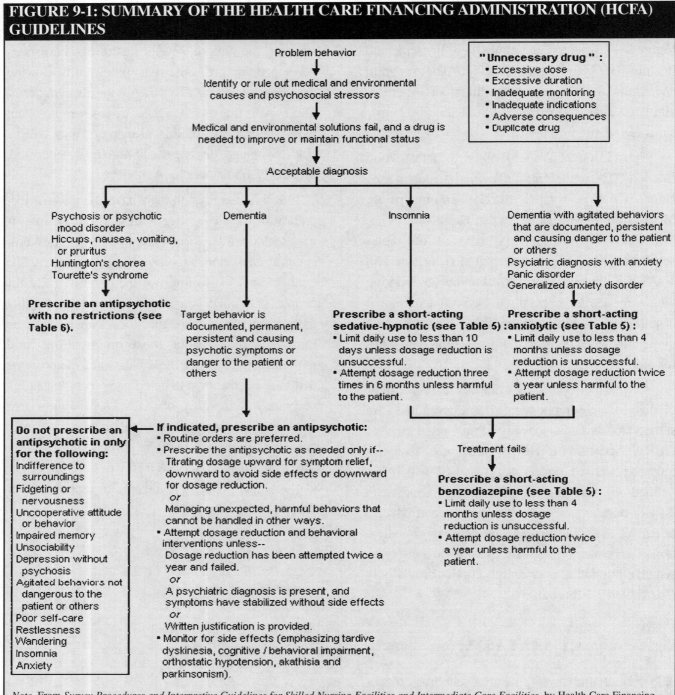

Note. From *Survey Procedures and Interpretive Guidelines for Skilled Nursing Facilities and Intermediate Care Facilities,* by Health Care Financing Administration, 1990. Baltimore: U.S. Dept. of Health and Human Services.

**** See Program Memorandum (2002), Department of Health & Human Services, SUBJECT: Provider Education Article: Psychotropic Drug Use in Skilled Nursing

TABLE 9-3: PROGRAM MEMORANDUM: DEPARTMENT OF HEALTH & HUMAN SERVICES (1 OF 3)

Intermediaries/Carriers

Centers for Medicare & Medicaid Services (CMS)

Transmittal AB-02-143 Date: OCTOBER 25, 2002

CHANGE REQUEST 2318

SUBJECT: Provider Education Article: Psychotropic Drug Use in Skilled Nursing Facilities (SNF)

An article is attached that will assist you in reminding the provider community about Medicare guidelines for psychotropic drug use in SNFs.

Include this article in your next regularly scheduled bulletin and post it immediately on any web sites or electronic bulletin boards you maintain. You are encouraged to include any additional information in your bulletin to supplement or complement the article.

The effective date for this Program Memorandum (PM) is October 25, 2002.

The implementation date for this PM is October 25, 2002.

These instructions should be implemented within your current operating budget.

This PM may be discarded October 25, 2003.

If you have questions, please contact the appropriate regional office.

Attachment

CMS-Pub. 60AB

Guidelines for Use of Antipsychotic Drugs

Attachment

Psychotropic Drug Use in Skilled Nursing Facilities (SNF)

In response to concerns expressed by the Senate Special Committee on Aging, the Office of Inspector General (OIG) studied the extent to which psychotropic drugs are being used in nursing homes as inappropriate chemical restraints. The OIG found that, in general, these drugs are being used appropriately. Where there are problems, they are related to inappropriate dosage, chronic use, lack of documented benefit to the resident, and unnecessary duplicate drug therapy. This article explains Medicare's guidelines for psychotropic drug use in SNFs including the definition of an unnecessary drug, justification for drug use outside guidelines, and antipsychotic drugs.

Definition of an Unnecessary Drug

Each resident's drug regimen must be free from unnecessary drugs. An unnecessary drug is any drug when used:

• In excessive dose (including duplicate drug therapy);

• For excessive duration;

• Without adequate monitoring;

• Without adequate indications for its use;

• In the presence of adverse consequences which indicate the dose should be reduced or discontinued; or

• Any combination of the above reasons.

NOTE: When a resident receives duplicate drug therapy, an evaluation should be completed for accumulation of the adverse effects.

NOTE: Adequate indications for use means that there is a valid clinical reason for the resident to receive the drug based on some, but not necessarily all, of the following:

• Resident assessment;

• Plan of care;

• Reports of significant change;

• Progress notes;

• Laboratory reports;

• Professional consults;

• Drug orders; or

• Observation and interview of the resident.

Justification for Drug Use Outside Guidelines

A drug used outside these guidelines must be based on sound risk-benefit analysis of the resident's symptoms and potential adverse effects of the drug. Some examples of evidence that would support a justification as to why a drug is being used outside these guidelines, but in the best interest of the resident, may include:

• A physician's note indicating that the dosage, duration, indication, and monitoring are clinically appropriate and the reasons as to why they are clinically appropriate. The note should demonstrate that the physician has carefully considered the risk/benefit to the resident in using a drug outside the guidelines.

TABLE 9-3: PROGRAM MEMORANDUM: DEPARTMENT OF HEALTH & HUMAN SERVICES (2 OF 3)

- A medical or psychiatric consultation or evaluation (e.g., Geriatric Depression Scale) confirming the physician's judgment that use of a drug outside the guidelines is in the best interest of the resident.
- Documentation of a physician, nursing, or other health professional indicating that the resident is being monitored for adverse consequences or complications of the drug therapy;
- Documentation confirming that previous attempts at dosage reduction have been unsuccessful;
- Documentation (including MDS documentation) showing the resident's subjective or objective improvement or maintenance of function while taking the medication;
- Documentation showing that the resident's decline or deterioration has been evaluated by the interdisciplinary team to determine whether a particular drug, a particular dose, or duration of therapy may be the cause; and
- Documentation showing why the resident's age, weight, or other factors would require a unique drug dose or drug duration, indication, or monitoring.

Guidelines for Use of Antipsychotic Drugs

SNFs must ensure, based on a comprehensive assessment of the resident, that:

I. When an antipsychotic drug has not been used in the past, it is not given unless antipsychotic drug therapy is necessary to treat a specific condition as diagnosed and documented in the clinical record. Antipsychotic drugs should not be used unless the clinical record documents that the resident has one or more of the following specific conditions:
- Schizophrenia;
- Schizo-affective disorder;
- Delusional disorder;
- Psychotic mood disorders (including mania and depression with psychotic features);
- Acute psychotic episodes;
- Brief reactive psychosis;
- Schizophreniform disorder;
- Atypical psychosis;
- Tourette's disorder;
- Huntington's disease;
- Organic mental syndromes (now called delirium, dementia, and amnestic and other cognitive disorders by DSM-IV) with associated psychotic and/or agitated behaviors which:
  - A. Have been quantitatively and objectively documented. This documentation is necessary to assist in:
    - Assessing whether the resident's behavioral symptom is in need of some form of intervention.
    - Determining whether the behavioral symptom is transitory or permanent.
    - Relating the behavioral symptom to other events in the resident's life in order to learn about potential causes (e.g., death in the family, not adhering to the resident's customary daily routine).
    - Ruling out environmental causes (e.g., excessive heat, noise, overcrowding).
    - Ruling out medical causes (e.g., pain, constipation, fever, infection).
  - B. Are persistent;
  - C. Are not caused by preventable reasons; and
  - D. Cause the resident to:
    - Present a danger to himself/herself or to others;
    - Continuously scream, yell, or pace and results in an impairment of functional capacity; or
    - Experience psychotic symptoms (e.g., hallucinations, paranoia, delusions) that are not exhibited as dangerous behaviors or as screaming, yelling, or pacing but result in distress or impairment of functional capacity.
- Short-term (7 day) symptomatic treatment of hiccups, nausea, vomiting, or pruritus. Residents with nausea and vomiting secondary to cancer or cancer chemotherapy can be treated for longer periods of time.

Antipsychotics should not be used if the only indication is one or more of the following:

- Wandering;
- Restlessness;
- Anxiety;
- Insomnia;
- Indifference to surroundings;
- Nervousness;
- Poor self care;
- Impaired memory;
- Depression (without psychotic features);
- Unsociability;
- Fidgeting;
- Uncooperativeness; or
- Agitated behaviors that do not represent danger to the resident or others.

TABLE 9-3: PROGRAM MEMORANDUM: DEPARTMENT OF HEALTH & HUMAN SERVICES (3 OF 3)

II. Unless clinically contraindicated, gradual dose reductions of the antipsychotic drug and behavioral interventions are considered in an effort to discontinue the drug. Close supervision should be provided when gradual dose reductions are carried out. If the gradual dose reduction causes an adverse effect on the resident and is discontinued, documentation of this decision and the reasons for it should be included in the clinical record. Gradual dose reductions consist of tapering the daily dose to determine whether symptoms can be controlled by a lower dose or the drug can be altogether eliminated.

NOTE: Behavior interventions is a modification of the resident's behavior or environment, including staff approaches to care, to the largest degree possible to accommodate the behavioral symptoms.

NOTE: Clinically contraindicated means that gradual dose reductions or behavioral interventions need not be undertaken if:

- The resident has a history of recurrence of psychotic symptoms (e.g., delusions, hallucinations) that have been stabilized with a maintenance dose of a antipsychotic drug without incurring significant side effects and has one of the following specific conditions:
    - Schizophrenia;Schizo-affective disorder;
    - Delusional disorder;
    - Psychotic mood disorders (including mania and depression with psychotic features);
    - Acute psychotic episodes;
    - Brief reactive psychosis;
    - Schizophreniform disorder;
    - Atypical psychosis;
    - Tourette's disorder; or
    - Huntington's disease
- The resident has organic mental syndrome, and gradual dose reductions have been attempted twice in one year that resulted in the return of symptoms for which the drug was prescribed to a degree that a cessation in the gradual dose reduction or a return to previous dose reduction was necessary; or
- The resident's physician provides a justification as to why the continued use of the drug and the dose of the drug are clinically appropriate. This justification should include:
    - A diagnosis that includes a description of the symptoms (not simply a diagnostic label or code);
    - A discussion of the differential psychiatric and medical diagnosis (e.g., why the resident's behavioral symptom is thought to be the result of a dementia with associated psychosis and/or agitated behaviors and not the result of an unrecognized painful medical condition or a psychosocial or environmental stressor);
    - A description of the justification for the choice of a particular treatment or treatments;
    - A discussion of why the present dose is necessary to manage the resident's symptoms.

Note. From *Survey Procedures and Interpretive Guidelines for Skilled Nursing Facilities and Intermediate Care Facilities,* by Health Care Financing Administration, 1990. Baltimore: U.S. Dept. of Health and Human Services.

**** See Program Memorandum (2002), Department of Health & Human Services, SUBJECT: Provider Education Article: Psychotropic Drug Use in Skilled Nursing

TABLE 9-4: 2002 CRITERIA FOR POTENTIALLY INAPPROPRIATE MEDICATION USE IN OLDER ADULTS: INDEPENDENT OF DIAGNOSES OR CONDITIONS (1 of 2)

Drug	Concern	Severity Rating (High or Low)
Propoxyphene (Darvon) and combination products (Darvon with ASA, Darvon-N, and Darvocet-N)	Offers few analgesic advantages over acetaminophen, yet has the adverse effects of other narcotic drugs.	Low
Indomethacin (Indocin and Indocin SR)	Of all available nonsteroidal anti-inflammatory drugs, this drug produces the most CNS adverse effects.	High
Pentazocine (Talwin)	Narcotic analgesic that causes more CNS adverse effects, including confusion and hallucinations, more commonly than other narcotic drugs. Additionally, it is a mixed agonist and antagonist.	High
Trimethobenzamide (Tigan)	One of the least effective antiemetic drugs, yet it can cause extrapyramidal adverse effects.	High
Muscle relaxants and antispasmodics: methocarbamol (Robaxin), carisoprodol (Soma), chlorzoxazone (Paraflex), metaxalone (Skelaxin), cyclobenzaprine (Flexeril), and oxybutynin (Ditropan). Do not consider the extended-release Ditropan XL.	Most muscle relaxants and antispasmodic drugs are poorly tolerated by elderly patients, since these cause anticholinergic adverse effects, sedation, and weakness. Additionally, their effectiveness at doses tolerated by elderly patients is questionable.	High
Flurazepam (Dalmane)	This benzodiazepine hypnotic has an extremely long half-life in elderly patients (often days), producing prolonged sedation and increasing the incidence of falls and fracture. Medium- or short-acting benzodiazepines are preferable.	High
Amitriptyline (Elavil), chlordiazepoxide-amitriptyline (Limbitrol), and perphenazine-amitriptyline (Triavil)	Because of its strong anticholinergic and sedation properties, amitriptyline is rarely the antidepressant of choice for elderly patients.	High
Doxepin (Sinequan)	Because of its strong anticholinergic and sedating properties, doxepin is rarely the antidepressant of choice for elderly patients.	High
Meprobamate (Miltown and Equanil)	This is a highly addictive and sedating anxiolytic. Those using meprobamate for prolonged periods may become addicted and may need to be withdrawn slowly.	High
Doses of short-acting benzodiazepines: doses greater than lorazepam (Ativan), 3 mg; oxazepam (Serax), 60 mg; alprazolam (Xanax), 2 mg; temazepam (Restoril), 15 mg; and triazolam (Halcion), 0.25 mg	Because of increased sensitivity to benzoadiazepines in elderly patients, smaller doses may be effective as well as safer. Total daily doses should rarely exceed the suggested maximums.	High
Long-acting benzodiazepines: chlordiazepoxide (Librium), chlordiazepoxide-amitriptyline (Limbitrol) clidinium-chlordiazepoxide (Librax), diazepam (Valium), quazepam (Doral), halazepam (Paxipam), and chlorazepate (Tranxene)	These drugs have a long half-life in elderly patients (often several days), producing prolonged sedation and increasing the risk of falls and fractures. Short- and intermediate-acting benzodiazepines are preferred if a benzodiazepine is required.	High
Disopyramide (Norpace and Norpace CR)	Of all antiarrhythmic drugs, this is the most potent negative inotrope and therefore may induce heart failure in elderly patients. It is also strongly anticholinergic. Other antiarrhythmic drugs should be used.	High
Digoxin (Lanoxin) (should not exceed >0.125 mg/d except when treating atrial arrhythmias)	Decreased renal clearance may lead to increased risk of toxic effects.	Low
Short-acting dipyridamole (Persantine). Do not consider the long-acting dipyridamole (which has better properties than the short-acting in older adults) except with patients with artificial heart valves	May cause orthostatic hypotension.	Low
Methyldopa (Aldomet) and methyldopa-hydrochlorothiazide (Aldoril)	May cause bradycardia and exacerbate depression in elderly patients.	High
Reserpine at doses >0.25 mg	May induce depression, impotence, sedation, and orthostatic hypotension.	Low
Chlorpropamide (Diabinese)	It has a prolonged half-life in elderly patients and could cause prolonged hypoglycemia. Additionally, it is the only oral hypoglycemic agent that causes SIADH.	High
Gastrointestinal antispasmodic drugs: dicyclomine (Bentyl), hyoscyamine (Levsin and Levsinex), propantheline (Pro-Banthine), belladonna alkaloids (Donnatal and others), and clidinium-chlordiazepoxide (Librax)	GI antispasmodic drugs are highly anticholinergic and have uncertain effectiveness. These drugs should be avoided (especially for long-term use).	High
Anticholinergics and antihistamines: chlorpheniramine (Chlor-Trimeton), diphenhydramine (Benadryl), hydroxyzine (Vistaril and Atarax), cyproheptadine (Periactin), promethazine (Phenergan), tripelennamine, dexchlorpheniramine (Polaramine)	All nonprescription and many prescription antihistamines may have potent anticholinergic properties. Nonanticholinergic antihistamines are preferred in elderly patients when treating allergic reactions.	High
Diphenhydramine (Benadryl)	May cause confusion and sedation. Should not be used as a hypnotic, and when used to treat emergency allergic reactions, it should be used in the smallest possible dose.	High
Ergot mesyloids (Hydergine) and cyclandelate (Cyclospasmol)	Have not been shown to be effective in the doses studied.	Low
Ferrous sulfate >325 mg/d	Doses >325 mg/d do not dramatically increase the amount absorbed but greatly increase the incidence of constipation.	Low
All barbiturates (except phenobarbital) except when used to control seizures	Are highly addictive and cause more adverse effects than most sedative or hypnotic drugs in elderly patients.	High

(continued)

TABLE 9-4: 2002 CRITERIA FOR POTENTIALLY INAPPROPRIATE MEDICATION USE IN OLDER ADULTS: INDEPENDENT OF DIAGNOSES OR CONDITIONS (2 of 2)

Drug	Concern	Severity Rating (High or Low)
Meperidine (Demerol)	Not an effective oral analgesic in doses commonly used. May cause confusion and has many disadvantages to other narcotic drugs.	High
Ticlopidine (Ticlid)	Has been shown to be no better than aspirin in preventing clotting and may be considerably more toxic. Safer, more effective alternatives exist.	High
Ketorolac (Toradol)	Immediate and long-term use should be avoided in older persons, since a significant number have asymptomatic GI pathologic conditions.	High
Amphetamines and anorexic agents	These drugs have potential for causing dependence, hypertension, angina, and myocardial infarction.	High
Long-term use of full-dosage, longer half-life, non–COX-selective NSAIDs: naproxen (Naprosyn, Avaprox, and Aleve), oxaprozin (Daypro), and piroxicam (Feldene)	Have the potential to produce GI bleeding, renal failure, high blood pressure, and heart failure.	High
Daily fluoxetine (Prozac)	Long half-life of drug and risk of producing excessive CNS stimulation, sleep disturbances, and increasing agitation. Safer alternatives exist.	High
Long-term use of stimulant laxatives: bisacodyl (Dulcolax), cascara sagrada, and Neoloid except in the presence of opiate analgesic use	May exacerbate bowel dysfunction.	High
Amiodarone (Cordarone)	Associated with QT interval problems and risk of provoking torsades de pointes. Lack of efficacy in older adults.	High
Orphenadrine (Norflex)	Causes more sedation and anticholinergic adverse effects than safer alternatives.	High
Guanethidine (Ismelin)	May cause orthostatic hypotension. Safer alternatives exist.	High
Guanadrel (Hylorel)	May cause orthostatic hypotension.	High
Cyclandelate (Cyclospasmol)	Lack of efficacy.	Low
Isoxsurpine (Vasodilan)	Lack of efficacy.	Low
Nitrofurantoin (Macrodantin)	Potential for renal impairment. Safer alternatives available.	High
Doxazosin (Cardura)	Potential for hypotension, dry mouth, and urinary problems.	Low
Methyltestosterone (Android, Virilon, and Testrad)	Potential for prostatic hypertrophy and cardiac problems.	High
Thioridazine (Mellaril)	Greater potential for CNS and extrapyramidal adverse effects.	High
Mesoridazine (Serentil)	CNS and extrapyramidal adverse effects.	High
Short acting nifedipine (Procardia and Adalat)	Potential for hypotension and constipation.	High
Clonidine (Catapres)	Potential for orthostatic hypotension and CNS adverse effects.	Low
Mineral oil	Potential for aspiration and adverse effects. Safer alternatives available.	High
Cimetidine (Tagamet)	CNS adverse effects including confusion.	Low
Ethacrynic acid (Edecrin)	Potential for hypertension and fluid imbalances. Safer alternatives available.	Low
Desiccated thyroid	Concerns about cardiac effects. Safer alternatives available.	High
Amphetamines (excluding methylphenidate hydrochloride and anorexics)	CNS stimulant adverse effects.	High
Estrogens only (oral)	Evidence of the carcinogenic (breast and endometrial cancer) potential of these agents and lack of cardioprotective effect in older women.	Low

Abbreviations: CNS, central nervous system; COX, cyclooxygenase; GI, gastrointestinal; NSAIDs, nonsteroidal anti-inflammatory drugs; SIADH, syndrome of inappropriate antidiuretic hormone secretion.

TABLE 9-5: 2002 CRITERIA FOR POTENTIALLY INAPPROPRIATE MEDICATION USE IN OLDER ADULTS: CONSIDERING DIAGNOSES OR CONDITIONS

Disease or Condition	Drug	Concern	Severity Rating (High or Low)
Heart failure	Disopyramide (Norpace), and high sodium content drugs (sodium and sodium salts [alginate bicarbonate, biphosphate, citrate, phosphate, salicylate, and sulfate])	Negative inotropic effect. Potential to promote fluid retention and exacerbation of heart failure.	High
Hypertension	Phenylpropanolamine hydrochloride (removed from the market in 2001), pseudoephedrine; diet pills, and amphetamines	May produce elevation of blood pressure secondary to sympathomimetic activity.	High
Gastric or duodenal ulcers	NSAIDs and aspirin (>325 mg) (coxibs excluded)	May exacerbate existing ulcers or produce new/additional ulcers.	High
Seizures or epilepsy	Clozapine (Clozaril), chlorpromazine (Thorazine), thioridazine (Mellaril), and thiothixene (Navane)	May lower seizure thresholds.	High
Blood clotting disorders or receiving anticoagulant therapy	Aspirin, NSAIDs, dipyridamole (Persantin), ticlopidine (Ticlid), and clopidogrel (Plavix)	May prolong clotting time and elevate INR values or inhibit platelet aggregation, resulting in an increased potential for bleeding.	High
Bladder outflow obstruction	Anticholinergics and antihistamines, gastrointestinal antispasmodics, muscle relaxants, oxybutynin (Ditropan), flavoxate (Urispas), anticholinergics, antidepressants, decongestants, and tolterodine (Detrol)	May decrease urinary flow, leading to urinary retention.	High
Stress incontinence	α-Blockers (Doxazosin, Prazosin, and Terazosin), anticholinergics, tricyclic antidepressants (imipramine hydrochloride, doxepin hydrochloride, and amitriptyline hydrochloride), and long-acting benzodiazepines	May produce polyuria and worsening of incontinence.	High
Arrhythmias	Tricyclic antidepressants (imipramine hydrochloride, doxepin hydrochloride, and amitriptyline hydrochloride)	Concern due to proarrhythmic effects and ability to produce QT interval changes.	High
Insomnia	Decongestants, theophylline (Theodur), methylphenidate (Ritalin), MAOIs, and amphetamines	Concern due to CNS stimulant effects.	High
Parkinson disease	Metoclopramide (Reglan), conventional antipsychotics, and tacrine (Cognex)	Concern due to their antidopaminergic/cholinergic effects.	High
Cognitive impairment	Barbiturates, anticholinergics, antispasmodics, and muscle relaxants. CNS stimulants: dextroAmphetamine (Adderall), methylphenidate (Ritalin), methamphetamine (Desoxyn), and pemolin	Concern due to CNS-altering effects.	High
Depression	Long-term benzodiazepine use. Sympatholytic agents: methyldopa (Aldomet), reserpine, and guanethidine (Ismelin)	May produce or exacerbate depression.	High
Anorexia and malnutrition	CNS stimulants: DextroAmphetamine (Adderall), methylphenidate (Ritalin), methamphetamine (Desoxyn), pemolin, and fluoxetine (Prozac)	Concern due to appetite-suppressing effects.	High
Syncope or falls	Short- to intermediate-acting benzodiazepine and tricyclic antidepressants (imipramine hydrochloride, doxepin hydrochloride, and amitriptyline hydrochloride)	May produce ataxia, impaired psychomotor function, syncope, and additional falls.	High
SIADH/hyponatremia	SSRIs: fluoxetine (Prozac), citalopram (Celexa), fluvoxamine (Luvox), paroxetine (Paxil), and sertraline (Zoloft)	May exacerbate or cause SIADH.	Low
Seizure disorder	Bupropion (Wellbutrin)	May lower seizure threshold.	High
Obesity	Olanzapine (Zyprexa)	May stimulate appetite and increase weight gain.	Low
COPD	Long-acting benzodiazepines: chlordiazepoxide (Librium), chlordiazepoxide-amitriptyline (Limbitrol), clidinium-chlordiazepoxide (Librax), diazepam (Valium), quazepam (Doral), halazepam (Paxipam), and chlorazepate (Tranxene). β-blockers: propranolol	CNS adverse effects. May induce respiratory depression. May exacerbate or cause respiratory depression.	High
Chronic constipation	Calcium channel blockers, anticholinergics, and tricyclic antidepressant (imipramine hydrochloride, doxepin hydrochloride, and amitriptyline hydrochloride)	May exacerbate constipation.	Low

Abbreviations: CNS, central nervous systems; COPD, chronic obstructive pulmonary disease; INR, international normalized ratio; MAOIs, monoamine oxidase inhibitors; NSAIDs, nonsteroidal anti-inflammatory drugs; SIADH, syndrome of inappropriate antidiuretic hormone secretion; SSRIs, selective serotonin reuptake inhibitors.

Note. From "Updating the Beers Criteria for Potentially Inappropriate Medication Use in Older Adults," by D.M. Fick, J.W. Cooper, W.E. Wade, J.L. Waller, J.R. Maclean, & M.H. Beers, 2003, *Archives of Internal Medicine, 163*(22), 2721. Copyright 2003 by the American Medical Association. Reprinted with permission.

TABLE 9-6: SUMMARY OF CHANGES FROM 1997 BEERS CRITERIA TO NEW 2002 CRITERIA

Medicines Modified Since 1997 Beers Criteria

1. Reserpine (Serpasil and Hydropres)*
2. Extended-release oxybutynin (Ditropan XL)†
3. Iron supplements >325 mg†
4. Short-acting dipyridamole (Persantine)‡

Medicines Dropped Since 1997 Beers Criteria

Independent of Diagnoses
1. Phenylbutazone (Butazolidin)

Considering Diagnoses
2. Recently started corticosteroid therapy with diabetes
3. β-Blockers with diabetes, COPD or asthma, peripheral vascular disease, and syncope or falls
4. Sedative hypnotics with COPD
5. Potassium supplements with gastric or duodenal ulcers

6. Metoclopramide (Reglan) with seizures or epilepsy
7. Narcotics with bladder outflow obstruction and narcotics with constipation
8. Desipramine (Norpramin) with insomnia
9. All SSRIs with insomnia
10. β-Agonists with insomnia
11. Bethanechol chloride with bladder outflow obstruction

Medicines Added Since 1997 Beers Criteria

Independent of Diagnoses
1. Ketorolac tromethamine (Toradol)
2. Orphenadrine (Norflex)
3. Guanethidine (Ismelin)
4. Guanadrel (Hylorel)
5. Cyclandelate (Cyclospasmol)
6. Isoxsuprine (Vasodilan)
7. Nitrofurantoin (Macrodantin)
8. Doxazosin (Cardura)
9. Methyltestosterone (Android, Virilon, and Testrad)
10. Mesoridazine (Serentil)
11. Clonidine (Catapres)
12. Mineral oil
13. Cimetidine (Tagamet)
14. Ethacrynic acid (Edecrin)

Considering Diagnoses
26. Long-acting benzodiazepines: chlordiazepoxide (Librium), chlordiazepoxide-amitriptyline (Limbitrol), clidinium-chlordiazepoxide (Librax), diazepam (Valium), quazepam (Doral), halazepam (Paxipam), and chlorazepate (Tranxene) with COPD, stress incontinence, depression, and falls
27. Propanolol with COPD/asthma
28. Anticholinergics with stress incontinence
29. Tricyclic antidepressants (imipramine hydrochloride, doxepin hydrochloride, and amitriptyline hydrochloride) with syncope or falls and stress incontinence
30. Short to intermediate and long-acting benzodiazepines with syncope or falls
31. Clopidogrel (Plavix) with blood-clotting disorders receiving anticoagulant therapy
32. Tolterodine (Detrol) with bladder outflow obstruction

15. Desiccated thyroid
16. Ferrous sulfate >325 mg
17. Amphetamines (excluding methylpenidate and anorexics)
18. Thioridazine (Mellaril)
19. Short-acting nifedipine (Procardia and Adalat)
20. Daily fluoxetine (Prozac)
21. Stimulant laxatives may exacerbate bowel dysfunction (except in presence of chronic pain requiring opiate analgesics)
22. Amiodarone (Cordarone)
23. Non–COX-selective NSAIDs (naproxen [Naprosyn], oxaprozin, and piroxicam)
24. Reserpine doses >0.25 mg/d
25. Estrogens in older women

33. Decongestants with bladder outflow obstruction
34. Calcium channel blockers with constipation
35. Phenylpropanolamine with hypertension
36. Bupropion (Wellbutrin) with seizure disorder
37. Olanzapine (Zyprexa) with obesity
38. Metoclopramide (Reglan) with Parkinson disease
39. Conventional antipsychotics with Parkinson disease
40. Tacrine (Cognex) with Parkinson disease
41. Barbiturates with cognitive impairment
42. Antispasmodics with cognitive impairment
43. Muscle relaxants with cognitive impairment
44. CNS stimulants with anorexia, malnutrition, and cognitive impairment

Abbreviations: CNS, central nervous system; COPD, chronic obstructive pulmonary disease; COX, cyclooxygenase; NSAIDs, nonsteroidal anti-inflammatory drugs; SSRIs, selective serotonin reuptake inhibitors.

*Reserpine in doses >0.25 mg was added to the list.

†Ditropan was modified to refer to the immediate-release formulation only and not Ditropan XL and iron supplements was modified to include only ferrous sulfate.

‡Do not consider the long-acting dipyridamole, which has better properties than the short-acting dipyridamole in older adults (except with patients with artificial heart valves).

Note. From "Updating the Beers Criteria for Potentially Inappropriate Medication Use in Older Adults," by D.M. Fick, J.W. Cooper, W.E. Wade, J.L. Waller, J.R. Maclean, & M.H. Beers, 2003, *Archives of Internal Medicine, 163*(22), 2722. Copyright 2003 by the American Medical Association. Reprinted with permission.

TABLE 9-7: DRUGS WITH A HIGH POTENTIAL FOR SEVERE OUTCOMES IN THE ELDERLY

Drugs	Comments
Psychotropics	
Amitriptyline (Elavil)	Strongly anticholinergic and sedating
Barbiturates	More side effects than most sedative-hypnotic drugs; should not be used except to control seizures (phenobarbital)
Long-acting benzodiazepines	Long half-life and, hence, prolonged sedation; associated with an increased incidence of falls and fractures
Doxepin (Sinequan)	Strongly anticholinergic and sedating
Meprobamate (Miltown)	Highly addictive and sedating
Analgesics	
Meperidine (Demerol)	Not effective when administered orally; metabolite has anticholinergic profile
Pentazocine (Talwin)	Confusion and hallucinations more common than with other narcotics
Miscellaneous	
Antispasmodic agents	Highly anticholinergic with associated toxic effects (gastrointestinal)
Chlorpropamide (Diabinase)	Serious hypoglycemia possible because of the drug's prolonged half-life
Digoxin (Lanoxin)	Decreased renal clearance; doses should rarely exceed 0.125 mg except when treating arrhythmias
Methyldopa (Aldomet)	Causes bradycardia and exacerbates depression
Ticlopidine (Ticlid)	More toxic than aspirin

Note. From "Explicit Criteria for Determining Potentially Inappropriate Medication Use by the Elderly. An Update," by M. Beers, 1997, *Archives of Internal Medicine, 157*(14):1531-36. Reprinted with permission of the American Medical Association.

TABLE 9-8: DRUGS WITH A HIGH POTENTIAL FOR LESS SEVERE OUTCOMES IN THE ELDERLY

Drugs	Comments
Analgesics	
Indomethacin (Indocin)	More central nervous system side effects than any other nonsteroidal anti-inflammatory drug
Propoxyphene (Darvon)	Few advantages over acetaminophen and has narcotic side effects
Antihypertensives	
Beta blockers	Can cause problems in patients with asthma or chronic obstructive pulmonary disease; may precipitate syncope because of negative inotropic and chronotropic effects
Reserpine*	Can cause depression, sedation, and orthostatic hypotension
Miscellaneous	
Antihistamines†	Highly anticholinergic
Cyclandelate (Cyclospasmol)	Generally ineffective for dementia or any other condition
Dipyridamole (Persantine)	Frequently causes orthostatic hypotension; beneficial only in patients with artificial heart valves
Ergoloid mesylates (Hydergine)	Generally ineffective for dementia or any other condition
Muscle relaxants	Increased cholinergic activity, sedation and weakness
Trimethobenzamide (Tigan)	Least effective antiemetic; can cause extrapyramidal symptoms

* Reserpine is available alone (in generic form) and is also found in combination drugs such as reserpine-trichlormethiazide (Metatensin).

† Over-the-counter and prescription first-generation antihistamines.

Note. From "Explicit Criteria for Determining Potentially Inappropriate Medication Use by the Elderly. An Update," by M. Beers, 1997. *Arch Intern Med, 157*:1531-6. Reprinted with permission of the American Medical Association.

TABLE 9-9: DRUGS RESTRICTED IN NURSING HOMES*

Barbiturates

- Amobarbital (Amytal)
- Amobarbital-secobarbital (Tuinal)
- Aspirin-butalbital-caffeine (Fiorinal)
- Butabarbital (Butisol)
- Pentobarbital (Nembutal)
- Secobarbital (Seconal) and other tranquilizers

Other

- Ethclorvynol (Placidyl)
- Glutethimide (Doriden
- Meprobamate (Miltown)

* In accordance with regulations relating to the Omnibus Budget Reconciliation Act of 1987, drugs listed in this table are not to be used unless started before admission to a nursing home, given as a single dose for a medical or dental procedure or used for the treatment of seizures (phenobarbital).

Note. From *Survey Procedures and Interpretive Guidelines for Skilled Nursing Facilities and Intermediate Care Facilities* by Health Care Financing Administration, 1990. Baltimore: U.S. Dept. of Health and Human Services.

TABLE 9-10: ANTIDEPRESSANT DRUGS AND PREFERRED DOSAGES FOR ELDERLY PATIENTS

Drugs	GERIATRIC DOSAGE (mg per day)		SIDE EFFECTS			
	Starting dosage	Maintenance dosage	Sedation	Agitation	Anticholinergic effects	Orthostatic hypotension
Tricyclic antidepressants						
Desipramine (Norpramin)	25	50 to 150	Low	Low	Low	Low
Nortriptyline (Pamelor)	10 to 25	40 to 75	Moderate	—	Low	Low
Selective serotonin reuptake inhibitors						
Citalopram (Celexa)	20	20 to 40	Low	Low	—	—
Fluvoxamine (Luvox)	50	50 to 200	Low	Low	—	—
Paroxetine (Paxil)	10	20 to 30	Low	Low	—	—
Sertraline (Zoloft)	25 to 50	50 to 150	Low	Low	—	—
Miscellaneous						
Bupropion (Wellbutrin)	100	100 to 400	—	Moderate	—	Low
Nefazodone (Serzone)	100	100 to 600	Moderate	—	Low	Low
Trazodone (Desyrel)	25 to 50	50 to 300	High	—	Low	Moderate
Venlafaxine (Effexor)	75	75 to 350	Low	Low	Low	Low

— = Very low or insignificant effects.

Note. From *Survey Procedures and Interpretive Guidelines for Skilled Nursing Facilities and Intermediate Care Facilities* by Health Care Financing Administration, 1990. Baltimore: U.S. Dept. of Health and Human Services.

TABLE 9-11: ANXIOLYTIC AND SEDATIVE-HYPNOTIC DRUGS COMMONLY USED IN THE ELDERLY

Drugs	Geriatric dosage (mg per day)*		Onset of action
	Anxiety	Insomnia	
Short-acting agents			
Benzodiazepines			
Alprazolam (Xanax)	0.75 mg	0.25 mg	Intermediate
Estazolam (Prosom)	0.5 mg	0.5 mg	Fast
Lorazepam (Ativan)	2 mg	1 mg	Intermediate
Oxazepam (Serax)	30 mg	30 mg	Slow
Temazepam (Restoril)	—	15 mg	Intermediate
Triazolam (Halcion)	—	0.125 mg	Fast
Antihistamines			
Diphenhydramine (Benadryl)	50 mg	25 mg	Fast
Hydroxyzine (Atarax)	50 mg	50 mg	Fast
Miscellaneous			
Zolpidem (Ambien)	—	5 mg	Fast
Long-acting agents			
Benzodiazepines			
Chlordiazepoxide (Librium)	20 mg	20 mg	Intermediate
Clonazepam (Klonopin)	1.5 mg	1.5 mg	Intermediate
Clorazepate (Tranxene)	15 mg	15 mg	Fast
Diazepam (Valium)	5 mg	5 mg	Very fast
Flurazepam (Dalmane)	15 mg	15 mg	Very fast
Halazepam (Paxipam)	40 mg	20 mg	Slow
Prazepam (Centrax)	15 mg	15 mg	Slow
Quazepam (Doral)	7.5 mg	7.5 mg	Intermediate

— = Not indicated.

* The dosages given in this table are as established by the Health Care Financing Administration guidelines for fulfilling the requirements of the Omnibus Budget Reconciliation Act (OBRA) of 1987. They are not the maximum dosages. When the OBRA-specified dosage of a drug is exceeded, documentation of necessity is required.

Note. From *Survey Procedures and Interpretive Guidelines for Skilled Nursing Facilities and Intermediate Care Facilities* by Health Care Financing Administration, 1990. Baltimore: U.S. Dept. of Health and Human Services.

EXAM QUESTIONS

CHAPTER 9
Questions 81-90

81. The nurses role in medication administration includes

    a. collecting data just after giving a drug.

    b. anticipating adverse effects and changing the dosage if adverse effects occur.

    c. delivering the correct dose and administering it safely.

    d. asking the physician if the drug did what it was supposed to.

82. Pharmacological treatments approved by the FDA for improving memory, enhancing cognition, and delaying the onset or slowing the progression of AD include

    a. CEIs.

    b. ginkgo biloba.

    c. hormones.

    d. barbituates.

83. A true statement regarding the adverse effects of CEIs is

    a. tachycardia is a common adverse effect.

    b. adverse effects are directly related to the rate of dose increase.

    c. nausea and vomiting are seldom seen as adverse effects.

    d. dose intervals should be started at a high level and then decreased until the optimal therapeutic dosage has been reached.

84. A change associated with aging that affects how the body uses drugs is

    a. a lower fat-to-lean ratio.

    b. more total body water.

    c. faster renal clearance.

    d. lower concentrations of serum albumin.

85. An anticholenergic effect from an antipsychotic agent is

    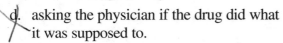

    p.164 answer found in glossary

    a. diarrhea.

    b. incontinence.

    c. lip smacking.

    d. urinary retention.

86. A true statement regarding prescribing and administering CEIs is

    a. treatment can be delayed until the second stage of the disease.

    b. treatment with CEIs should be started at the time of the diagnosis of AD.

    c. the more severe the deterioration of AD, the more effective the CEI.

    d. delays in administering the medication do not reduce the maximum possible response to CEIs.

87. Liver toxicity is a major adverse effect in the CEI

    a. tacrine.

    b. galantamine.

    c. rivastigmine.

    d. donepezil.

88. A rare, yet potentially fatal side effect of antipsychotic medication is

    a. neuroleptic malignant syndrome.
    b. tardive dyskinesia.
    c. orthostatic hypotension.
    d. photosensitivity.

89. Research and development in the field of AD can best be described as

    a. a cure for AD has been found.
    b. little research is being performed.
    c. drug development is an expensive and lengthy process.
    d. there is little information in the media about new drugs for AD.

90. A consideration for discontinuation of CEIs is

    a. taper off the drug by reducing the dose every few weeks.
    b. once therapeutic benefits are seen, the drug should be stopped.
    c. the drug should never be given for more than a year.
    d. abruptly withdraw the drug, all at once.

CHAPTER 10

CAREGIVER ISSUES

CHAPTER OBJECTIVE

After completing this chapter, the reader will be able to identify issues faced by caregivers of people with Alzheimer's disease (AD) as well as interventions designed to improve their quality of life. The reader will also be able to recognize the effects of stress, depression, and other demands on the risk of abuse or neglect of AD patients and measures that may be necessary to protect these patients.

LEARNING OBJECTIVES

After studying this chapter, the reader will be able to

1. specify the three keys of managing nursing care for patients with AD.

2. recognize three stages of caregiving and nursing interventions for caregivers at each stage.

3. specify the purpose, arrangement, and benefit of special care units (SCUs) for dementia.

4. identify alternatives to nursing home placement, and the advantages of each service.

5. specify differences between Medicare and Medicaid and the financial assistance to caregivers (if any) provided by these federal agencies as well as by community agencies.

6. discuss the importance of the Patient Self-Determination Act and living wills for people with AD and their family members.

7. distinguish the central focus of support groups for caregivers.

8. recognize the importance and availability of educational programs for caregivers.

9. analyze the correlation between caregiver feelings and the potential for violence or abuse of people with AD and the associated interventions to aid caregivers with their feelings.

10. demonstrate comprehension of the interventions that create better outcomes for traveling with people who have AD.

INTRODUCTION

As the population of the United States ages, the need to provide nursing support and increase knowledge about family caregiving grows. The Omnibus Budget Reconciliation Act of 1987 focused the nation's attention on the long-term care needs of the elderly. Much of the emphasis since this legislation has been on providing quality care at home. The burden of this care falls mostly on family members, who may be the primary caregivers for many years. The toll of dementia and AD on caregivers has been well documented (Covinsky, Eng, Lui, et al., 2001; Janevic & Connell, 2001; Meuser & Marwit, 2001).

This chapter focuses on the role of nurses as caregivers as well as their role in supporting and facilitating family caregivers. It also discusses family or extended family members as caregivers for demented patients who live either at home or in a health care facility and how nurses can recognize common reactions to caregiving and ease family caregiver burdens.

Furthermore, it explores the importance of the environment for patients with dementia and compares care at home to that of care in nursing homes, including how to help families choose nursing homes, the legal and financial implications for family caregivers, and information on advanced directives and use of Medicare and Medicaid funds.

NURSES AS CAREGIVERS

Home care providers are usually the first people to identify dementia in elderly patients. Due to consistent interaction with loved ones, family members may be the first to notice cognitive decline. Once diagnosed, fear, anger, disbelief, and grief are the typical reactions of family caregivers to the experience of caring for a person who has AD or any other dementia. Although the process of identification may differ, the nursing care, the behaviors, and the activities to be provided are essentially the same for all types of dementia. Nurses and other health care staff members, whether in homes or in facilities, may be frightened when the behavior of a demented patient is bizarre, aggressive, and hard to understand.

Three keys to managing the care nurses provide in nursing homes were suggested in 1985 (Gwyther, 2001) and remain pertinent today:

1. Symptom management
2. Adaptations for a therapeutic environment
3. Support for the caregivers, families, and other staff or personnel.

These ideas can be expanded to encompass the role of nurses as caregivers at home or in any setting where health care is provided. Managing patients' signs and symptoms and behaviors and taking steps to create a therapeutic environment are key no mat-

ter where the person with dementia lives or receives care. Most nurses encounter patients with AD or another type of dementia in daily practice.

Supporting caregivers is a major role of professional nurses. Access to current information and the ability to convey that information to caregivers is essential. Much new information has become available, as well as a great deal of misinformation. For instance, it is now known that AD is not a mental illness, and the disease is not a result of the life the person has lived. A better understanding of what is known and unknown about AD can relieve the fears of caregivers.

FAMILY CAREGIVERS

Imagine living with a person who goes to the hardware store to buy some household repair items, only to return hours later with no recollection of where he or she has been or where they left the car. Or kissing your loved one of 40 years only to hear them ask in return, "Who are you?" For the 18 to 20 million Americans who provide home care for their loved ones who have AD, these experiences can be frightening and can become commonplace over time.

Families must adapt every day to living with ambiguity and uncertainty. Each day with a person who has AD is different, with different behaviors, and what worked yesterday may not work today. Many caregivers have never experienced the personal and interpersonal conflicts associated with caring for someone with AD. Attempting to reason with someone who is unreasonable and argumentative and who behaves in a bizarre manner is disconcerting to a person who thinks that love and openness can take care of most situations.

WHO ARE CAREGIVERS?

Who are the caregivers and how does caring for a loved one with AD impact their lives? Home care is made up mainly of family members, and these family members have been called the hidden victims of AD. It is not hard to comprehend how AD victimizes those it afflicts, but many people do not appreciate the other victims of the disease, such as family members, friends, and caregivers.

The reaction of caregivers to the diagnosis of AD varies — from attempts to obtain information on the disease to panicked attempts to find a less fearsome explanation for the changes they are seeing in their loved ones (Yaffe et al., 2002).

It is also easy to understand how family members can dismiss, in the very early stages of AD, the forgetfulness, personality changes, and confusion as simply part of the aging process or depression. It may not be until their loved one cannot put sentences together, cannot remember how to make coffee, or gets lost going to the grocery store that the family realizes. At this point, they can feel helpless, realizing that they can no longer do anything to stop AD from taking their loved one away from them. They can no longer deny the diagnosis of AD. This is also the time when they may seek help from professionals.

Grief is one of the emotions to be anticipated in family members and caregivers of AD patients. People with AD still look the same, walk the same, look healthy, and even act the same from time to time. Remember that the degeneration process of AD can last up to 15 years and, as a result, some family members call it "the funeral that never ends." AD patients can go from walking, to wheelchairs, to reclining wheelchairs, to being bedbound, to being nonresponsive. Each of these changes is a crisis with individual issues of care. Families have referred to this series of crises as "little deaths." They have also referred to their loved ones as "the walking dead" (Hurley & Volicer, 2002). With a loved one with AD still in their midst, it is extremely hard to grieve outwardly and even get other people to understand or acknowledge their loss.

Many family members must care for their loved ones 24 hours a day. The language of this caregiving is often described in negative terms, such as caregiver burden or stress. "Caregiver burden" is the stress of caring for someone with AD; it increases the risk of morbidity among caregivers. As AD progresses, caregiver burden spirals, sometimes out of control (Yaffe et al., 2002).

Mahoney et al., (2003) have used a more neutral term, "vigilance," to describe caregivers' perceptions of caring for a loved one with AD. Vigilance is caregivers' continual supervision over their loved ones' care. Mahoney et al. point out that there are five components of vigilance: watchful supervision, protective intervening, anticipation, always being on duty, and being there. Caregivers who are vigilant see themselves as "on duty" even when they are sleeping or not providing direct care.

Nurses need to be aware that caregivers who are "vigilant" remain so even with interventions of professional care services or institutionalization. Nurses need to talk at length with family members to discover the unique care practices or strategies family members have employed in the care of their loved ones at home. Incorporating these practices into caregiving by nurses is essential for building family trust and reducing family vigilance.

Eventually, the daily tasks of bathing, dressing, toileting, grooming, and feeding can be met with anger, resistance, and even abuse. The demands can be so great that family members must give up their jobs, their social lives, and any form of physical recreation in order to provide care.

Researchers have looked at the reactions of caregivers and families who care for patients with dementia. A recent study (Covinsky et al., 2001) looked at the economic impact on caregivers of providing home care for frail elders. The ability of individuals to stay at home is largely due to the unpaid care given by family caregivers, who are usually women. When the amount of care required rises to more than 40 hours a week, not surprisingly, this interferes with employment outside the home. The study showed that 22% of caregivers reduced their number of hours working or quit working.

The risk of reduced employment was found to depend on ethnicity and clinical characteristics. Caregivers of African American and Hispanic individuals are more likely to live with their families, report lower amounts of caregiver burden, and demonstrate a willingness to reduce employment in order to care for family at home.

Janevic and Connell (2001) reviewed published studies to compare ethnic, racial, and cultural differences in dementia caregiving. They found that African American and Hispanic caregivers are less likely than Caucasians to be spouses and more likely to be another family member. Among Korean, Chinese, and Korean-American groups, stress and burden from caregiving was not as customary. However, the authors emphasize the scant amount of research on Asian-American caregivers in light of reports of dementia symptoms being a source of shame among people of Asian culture. This study has increased interest in cultural differences in dementia caregiving. The findings have the potential to affect public policy decisions about costs for nursing home placement because they imply that African American and Hispanic families bear a larger share of the cost of caregiving in the home and utilize more formal home care.

The reactions of caregivers and families who care for patients with dementia can also be demonstrated in the following scenario. Mrs. White, who was diagnosed several years ago with AD, lives with her daughter and family. It is Sunday, and the family is hurrying to get ready for church. Mrs. White's daughter encourages her mother, who has always dressed herself, to get dressed and be ready to go in 15 minutes. On this Sunday, her daughter finds her in her room crying, and saying she does not want to go to church. The daughter is feeling hurried so she insists, picks out two dresses, lays them on the bed,

and tells her mother to hurry. A few minutes later, the family hears the sound of Mrs. White screaming and ripping up her dresses. Her daughter becomes upset with her and starts trying to dress Mrs. White. Mrs. White really begins to yell.

Expecting either too much or too little capability for self-care can have a negative effect. The functional status of the demented person affects the caregiver. The cognitive losses of the elderly person seem to have less effect on the health and depression of the caregiver than the demented person's limitations in functional abilities, such as the ability to perform activities of daily living (ADLs). Yet, much of public policy and funding do not recognize the need for in-home assistance with ADLs unless skilled care is needed, such as after hospitalization for a major illness or injury. Some self-insured companies are beginning to recognize the need for in-home assistance that is not nursing care. These companies are also aware of the dollar savings associated with keeping people in their homes for as long as possible.

The concept of home care is very loosely defined. In 1994, the World Health Organization defined it as "an array of health and social support services provided to clients in their own residence. Such coordinated services may prevent, delay, or be a substitute for temporary or long-term institutional care" (Thome, Dykes, & Hallberg, 2003, p. 861). These researchers found that the basis for planning and implementing care has been focused on the level of individual needs and their predictors. The variety of activities included preventing decreased functional abilities, maintaining independence, increasing quality of life, and allowing death to occur in the home. Those providing the care included every concept of care provider from informal family members, to social caregivers, to certified nursing assistants, to nurses, to advanced practice nurses, with an occasional mention of physician home visits.

STAGES OF CAREGIVING

Research have examined the role of caregivers in the care of patients with AD (Lindgren, 1993; Lindgren, Connelly, & Gaspar, 1999; Wisniewski, Belle, Coon, et al., 2003). The role of caregiver was conceptualized as a period in a spouse's life when the focal point is caregiving. The active, focused role of the caregiver is similar to the role a person takes when managing his or her career. Three stages of the caregiving career were developed:

1. The encounter stage
2. The endurance stage
3. The exit stage.

The career begins with the encounter stage, which involves receiving and understanding the diagnosis and adjusting to the impact of the diagnosis while learning new care skills and making lifestyle changes. The middle stage, or working stage, is the endurance stage. During this stage, the heaviest workload is common as routines become established. The final stage is the exit stage, in which decisions, activities, and adjustments are made in association with the end of life.

Each stage is associated with different experiences. The encounter stage involves caregiver grief for the loss of the loved one. During this stage, the need for information and the development of new skills for providing adequate personal care can be overwhelming. Educational and caregiving classes and one-to-one teaching by nurses are important.

In the endurance stage, signs of both mental and physical stress are apparent as caregivers struggle through years of caregiving burdens. During this time, caregivers often have more health problems, use more prescription medications, limit social activities, take fewer vacations than before, visit less with friends, and have fewer opportunities to attend church or engage in other meaningful activities. Generally, caregivers experience a lessening of their quality of life during this stage.

Finally, in the exit stage, some caregiver responsibilities decrease as the demented patient is admitted to a health care facility and death approaches. Looking at the needs of caregivers as a continuum of stages can help staff determine nursing interventions along the way.

Caregivers can also move through stages of acceptance throughout the course of their family members' illness. The first stage is denial, which is seen as disbelief, trying to minimize the diagnosis of AD, thereby avoiding the implications associated with it. The next stage is resistance, during which caregivers speculate that the disease will not "get" to them. Resistance is particularly apparent in caregivers who have always had good health. Next is affirmation, in which caregivers accept help and begin to discuss their feelings more openly. It is during this stage that nurses may be able to help caregivers address difficulties in adjusting to the disease. From affirmation, caregivers move to acceptance. During this stage, they come to terms with the illness and move on with daily life in a matter-of-fact way. Finally, growth and healing occur as a new sense of hope and determination arises. Caregivers begin to talk about the future beyond the death of the person with AD. Many caregivers experience a sense of having learned and grown from their situation. Not everyone experiences all of these stages or experiences them in the sequence described here.

CARE OF CAREGIVERS

Caregiver education is essential and improves patient outcomes. It is important to understand what has been tried and what has been successful in the education of both family and staff caregivers. One positive outcome of educational programs in long-term care facilities (LTCFs) is a reduction in the need for antipsychotics in AD patients.

The majority of the time, informal care is provided by family members. To these family members, caregiving is a profession. Much of the care of AD patients is provided by unpaid health care and home-maker services. Most caregivers receive no assistance, work an average of 20 hours per week, and put in more than 5 years of service. Many of these individuals also work at part-time or full-time jobs. The unpaid care of AD patients totals between 115 and 288 billion dollars a year, in both health care and homemaker services (Koppel, 2002).

As is most often the case, there comes a time when the family must relinquish home care. They either lack the resources to provide 24-hour care or are no longer able to manage problematic behaviors. At this time, families seek care from some form of nursing home or LTCF. In making the decision to place a loved one in an LTCF, two concerns arise: (1) locating the right facility and (2) managing the guilt of giving up primary responsibility for the person with AD.

Education

Care problems faced by caregivers are well documented in the research literature. Research is still ongoing about what caregivers need to know about AD and how that knowledge should be communicated to them.

Much of the stress associated with care of people with AD can be directly related to ignorance of the disease and what courses of action to take for specific problems of AD patients (Robinson, Adkisson, & Weinrich, 2001). The use of theory-based stress and coping education has provided positive outcomes for caregivers by providing information, links to resources, and role coaching. Having access to information, coaching, and knowing where to go for additional information were associated with decreased burden of providing care and decreased depression among caregivers (Hepburn, Tornatore, Center, & Ostwald, 2001).

Many studies have shown that education alone does not always have a significant impact on patient outcomes and caregiver burden. It is important to educate caregivers at appropriate times as the dis-

ease progresses and provide them with additional resources.

Short-term educational programs have been successful and are well-liked by family caregivers. These focused educational sessions assist in increasing disease-based knowledge and increase caregivers' confidence in caring for loved ones.

Nurses must recognize that although the caregiving experience might be seen as one-dimensional, it is neither all negative nor all positive. Nurses can help caregivers reframe their perceptions or consider a different meaning for the experience. Providing education and support for caregivers includes education about roles, patient safety, and community resources (Cuellar, 2002). (See Appendix B: Resources for AD Patients and Caregivers.)

COMMUNITY FACILITIES AND CAREGIVERS

Alternatives to nursing home placement were not always available to help families when caring for a demented patient became overwhelming. However, choices now exist, and nurses must be able to help families make informed decisions. Costs and specific needs, which vary depending on the stage of the illness, are usually major concerns.

Respite Care

Respite care refers to various forms of in-home help available to families, including adult day-care and short-term residential care. The providers of these services assume intermittent supervisory, personal, and nursing care responsibilities for impaired adults. Temporary help may allow a family caregiver to take a vacation or trip or to rest up and then resume caring for the patient with renewed enthusiasm. Nonprofessionals who have special training in dealing with individuals with dementia supplied through a local Alzheimer's Association chapter can provide respite care. Although there is little research to validate the effectiveness of respite care in relieving caregiver stress or burden, the Alzheimer's Association has supported and politicized government provision of respite care (George, 2001).

Respite care can also be offered in adult day-care centers designed specifically for confused people. Families can avail themselves of the services daily or several times per week. The emphasis is on keeping the individual with dementia active as long as possible. Daily fees range from $15 to $80. Nurses can assist family caregivers by becoming informed about local day-care services, especially if the services center their programs on patients with AD. If wandering is a problem, special programs should be in place to curb the behavior. Low staff-to-patient ratios and active, stimulating but calm environments should be provided. Respite care at home can be arranged through health care agencies or other community-based agencies.

Another in-home service is the provision of equipment, such as wheelchairs and walkers, by community and fraternal groups. Services such as transportation and Meals on Wheels are available to those living at home. Nurses should be aware that nonprofessionals provide most respite care. Therefore, if a patient with AD has complex needs, respite care in the home may not be advisable; home care may be needed instead. Some organizations offer financial support to families who need this type of in-home care.

Nursing homes, hospitals, and other care facilities can offer respite care for several days or weeks in an emergency or during a vacation by the caregiver. Nurses should be informed about local nursing homes and residential care facilities that offer this care. Nurses should also be familiar with both federal and state regulations on respite care, because each state may enact its own regulations and laws. An added benefit of residential respite care for patients in the advanced stages of AD is that their caregivers may then realize that it is time to arrange for long-term care in a nursing home.

Assisted Living

Foster care homes, board and care homes, assisted living facilities, and adult congregate living facilities are additional options for families of patients with AD. When a less restrictive and less intensive form of care is needed and a mix of services is required, these options provide choices (Centers for Medicare and Medicaid Services [CMS], 2000). Nurses should know if state regulations govern the type and extent of services that can be offered.

Facilities offer assisted living for patients with a wide variety of needs. In most facilities of this type, the patient or family pays a flat rate for certain contracted services, such as meals. Any additional services are paid for as needed. Nurses should be aware of facilities such as this in their area. They should find out if the services a facility advertises or promises families of patients with AD can be legally offered and are truly provided by the facility. Families should avoid facilities that charge exorbitant prices merely to "lock up" patients with dementia in a unit with few or no programs to retain the functional abilities the patients still have.

Many facilities are developing special programs for patients with dementia. Currently, little or no public funding is available for the assisted living level of care, so families often assume the financial burden. As advocates, nurses can ask questions about programming and use their position in the community to verify what is being advertised about facilities of this type. When the nurse encounters someone who has used a service or visits regularly, the nurse can get the person's opinion and recommendations. Nurses are in a unique situation to learn about community resources and become an authority on their community.

When a patient with AD needs 24-hour care and supervision, home care services for seniors, such as Home Instead Senior Care, can be a relatively inexpensive option. These professional services bring care, meal planning, housekeeping, companionship, medication reminders, and transportation to home-bound older adults; however, they do not provide nursing care per se. When people with AD advance to the point where nursing care is required, a combination of the two services is one viable option. Eventually 24-hour nursing care may be required and a nursing home may be the best or only option.

CHOOSING A NURSING HOME

In 1999, there were approximately 16,000 nursing homes in this country and 1.5 million individuals living in them (Jones, 2003). On any given day, nursing homes care for about 4.2% of, or one of every 23, Americans over age 65. At least one-half of people admitted to nursing homes have some type of dementing illness, such as AD. Many times, the choice of a nursing home is made in a crisis. Nurses can help caregivers and patients with AD consider the options in advance. The Caregiver's Checklist is a tool that can help caregivers look at future needs of patients with AD. (See Table 10-1 for a sample Caregiver's Checklist.) Caregivers may never employ the help of a nursing home, but the problems of trying to locate a good nursing home quickly are monumental. Families can end up losing money or using facilities they do not like because they did not anticipate the need.

If a caregiver has time, and the patient with AD is not hospitalized or does not need immediate placement, the caregiver can talk to the local Alzheimer's Association chapter and ask friends or relatives for suggestions. Another source of information on good nursing homes is the local library, ombudsman, or nursing home advocacy group. Caregivers must be sure, however, that survey results available in the library reflect the current condition of local nursing homes. Seeking referrals can help caregivers avoid frustration and focus their search.

Key Questions to Ask

As the search continues, caregivers can make telephone calls, which can help to eliminate some facilities. The following are key questions to ask (CMS, 2000):

1. Is the nursing home certified to participate in Medicare and Medicaid programs? And will a Medicaid or Medicare "bed" be available when it is needed?

2. What are the facility's admission requirements for residents?

3. What is the typical resident in the facility like? (For example, if the facility specializes in rehabilitation of older adults and the family needs a facility to assist in wandering then the rehabilitation facility might not be a good one.)

4. Does the nursing home require signing over of personal property or real estate in exchange for care? What charges does the basic rate not cover, such as haircuts, telephones, and television?

5. Does the facility have a waiting list, or does it have immediate vacancies?

6. Does the facility offer cultural and religious diversity or is there a facility-wide preference? What languages do the staff members speak? If the staff speaks another primary language, the resident may feel cut off or lonely.

The location of a nursing home is another consideration. Many elderly caregivers prefer not to drive at night, so having their family member in a facility near their own home is important to them.

Quality of Life in Nursing Homes

In the 1980s, researchers recognized problems with the quality of life in many nursing homes in the United States. Consequently, nursing home reforms went into effect in 1990 that were designed to enhance both the quality of care and the quality of life for residents in nursing homes. In the mid-1990s, enforcement regulations were enacted that provided

TABLE 10-1: CAREGIVER'S CHECKLIST

This checklist is designed to serve as a reminder of medical, legal and financial concerns caregivers will need to consider when a loved one has been diagnosed with Alzheimer's disease.

Medical
☐ Referral to a physician (neurologist, psychiatrist or geriatrician) knowledgeable about Alzheimer's disease.
☐ Complete diagnostic work-up.
☐ Discussion with the physician regarding what is happening and what to expect.
☐ Regular medical checkups.
☐ Determine the individual's current level of functioning.
☐ Know patient's medical history, medications and dosages.

Caregiving
☐ Learn as much as you can about the disease and caregiving techniques specifically helpful in coping with this disease.
☐ Identify/attend local support group meetings.
☐ Attend caregiver training.
☐ Develop knowledge of community resources.
☐ Develop caregiving plans, including alternate plans for care of the patient in the event of your illness.
☐ Determine what you are emotionally/physically able to do. Arrange for additional assistance through family, volunteers, respite care (home health care, adult day care or short-term respite care in a facility).
☐ Make the home safe for the patient (accident-proofing).
☐ Schedule regular medical care for yourself, reporting any changes in your health to your physician.

Legal
☐ Determine if the patient needs assistance to manage his or her legal/financial affairs.
☐ Consult an Elder Law Attorney knowledgeable in issues such as Medicaid, Medicare, Guardianships, Estate Planning, Trusts and Advanced Directives. (The Florida Bar at 1(800)342-8060 can give you a list of Elder Law attorneys.)
☐ Contact attorney for advice regarding:
  • Durable Power of Attorney
  • Health Care Surrogate Power of Attorney
  • Living Will
  • Will
  • Trusts
  • Guardianship
☐ If documents have been prepared previously, know location and check that they are up to date with current state laws.
Financial
☐ Someone should assume the responsibility for:
  • Checking Account (bill payments)
  • Savings Account
  • Other Assets (Money Market, Stocks, Bonds, CDs)
  • Real Estate and other property (location of deeds)
  • Safety Deposit Box — Co-signer for box access (location of box and keys)
  • Security Box or home safe (location and key combination.)
☐ Review and determine the location of all insurance policies (Medical, Disability, House, Car, Long Term Care, Life Insurance, VA.)
☐ Check for Waiver of Premium Clause on insurance policies.
☐ Investigate patient's eligibility for financial assistance programs (see Section IV).
☐ Determine the amount and source of all monthly income. Are any checks (Social Security, Retirement, etc.) sent direct deposit?
☐ If the patient is receiving Social Security, do you want to be designated as the Representative Payee?
Funeral/Burial Arrangements
☐ Know previously made arrangements for cemetery lot, funeral, etc.
☐ Are wishes known regarding burial/cremation?
☐ Autopsy arrangements.

Other
☐ Driving (You must judge when the patient can no longer safely operate a motor vehicle.)
☐ ID Bracelet for Alzheimer's disease patient, particularly if wandering becomes a problem.

Note. Reprinted with permission from "Caregiver's Checklist," by Area Agency on Aging of Pasco-Pinellas, Inc., n.d. Retrieved May 16, 2004 from http://www.agingcarefl.org/caregiver/alzheimers/checklist

for increasing monetary penalties for failure to comply with federal regulations for nursing homes.

Each nursing home has an unannounced survey every 9 to 15 months conducted by the designated state agency. The most frequently cited deficiencies are food sanitation, comprehensive assessments, comprehensive care planning, hazard-free environment, pressure ulcers, physical restraints, housekeeping, dignity, and accident prevention. Federal law requires the disclosure of information about nursing homes that have not met minimum standards.

Caregivers should visit several nursing homes, ideally more than once. At least one visit to each home should be made in the late morning or at noontime so they can observe whether residents are out of bed and whether a meal is being served. Visiting on a weekend provides good information on the staffing ratio. Preparing and serving meals are two of the most important functions provided by nursing home staff. Caregivers should take the time to observe serving of a meal. They should look at how residents are assisted with eating, how special adaptive equipment is used, and how much time is allowed for residents to eat. For patients with AD, cueing and suggestions by staff for recalling lost abilities such as how to use utensils are important. Caregivers should ask to sample the food and should observe whether residents appear to be enjoying the meal.

If the residents of a nursing home are in physical restraints, representatives of the facility should be asked about the home's philosophy on using restraints and about what activities and rehabilitation are available to keep residents free from restraints. The use of both physical and chemical restraints is strictly limited by federal regulations. A restraint cannot be used because of lack of staff and must be ordered by a physician. When a medication is used, staff personnel must monitor the behaviors that justified the use of the chemical restraint and must make a record of any side effects.

While visiting nursing homes, caregivers should talk to residents and staff members. Questions to ask include: what do the residents and staff members like about their home; what would they change if they could; and what do they do if they dislike something and to whom should they talk about their dislikes? The answers to these questions can provide valuable insight into the quality of life in the home. After touring various homes, talking to residents and staff, and observing the conditions of the home, caregivers can form their own impression. Caregivers should trust their own instincts and perceptions.

SPECIAL CARE UNITS FOR PATIENTS WITH DEMENTIA

Before a patient with AD is admitted to a nursing home, it is essential to inquire about the environment and systems in place in the nursing home to support patients with dementia. Table 10-2 lists common concerns about the care of nursing home residents with dementia. Placing confused residents with alert and oriented, frail elderly residents can lead to confrontations between demented patients and other residents, staff members, and family and can lead to the tendency to use physical and chemical restraints on the AD residents for safety and peace (Ronch, 1987).

Special Care Units (SCUs) have been developed to address the care issues of people with dementia and to meet their special needs. The literature suggests that SCUs facilitate interaction between people with dementia and their new living space. As compared to nursing homes, SCUs have been found to offer a more individualized care setting with more activation and supervision and to be more relationship oriented (Ronch, 1987; Zingmark, Sandman, & Norberg, 2002).

The literature on the effectiveness of SCUs for AD patients is controversial. In the late 1980s, some people argued that patient outcomes improved by

TABLE 10-2: FREQUENTLY CITED COMPLAINTS AND CONCERNS ABOUT THE CARE PROVIDERS FOR NURSING HOME RESIDENTS WITH DEMENTIA

- Dementia in nursing home residents often is not carefully or accurately diagnosed and sometimes is not diagnosed at all.

- Acute and chronic illnesses, depression, and sensory impairments that can exacerbate cognitive impairment in individuals with dementia are frequently not diagnosed or treated.

- There is a pervasive sense of nihilism about nursing home residents with dementia; that is, there is a general feeling among nursing home administrators and staff that nothing can be done for these residents.

- Nursing home staff members frequently are not knowledgeable about dementia or effective methods of caring for residents with dementia. They generally are not aware of effective methods of responding to behavioral symptoms in residents with dementia.

- Psychotropic medications are used inappropriately for residents with dementia, particularly to control behavioral symptoms.

- Physical restraints are used inappropriately for residents with dementia, particularly to control behavioral symptoms.

- The basic needs of residents with dementia, such as hunger, thirst, and pain relief, sometimes are not met because the individuals cannot identify or communicate their needs, and nursing home staff members may not anticipate the needs.

- The level of stimulation and noise in many nursing homes is confusing for residents with dementia.

- Nursing homes generally do not provide activities that are appropriate for residents with dementia.

- Nursing homes generally do not provide enough exercise and physical movement to meet the needs of residents with dementia.

- Nursing homes do not provide enough continuity in staff and daily routines to meet the needs of residents with dementia.

- Nursing home staff members do not have enough time or flexibility to respond to the individual needs of residents with dementia.

- Nursing home staff members encourage dependency in residents with dementia by performing personal care functions, such as bathing and dressing, for them instead of allowing and assisting the residents to perform these functions themselves.

- The physical environment of most nursing homes is too "institutional" and not "home-like" enough for residents with dementia.

- Most nursing homes do not provide cues to help residents find their way.

- Most nursing homes do not provide appropriate space for residents to wander.

- Most nursing homes do not make use of design features that could support residents' independent functioning.

- The needs of families of residents with dementia are not met in many nursing homes.

Note. Adapted from *Surveyor's Guidebook on Dementia* (Pub. No. 386-897/33457) by Health Care Financing Administration, 1997. Washington, DC: U.S. Government Printing Office.

segregating demented patients. This segregation also improved family and staff satisfaction and improved the stay of nondemented patients (Maas, Specht, Weiler, Buckwalter, & Turner, 1998; Ronch, 1987). In the late 1990s, however, some of the same authors found little difference in the rate of functional decline by segregating the AD patients and even suggested that some LTCFs use the SCUs as ploys to increase revenues (Maas, Swanson, Specht, & Buckwalter, 1994; Maas et al., 1998). In 2001,

Gerdner and Beck conducted a survey in Arkansas. They found only 24 SCUs in the 147 LTCFs in the state, and none of these met the state codes.

Most units have approximately 30 to 34 residents (40% in single-occupancy and 60% in double-occupancy rooms). At least five characteristics make dementia units special:

1. Staff selection and training — staff members in the SCUs reported less stress as compared with those who worked in traditional units

2. Activity programs developed for patients with dementia

3. Programs for the families of patients with dementia

4. Environmental alterations, including décor and reduced use of chemical and physical restraints

5. Admission criteria that specify patients must have AD or some other dementia.

(Gerdner, Buckwalter, & Reed, 2002).

Although the literature is mixed on the effectiveness of SCUs, the important notion is that a facility should be thoroughly analyzed before a person with AD is placed into that environment. It is not always the environmental structures that provide a good life for people with AD; rather, it is reflected by the caregivers who are associated with that facility and the things they do should exemplify nursing care that promotes a meaningful living situation in the midst of dying.

FINANCIAL AND LEGAL IMPLICATIONS OF CAREGIVING

Caregivers make tremendous financial sacrifices to care for patients with AD. As dedicated and determined as most caregivers are, the burden is often too much to bear alone. Help for caregivers is fragmented, not always available, and sometimes expensive. For most caregivers, finding ways to finance nursing home care is a major concern. Four basic methods are used:

1. Personal resources: About 25% of nursing home residents pay for their care from their own resources (Jones, 2003). When their resources are depleted, they apply for Medicaid.

2. Private insurance: Purchasing long-term care insurance is another option. If this option is being considered, caregivers should check the length of time that preexisting conditions are excluded and, of course, whether the insurance has any permanent exclusions for AD.

3. Medicaid.

4. Medicare.

Medicare and Medicaid, the major government reimbursement programs for the care of older people, spend most of their dollars on nursing homes and hospitals. Much less Medicare spending goes to cover in-home costs of care. Medicare is designed to cover acute care, not long-term care (Mace & Rabins, 2001). Medicare may pay for at least part of nursing home costs for up to 100 days per benefit period for patients who require intensive rehabilitation or skilled nursing care (Pouncey, 2003).

In September 2001, the Centers for Medicare and Medicaid Services (CMS), formerly the HCFA, issued a program memorandum prohibiting the automatic denial of claims for medical services based solely on a diagnosis of dementia. The policy clarification corrected the serious problem of payment denials that occurred solely because the individual had dementia. The assumption has been that people with dementia could not benefit from various interventions. Medicare now covers evaluations, management, and therapies, if they are reasonable and necessary. One example is payment for physical therapy gait training for a patient with dementia and an unsteady gait. A convenient appeal process is available to residents in nursing homes who think they have been wrongly denied Medicare benefits.

Qualifying for Medicaid benefits can be frustrating and complicated, but Medicaid can pay for nursing facility care when more than room and board, but not skilled care, is required. However, the patient must meet income and resource eligibility guidelines. Financial criteria vary from state to state, so nurses should help caregivers contact the local state Medicaid agency as early as possible. Recent changes in Medicaid law related to "spousal impoverishment" provisions protect a certain amount of income and resources for a spousal caregiver still living at home when the partner needs nursing home care.

Community agencies can also lessen the financial burden on caregivers. Caregivers can contact the local Area Agency on Aging (listed in the telephone book) or their state's department of elder affairs on aging. These agencies can refer caregivers to community resources or to the information hotlines of local age-related services. The Alzheimer's Association and local churches are other sources for community support services. See Appendix B for online resources for professional and family caregivers. Financial planners, accountants, and tax professionals can help caregivers make prudent decisions about money management.

Caregivers should also consult an attorney about legal strategies before nursing home care is needed for a patient with AD. Discussions should include legal arrangements, such as joint checking and savings accounts, power of attorney agreements, and guardianships or trusts.

PATIENT SELF-DETERMINATION ACT

When the Patient Self-Determination Act went into effect in 1991, it ensured that individuals have the final say about how much and what kind of medical treatment they receive. Almost 50% of nursing home residents have completed some form of advanced directive, such as a living will or durable power of attorney for health care (Bottrell, 2001). Most states now require that health care facilities ask each patient if they have an advanced directive and must record the patient's response. Additionally, facilities and agencies must educate their staff, patients, and the public about having and implementing advanced directives. Simply having an advanced directive is not sufficient to ensure that the individual's wishes will be respected.

Laws on drawing up and implementing living wills vary from state to state. Nurses should familiarize themselves with the laws of the state in which they practice. In general, a living will outlines a person's wishes for initializing and maintaining medical treatments and nutrition in the future. For a person who becomes demented, the living will assists the designated health care surrogate or proxy to make decisions based on the person's wishes. Many people have voiced specific desires about the use of feeding tubes or cardiopulmonary resuscitation.

By planning ahead, patients with AD can discuss their wants and desires with their caregivers, and together with their caregivers can prepare a durable power of attorney for health care. Many states have preprinted forms that are easy to use and readily available. Caregivers should not use a standard power of attorney form, because this form is related to managing property, not making decisions about health care.

As dementia progresses, the designated person can make all the health care decisions in collaboration with health care providers. When a person with AD is dying, the decisions of the designated person, based on knowledge of the demented patient's wishes, take legal precedence over the decisions of others involved with the patient. Families sometimes find it difficult to face these decisions. Nurses occupy a unique place in offering guidance and support to family caregivers and to patients with AD. They can encourage caregivers and patients to discuss these issues and plan ahead.

Attorneys and the Alzheimer's Association can help demented patients and their families plan for the eventuality of needing someone to act in the demented patient's best interests. Some states specify by law which close relatives can make medical decisions without a guardianship. If needed, a petition may be filed with the court to request a guardian of the person with dementia. Making formal arrangements can prevent serious problems for families when disputes or conflicts occur.

CAREGIVER HEALTH

Taking care of an AD patient who needs full-time supervision and care puts caregivers at high risk for burnout. The vigilance associated with the care of persons with AD can bring on depression, increased stress, physical illness, and frustration in caregivers. These can all lead to feelings of inadequacy, which in turn can lead to suffering by both the person with AD and the caregiver.

Common Problems

Common problems among caregivers are depression, heightened stress, physical illness, and frustration. The single strongest predictor of impaired well-being of the caregiver is emotional lability (Croog, Sudilovsky, Burleson, & Baume, 2001; Wisniewski et al., 2003). The higher the level of destructive behavior in the person with AD, the higher the level of depression and anxiety and the lower the level of positive well-being in the caregiver. Caregivers often feel unappreciated, mainly because people with AD cannot appreciate what their caregivers are going through. Social isolation is also common among caregivers. Friends and other family members drift away as AD progresses. Caring for a person with AD is not just a short-term problem; remember that this can go on for many years. These conditions often lead to depression in the caregiver.

Emotional Health

The majority of caregivers indicate that they and their families experience emotional stress and depression, although stress varies according to the phase of the illness. Depression can manifest as a feeling of sadness and discouragement. Distinguishing between depression, worry, grief, and helplessness is difficult. Caregivers can feel apathetic, listless, irritable, or anxious, and the feeling can last day after day and week after week (Mace & Rabins, 2001). Table 10-3 is a tool that can be used with caregivers to help quantify their level of anxiety.

Nurses can be the most important people in caregivers lives. Nurses provide care to their loved ones and care to them. Caregivers often seek out nurses for education and personal physical and psychological assistance. Nurses in this situation should focus on the caregiver's emotional health by asking:

- How are you doing?
- What are your plans for next week or next holiday?
- Has the patient done anything unusual lately?
- Do family members come to visit you much?
- Are you experiencing any pains, headaches, or digestive problems?
- How is your family or spouse?
- Is there anything new that you are worried about?
- When was the last time you did some gardening, went out to dinner or lunch with a friend, worked on your hobby, or read a book?
- What time did you go to bed last night and what time did you first awaken?

Observe for nonverbal cues of depression, anxiety, or stress, including:

- excessive head shaking or crying and hand wringing
- gain or loss of weight
- excessively tired look

TABLE 10-3: THE ANXIETY SCALE

This questionnaire is designed to measure how much anxiety you are currently feeling. It is not a test, so there are no right or wrong answers. Answer each item as carefully and as accurately as you can by placing a number beside each one as follows:

1 = Rarely or none of the time

2 = A little of the time

3 = Some of the time

4 = A good part of the time

5 = Most or all of the time

_____1.   I feel calm.

_____2.   I feel tense.

_____3.   I feel suddenly scared for no reason.

_____4.   I feel nervous.

_____5.   I use tranquilizers or antidepressants to cope with my anxiety.

_____6.   I feel confident about the future.

_____7.   I am free from senseless or unpleasant thoughts.

_____8.   I feel afraid to go out of my house alone.

_____9.   I feel relaxed and in control of myself.

_____10.   I have spells of terror or panic.

_____11.   I feel afraid in open spaces or in the streets.

_____12.   I feel afraid I will faint in public.

_____13.   I am comfortable traveling on buses, subways, or trains.

_____14.   I feel nervousness or shakiness inside.

_____15.   I feel comfortable in crowds, such as shopping or at a movie.

_____16.   I feel comfortable when I am left alone.

_____17.   I rarely feel afraid without good reason.

_____18.   Due to my fears, I unreasonably avoid certain animals, objects, or situations.

_____19.   I get upset easily or feel panicky unexpectedly.

_____20.   My hands, arms, or legs shake or tremble.

_____21.   Due to my fears, I avoid social situations whenever possible.

_____22.   I experience sudden attacks of panic that catch me by surprise.

_____23.   I feel generally anxious.

_____24.   I am bothered by dizzy spells.

_____25.   Due to my fears, I avoid being alone whenever possible.

Note. From "Clinical Anxiety Scale. University of Georgia School of Social Work" by B. Thyer, 1986. In K. Corcoran & J. Fischer (Eds.), *Measures for Clinical Practice: A Source Book* (4th ed.) (p. 187). New York. Reprinted with permission.

- inability to listen to the speaker (part of participating in a conversation).

Support of Family Members and Caregivers

The initial sadness or grief that occurs with diagnosis of AD is later replaced by myriad emotions. Unfortunately, sadness and grief can return upon transferring the patient to an LTCF. The family can feel they have failed the person with AD. Upon admission to a facility, nurses need to remember this fact and provide emotional support to family members. Remind the family that it now takes a staff of nurses and support personnel who take shifts around the clock, 7 days a week, to do the job they have been doing at home. Regrettably, nurses must also remind the family that no matter who provides the services or how good these services are, AD will progress relentlessly and the patient's condition will continue to deteriorate until the patient dies from either a consequence of AD or from another illness.

"An important aspect of family support is acknowledgment that the wish for the victim's death may be the ultimate expression of love as well as a wish for relief from the pain of observing its process. Families must be helped to anticipate death and learn to live with the mixture of joy and rage at the prolongation of the dying process. Grief and mourning seem never ending" (Hurley & Volicer, 2002). As the disease progresses, nurses recognize that grieving accelerates. Nurses need to recognize the need for and benefit of services from a bereavement counselor.

The majority of family members remain involved in care of AD patients after admitting loved ones to LTCFs. Just because a loved one has been institutionalized does not mean that the level of stress experienced by the caregiver is reduced.

Another common reaction related to caregiving is anger. The caregiver may be angry at what has happened to him or her, angry that life has changed, angry with others who cannot or do not help, angry for being trapped in this situation and, finally, angry at the person who is sick because of the person's irritating behavior. Financial worries and family duties are two common contributors to anger against the AD patient. It is important for nurses to help family caregivers differentiate between being angry at the patient's behaviors and being angry with the patient. The behaviors can be aggravating, but they are not aimed at the caregiver personally and are part of the dementing illness.

Nurses must be aware of the potential for violence in caregiving situations. Most violence occurs when the caregiver is the patient's spouse; this may be related to cultural norms of violence toward spouses. The exact nature and dynamics of violence in a caregiving relationship are not known. One study found that a poor premorbid relationship, caregiver anxiety, and the perception of not receiving help were strongly associated with physical abuse (Compton, Flanagan, & Gregg, 1997).

Interventions for Caregivers

How much psychosocial support should nurses provide or do caregivers need? Support of caregivers may become more important once a loved one is institutionalized. The caregiver may now experience feelings of guilt, grief, anger, and depression. Anxiety may now develop concerning the quality of care given at the institution.

Support Groups

Geriatric nurses have come to recognize that many caregivers live lives with a roller coaster of emotions, and interventions need to be developed that meet individual caregiver needs. Support groups are recommended to help address these feelings and concerns. Social support groups can provide the coping mechanisms necessary to manage life stressors (Larrimore, 2003). Group support can help caregivers find ways to get help, discover new ways of relating to their family member with dementia, and find new ways to cope with the problems they encounter.

Even after AD patients are placed in LTCFs, caregivers benefit from participation in support groups. The outcome of participation in a support group is a reduction in stress levels of the caregiver, which can have a positive impact on the person with AD.

Subject matter of support group meetings or community resources should vary, considering the many different needs of the participant family members. When considering joining a group, family members should survey groups for their specific needs. Topics such as nutrition, research, exercise, coping strategies, finances, professional services, and selection of an LTCF should be discussed. Various speakers and methods of presentation should be utilized. Many family members feel they cannot attend meetings on a routine basis, and some prefer online support. Online support networks have been shown to benefit homebound caregivers, especially older adults and nurses, by providing support and assurance and building self-confidence. Nurses should be aware of the array of online services and recognize which sites are the most effective at providing the various types of information. (See Appendix B: Resources for AD Patients and Caregivers, for more information.)

Technology can be used to provide support to caregivers and increase the quality of life for both caregivers and people with AD. Online discussion groups, email, and web-based programs are all means of linking caregivers to support systems. Telecommunication systems facilitate family caregivers in communicating with other family members, who may live far away or just next door; other caregivers across the country; therapists; and others at any hour of the day. The freedom of "any hour of the day" is of particular help to families caring for people with AD in their homes because caregivers are not constrained by geographics, substitute caregivers, or other incapacities.

Telecommunication is particularly helpful to enhance service delivery in rural and underserved communities. Caregivers can receive guidance, information, encouragement, and even formal training through telecommunications and can become empowered through such support (Buckwalter, Davis, Wakefield, Kienzle, & Murray, 2002; Czaja & Rubert, 2002; White & Dorman, 2003).

Although the universality of the experience of caregiving is the central theme of support groups, remember that the key to the success of support groups can depend on when and where they are offered. In the early stages of AD, support groups are more likely to be selected by and benefit caregivers. Levels of dementia in the person with AD, levels of caregiver stress and time, caregiver goals, and individual caregiver learning styles help to determine the success of such programs.

Groups can be located through the Alzheimer's Association or listings in newspapers. People in support groups for families of Alzheimer's patients know what others are going through. Grief, bizarre behavior, exhaustion, and frustration are common experiences for all types of caregivers. Minority cultures may find it more difficult to find a support group with which they feel comfortable. Nurses can encourage caregivers to seek out established organizations and can assist in setting up groups in the community that meet the caregivers' special needs.

Professional Caregiver Support and Education

Research on caregivers has focused on what happens to both family caregivers and nursing care staff (Gwyther, 2001). Investigators have examined the effectiveness of care techniques taught in educational and group settings. Earlier studies examined the burden on family caregivers, and now research is beginning to scrutinize the stress or burden leading to burnout put on professional caregivers (nurses and nursing assistants) who care for patients with AD.

The extent of knowledge of AD among health care providers remains limited, even despite the proliferation of research and information on AD and the increasing number of individuals with AD. To develop an educational program for health care providers, it is first essential to identify what staff members currently know. Sadly, studies have shown that educational programs do not reach those working directly with AD patients. Historically, nurses have received very little education on AD or the care of AD patients and their families in their programs.

The importance of education of nursing staff is demonstrated by a classic research study by Hagen and Sayers (1995). These researchers studied the incidence of physical aggression by AD patients against staff and the effects of an educational program directed at this behavior on staff and patients. The educational program consisted of 30-minute modules. The first addressed the dementia of AD, including how memory loss created stress in the AD patient and how the stress was manifested as aggression. The second module addressed preventing aggression through comfort measures, resident safety, and individual patient sense of control and pleasure. The last session reviewed effective nursing staff responses to physical aggression displayed by the person with AD. After the sessions, reported incidences of aggression by residents dropped by 50%.

Nurses have a major responsibility in learning about diseases and educating families and other health care providers. Nurses must communicate what they know about AD to family members and staff to assist in the reduction of caregiver burden. They must remain abreast of the most recent and pertinent advances in AD (Hepburn et al., 2001).

Education of caregivers can be a positive source of changing perceptions about AD. Research continues to evaluate why recipients of educational programs do not consistently change their behavior or use what they have learned. Some areas under investigation relate directly to working conditions. Low wages, poor benefits, and minimal training have traditionally been the experience of nursing home workers and certified nursing assistants, the people who give 80% to 90% of the hands-on care

(Kerley & Turnbull, 1998). For professional caregivers, burnout is a process they become accustomed to as a result of psychological, physical, and emotional job stressors. Signs can include:

- frequent tardiness or absenteeism
- feeling overwhelmed at the thought of going to work
- a feeling of failure
- resentment toward supervisors, the facility, and sometimes even the residents
- a tendency to go by the book and do only the minimum.

Job satisfaction for professional caregivers depends on individual and organizational attention. Many of the same techniques taught to family caregivers help professionals as well. Taking time-outs, managing workload, and sharing concerns and ideas can be beneficial. The response of caregivers to their tasks and effective interventions for demented patients are important for nurses and can make a difference in the lives of all caregivers. More research is needed in these areas.

Universal pitfalls of caregiving for AD patients, which can be apparent in nursing staff as well as in family caregivers, may include:

- not allowing the patient to do as much as he or she is capable of doing
- always putting the needs of the patient first
- trying to protect the patient by limiting his or her activities
- using reason or logic to assure the patient
- holding expectations for the patient that are unrealistic.

Not every family caregiver, or every nurse helping a caregiver, faces the same problems. The nature and extent of the problems encountered are related to the signs and symptoms of the disease that occur, the personality of the caregiver, and the personality of the person who has AD (Gwyther, 2001)

Caregiver Coping

How can the caregiver cope? Nurses, family members, and current caregivers can watch for the warning signs of burnout. Watch nonverbal cues and ask the following questions:

- Does the caregiver, have trouble getting organized?

- Does the caregiver cry for no reason?

- Is the caregiver short-tempered?

- Does the caregiver feel numb and emotionless?

- Are everyday tasks getting harder to accomplish?

- Does the caregiver feel constantly pressed for time?

- Does the caregiver feel an inability to do anything right?

- Does the caregiver feel a lack of time for himself or herself?

- Does the caregiver have aches and pains?

- Does the caregiver increasingly demonstrate anger or sarcasm?

- Does the caregiver constantly worry or show anxiety?

- Does the caregiver experience headaches?

- Does the caregiver have feelings of hopelessness?

- Does the caregiver show lack of emotional affect?

- Does the AD patient strike out at the caregiver? When an AD patient becomes violent, it is generally a sign that the caregiver is suffering from stress or burnout. Look for bruises and scratches on the caregiver as a sign of the AD person's aggression.

- Is the AD patient incontinent? Fecal incontinence is especially difficult to deal with for many caregivers, and it might just be enough to create a crisis that leads to abuse.

- Are social workers involved in the care of the AD patient? This involvement can be a sign that something has changed with the AD patient or the caregiver that has caused a crisis.

If the answer is "yes" to any of the above questions, some degree of caregiver burnout may be present or the caregiver may be heading for it.

Reducing Caregiver Burnout

The following is a list of suggestions that can make caregivers' days easier and help to decrease burnout:

1. Teach the caregiver coping strategies soon after the diagnosis of AD.

2. Stay informed. Learn as much as possible about dementia. Behavioral management becomes more effective with more knowledge.

3. Get enough rest. Exhaustion amplifies the pressures faced and ability to cope. Set aside the time caregivers feel they need for rest, and upon retiring do not replay the day's events; problems are not generally solved at bedtime. Strenuous activity during the day assists in promoting sleep.

4. Eat well. Regular, well-balanced meals help to maintain sufficient energy levels to carry out the daily routine as well as maintain or increase resistance to illness. Skipping meals can lead to vitamin deficiencies that deplete strength and contribute to exhaustion.

5. Learn to recognize how you, as a caregiver, respond to stress. Do you get angry, cry, withdraw, or get very busy? Dealing with feelings can be stressful, but it helps to be aware of how you cope.

6. Take care of yourself. Develop a repertoire of activities that rejuvenate you enough to enable to continue. Use proactive stress-reducing rituals that work for you: swimming, walking, meditating, or anything that has a calming effect on you. Learn to delegate tasks. Know when to hire extra care workers or coordinate other family members' care of the person with AD.

7. Recognize that other family members may have

different reactions in the same circumstances.

8. Maintain meaningful friendships. Help others in your support system understand the changes as the changes appear. Confiding in them can help resolve conflicts. If a person cannot overcome being negative or depressing, avoid that person.

9. Keep the hassles small. Decide what small daily irritant you can handle today, and ignore the rest. Practice this method and it will become easier, more like a habit.

10. Use common sense and humor. These are your best tools. Share your experiences with other members of your family and with other families of patients with AD. In a group, what seemed sad or frustrating may seem humorous. Let it.

11. Know what local services are available from the Alzheimer's Association, area aging agencies, Council on Aging, local universities, and other groups that offer services. This will help in the event of an emergency or another problem. Universities may offer conferences or participation in research that generally provides free in-home services.

Changes in appetite and sleep can occur in family caregivers. Being depressed is painful. Time spent alone participating in satisfying activities or in a support group may be the answer. Counseling may relieve the depression. At other times, medical help from a physician or nurse practitioner may be necessary. For some caregivers, feelings of discouragement may go beyond the typical feelings of sadness, and antidepressant medications may be required.

ABUSE OR NEGLECT OF THE AD PATIENT

Abuse and neglect are serious and prevalent problems for older people in general in private homes, the community, and institutions. It is estimated that 10% of adults over age 65 have been vic-

tims of abuse or neglect. Elderly female patients are more at risk for all types of abuse than elderly males. Adults over age 80 have the highest level of risk. Abuse or neglect involves both sexes, well and frail, and occurs in all racial, ethnic, and socioeconomic groups. Ignorance, disability, poverty, limited access to care, and poor caregiver training all contribute to abuse or neglect.

Abuse always involves specific actions against the person that knowingly cause harm. Neglect involves failure to provide adequate care in the form of treatments, care, and goods or services, that can then lead to harm. Neglect and abuse can be physical, emotional, sexual, or psychological; abandonment, financial exploitation, and self-neglect are also considered forms of abuse.

Cognitive impairment, such as dementia, and shared living arrangements are risk factors that place older adults at the highest level of risk for mistreatment. Extreme psychological and physical demands placed on caregivers of people with AD (who may be aggressive, disruptive, or hostile toward caregivers) predispose AD patients to mistreatment by stressed or fatigued caregivers. With increased stress or depression and other demands of life and family, the risk of abuse or neglect of the AD patient increases. Caregiver behavior may lead to abuse. Abuse can occur when the caregiver reaches a crisis point in the care of a person with AD. When a nurse notices a caregiver exhibiting signs of stress or burnout, increased stress on the caregiver may lead to abuse, he or she should suggest placement of the patient with AD in an alternative care setting.

Case Study

The following case is an example of possible abuse. It takes place in an LTCF; however, this situation could occur in any setting, even a private home.

Mrs. Jensen is an 84-year-old woman with moderately advanced AD who has remained fairly active, visiting with family, moving about the SCU, participating in unit activities, and still communicating with staff and other residents. She has lived in a nursing home for 2 years and, as one would anticipate, her cognition is steadily deteriorating. She is experiencing ambulation problems, as seen in her unsteady gait. She has been known to fall but never sustains more than a couple of bruises. You have just returned from a 2-week vacation and go in to do your morning assessment of Mrs. Jensen. You find her in a fetal position, not responding to your presence and resisting your attention. You quickly review the last couple of weeks entries in her chart and find that she has lost 5 pounds over the last month, but there are no other indications of any illnesses or reasons for this acute change in Mrs. Jensen.

You are able, after some coaxing, to do a physical exam on Mrs. Jensen and are startled by your findings. The assessment of her major organs and vitals signs revealed no abnormalities, but when you perform your exam you find several bruises on her chest and anterior aspect of her arms. Some of the bruises on her anterior arms are purple, and the bruises on her chest are yellow-green. You quietly and reassuringly question Mrs. Jensen about these bruises but, because of her dementia, she is unable to tell you about the bruises or what happened to her. After comforting Mrs. Jensen, and urging her to get up and move about, you return to speak with the staff. In response to your questioning, one member of the nursing staff states that Mrs. Jensen fell or bumped herself as a result of her unsteady gait. What do you think?

Signs of Abuse

Physical abuse can be difficult to detect because of the similarities in age-related physical changes and physical abuse signs: bruising, weight loss, depression, and even fractures from falls. How does a nurse decide if these signs and symptoms are evidence of abuse?

Several factors point toward abuse in the case of Mrs. Jensen. She has had a significant change in her physical, cognitive, and psychological status. In addition to these functional changes, there is physical evidence of abuse.

Although bruising is certainly a common phenomenon among nursing home residents, Mrs. Jensen's case raises suspicion for a number of reasons:

- The location of the bruising is unusual; it is difficult to bump the anterior aspect of one's arm.

- The bruising may reflect marks that result when a resident is grabbed too hard.

- The fact that the bruises varied in color indicate that they were not likely inflicted at the same time.

Neglect is another sign of abuse in elders. It is an act of omission that leads to pain or injury. Signs of neglect may be very difficult to distinguish from signs of unavoidable outcomes, particularly in patients who are severely debilitated and may be in the terminal stages of life. In fact, the signs may be the same: contractures, pressure ulcers, malnutrition, and dehydration. When these signs are present, the nurse must investigate to rule out neglect as a cause (Mosqueda, Heath, & Burnight, 2001).

Risk Factors for Abuse

Various factors can make an individual vulnerable to abuse. Residents who have combative, aggressive, or resistive behaviors are more likely to be physically abused by staff. Neglect is due to multiple, interacting factors. Residents without advocates (those who are unable to speak for themselves and have no family or visitors) may be more prone to neglect. Residents who are more dependent and more difficult to care for, and therefore require more assistance, may be at higher risk as well. Regardless of how difficult a patient is considered, no resident within any setting should ever endure maltreatment from those whose jobs it is to provide appropriate care (DeLaine, Scammell, & Heaslip, 2002; Mosqueda, Heath, & Burnight, 2001).

Abuser Profiles

Two types of abusers can be found in our communities: "reactive abusers" and "sadistic abusers."

Caregivers who are unable to control their impulses (for example, when a person with AD resists getting undressed and the caregiver strikes the resident) are reactive abusers. In contrast, a sadistic abuser methodically and repeatedly abuses a person with AD. Other factors that are extrinsic to the person with AD that may contribute to abusive behavior include physical or emotional exhaustion and a lack of knowledge or understanding of behavioral problems on the part of the caregiver. Inadequate staffing ratios, poor teamwork and communication, and staff burnout may also lead to neglect in LTCFs (Mosqueda, Heath, & Burnight, 2001).

If abuse or neglect is suspected, it must be reported to the state regulatory body. The state investigates and intervenes as necessary. This may be in the form of additional education of the caregiver or through an alternative care setting for the AD patient.

TRAVELING WITH AD PATIENTS

When considering a trip with a person with AD, caregivers are presented with special challenges. Traveling with people with AD can be very difficult and frustrating if not planned thoroughly in advance. Caregivers need to keep in mind how changes in environment (location, time zones, noise) affect someone with AD. They also must keep in mind that the normal cues that help keep the patient in touch with their reality are not present and unfamiliar places do not have those same cues. The outcome can be fear or anger when those cues are missing.

The old adage "plan for the worst but hope for the best" can be true in planning a trip. Confusion will most likely worsen for the duration of the trip. Some people become agitated or violent and may even demand to go home upon arrival. If such behavior does occur, caregivers must remember that AD patients cannot control their behavior and they need to have a plan made for behavioral changes that may occur during the trip. Caregivers should be aware of the early warning signs of increased anxiety because these behaviors may be the first indicators of loss of control of emotions. Indications of increasing anxiety include statements by the person with AD about the crowds, the menu, or things going on in the environment; attempts to leave the situation; anxious statements about needing to go home or to the toilet; loss of eye contact; crying; physical illness; urinary or fecal incontinence; or wanting to lie down.

Family caregivers may travel by themselves or with additional caregivers. Nurses traveling as hired caregivers for a trip should ask the following questions in preparation for the travel:

- Have all of limitations been noted?
- What is the trip location?
- What is the expected mode of travel?
- How long is the trip?
- If overnight travel is expected, is the person with AD capable of spending nights away from familiar people or things?
- Where will everyone be staying during the trip and upon arrival at the final destination?
- What activities will take place once at the final destination?
- Will there be special resources or needs during the trip?

In order to have a successful trip with limited difficulties, all caregivers, family or hired, must plan for emergencies and make sure that everyone traveling with them understands those plans. They also need to assess the traveling party's limitations and ask:

- Are they able to handle stress well?
- Are they embarrassed by the AD patient's behavior?
- Are they embarrassed to go into "opposite sex" bathrooms?

- Are they able or willing to make significant adaptations during the trip?

- Do they plan well in advance?

- Will they resist seeking help as needed?

Here are other tips to consider when planning a trip:

- Be flexible.

- Give others a copy of the itinerary.

- The process of "getting there" should be short and generally include a single destination.

- Try to stick with familiar routes or means of travel.

- When planning to travel overnight, a trial overnight trip can be very beneficial and a good indicator of the individual's limitations and planning needs.

- During the actual travel, remember to travel during the patient's best time of day.

- Use disabled citizens services.

- Stay away from large groups of people because their noise and confusion can impact behaviors by the person with AD.

- Never allow an AD patient to travel alone. Newspaper articles are full of stories about lost AD patients who thought they could travel alone or how airlines "lost" a family's loved one because the person with AD "wandered away." This should remind caregivers to never leave an AD patient alone, not even for a very short period of time, especially in unfamiliar surroundings or situations.

If the travel requires that the person with AD stay in a hotel, consider these tips that can reduce potential catastrophes:

- Ask for a large, quiet room.

- Take familiar clothes, pillows, and other items.

- Use room service for the night you arrive.

- Take night-lights.

- Be on guard for wandering.

- Allow extra time for everything.

- Provide nap times.

Airline travel can remove the time element associated with distance traveling, but it brings with it a whole host of problems. Some ideas that will reduce those potential problems include flying during the patient's best time of day. Before you leave, be sure to register with the Alzheimer's Association Safe Return Program at your destination. Make sure the patient has identification on at all times. Minimizing carry-on luggage allows the caregiver to give full attention to the person with AD. Avoid caffeine and limit fluid intake before and during the flight. Bring familiar things as distractions. Bring a tranquilizer "just-in case:" it can save even the best planned trip. Bring the AD patient's favorite snack because airlines rarely provide much more than drinks and small snacks. Plan for the arrival as part of planning the trip to help eliminate travel surprises and behavior problems. Make sure there is someone to meet you.

When airplane travel is not feasible, travel by automobile is the alternative. Consider these tips for automobile travel:

- Never leave an AD patient alone in the car.

- Plan travel activities, including pictures, games, and music.

- Prepare for spills and soiled garments.

- Bring a covered cup and straw for drinking.

- Do not plan activities for the night of arrival because the person with AD may be tired, confused, or agitated and these activities will increase the possibility of behavior problems. Adequate rest after the trip will decrease the risk.

- Keep the seat belt on and the doors locked at all times.

- Plan the itinerary well in advance and leave copies with family and friends.

- If the AD patient becomes confused or problem

behavior escalates, stop at the first available place.

• Make sure the AD patient has identification on at all times.

Family and friend's weddings are another opportunity for the person with AD to interact in social environments. It is really important to contact the host to know what to expect during the wedding. Do not let "should's" make the decision, such as "Grandpa should attend because the groom is his only grandson." If Grandpa does not handle crowds or sitting still for periods of time well, the entire wedding can be impacted and the outcome of attending can become a negative one for all concerned. Be sure that both the caregiver and the person with AD rest before and during the event and remember that lack of rest is a major contributor to agitation. Be realistic about what events to attend. If the caregiver wants to attend all events or certain events without the person with AD, it is imperative to find suitable substitutes for the primary caregiver (Hall, 2003a).

SUMMARY

Planning ahead is the best way to avoid some of the stresses of caregiving for patients with AD. Nurses offer services throughout the community to assist and support family caregivers in taking care of not only the patients but also the caregivers themselves. The concerns of family caregivers and the problems encountered by nursing staff caregivers are similar. Research is determining strategies for managing stress and techniques for successfully managing the behavioral issues of demented patients. Making choices about the available continuum of care is complicated, and nurses should be informed about the choices caregivers must make as they maneuver through financial and legal decisions.

Stress experienced by caregivers can produce negative outcomes for people with AD, such as abuse. Nurses must recognize the signs and symptoms of abuse and find ways of educating caregivers on the possibility of abuse.

Much of the stress associated with care of people with AD can be directly related to ignorance of the disease and the proper course of action to take for specific problems of AD patients. Education is the best intervention possible; support groups are also important. In the absence of formal support groups, new telecommunication systems can often provide easy access to various forms of education and support.

EXAM QUESTIONS

CHAPTER 10
Questions 91-100

91. The keys to managing the care nurses provide in nursing homes include

    a. supporting staff, managing symptoms, and creating a therapeutic environment.

    b. creating a therapeutic environment, managing behaviors, and increasing profits for LTCFs.

    c. managing symptoms, providing access to current information for caregivers, and increasing the profits for LTCs.

    d. creating a therapeutic environment, segregating specialized personnel, and managing troublesome behaviors.

92. The role of the caregiver is broken down into three stages. The most helpful nursing intervention during the 'encounter stage' would be

    a. providing support and education on caregiving.

    b. determining how the caregiver reacts to stress.

    c. finding respite care in a residential facility.

    d. assisting with hospice and end-of-life.

93. A suggestion to prevent caregiver burnout is

    a. avoid complaining to others about your situation.

    b. recognize how you respond to stress.

    c. recognize that everyone generally reacts the same in the same circumstances.

    d. avoid using humor to lighten the situation.

94. Which of the following statements is true regarding respite care?

    a. Respite provides temporary relief for caregivers.

    b. A high staff-to-patient ratio is recommended in adult day cares.

    c. Respite is only performed by skilled nursing professionals.

    d. For insurance reimbursement, respite must be provided in the home.

95. Appropriate strategies that should be employed by family caregivers prior to placement of a person with AD into an LTCF include

    a. finding the facility nearest to all family members that seems clean and cheap and visiting during later evening hours when residents are in their rooms and quiet.

    b. one visit to the facility, which is usually sufficient for the decision-making process and should be conducted early in the morning to see the morning routine.

    c. visiting a facility several times around meal times, inspecting for cleanliness and the use of restraints, and visiting with current residents.

    d. trying to visit a facility during the early daytime, visiting with the administrators of the facility, and looking at parking access and the outside grounds.

96. A correct statement about Medicare and Medicaid is

    a. Medicare is not designed to handle acute care needs.

    b. Residents in nursing homes can appeal decisions about Medicare payments for services.

    c. Medicaid financial eligibility criteria are established by the federal government.

    d. The spouse of the person attempting to qualify for Medicaid must spend all remaining money before Medicaid funds are provided.

97. The Patient Self-Determination Act requires that

    a. all terminally ill patients have advance directives.

    b. health care facilities educate staff members and patients about advance directives.

    c. all nursing home residents have some form of advance directive.

    d. spouses be allowed to make decisions for patients with AD.

98. Support groups help caregivers of patients with AD focus on

    a. the uniqueness of each person.

    b. common experiences that every caregiver encounters.

    c. how to limit the activities of the person with AD.

    d. how to explain things to a person who has AD.

99. Violence or abuse in a caregiving situation is more likely to occur when

    a. the person with AD is combative, aggressive, or resistive, and the caregiver of the person with AD is the person's spouse.

    b. there is decreased stress and depression and increased family presence.

    c. there is cognitive impairment such as dementia, and the person with AD is living alone.

    d. the person with AD is unable to speak for themselves and there are never any family or friends who visit or care for the person with AD.

100. Stephen, who has AD, lives with his sister and her husband. His sister is planning a trip with Stephen to visit another sister. The advice that would be most appropriate to provide to Stephen's sister regarding the upcoming trip is

    a. Go with a plan and do not deviate from it, even if it means several destinations along the way.

    b. Be flexible as you travel but keep the trip time to a minimum.

    c. It would be much easier to send just Stephen on a plane to the destination.

    d. Wait until the last minute to plan the trip and do it alone with Stephen.

This concludes the final examination.

APPENDIX A

THE MOSES SCALE
Multidimensional Observation Scale for Elderly Subjects

INTRODUCTION

The Multidimensional Observation Scale for Elderly Subjects (MOSES) was designed to evaluate the major aspects of functioning in elderly residential patients. The scale is appropriate for use in many settings, such as continuing care facilities, homes for the aged, nursing homes, and psychiatric facilities for older persons.

The five areas of functioning assessed by the scale are:

1. Self-care functioning (items 1 to 8)
2. Disoriented behavior (items 9 to 16)
3. Depressed or anxious mood (items 17 to 24)
4. Irritable behavior (items 25 to 32)
5. Withdrawn behavior (items 33 to 42).

INSTRUCTIONS FOR RATERS

1. READ OVER THE SCALE

Before starting to observe any residents, you should read over the 42 questions that make up the scale several times, so that you will know the types of behaviors to watch for. The best way to do this is to read over the questions once quickly, and then go through them again in more detail with a particular resident in mind.

Many of the questions include examples that should help to make the questions clearer. Also, in many of the questions, when a word referring to the number of times a behavior occurs (for example,

"Seldom" or "Often") is used, a more specific meaning for the word is given right below it. This is to help different raters to use the words in the same way. So please read these defining phrases carefully as you use the scale.

2. PERIOD OF OBSERVATION

Usually, the period of observation is 4 to 6 days. It is this period of observation that is meant in all the questions when we say "during the past week." Only the resident's daytime behaviors (those he engages in from early morning [about 7 a.m.] until he goes to bed at night [about 9 p.m.] should be considered. Note: the word "he" (rather than "he/she) is used for all residents, male or female, in the interest of saving time.

You should only rate behaviors that you have seen (or that were reported to you) during the period of observation. Behavoirs that occurred before this time, or behaviors that you think the resident might be capable of, should not be considered. Only behaviors the resident actually displays during the period of observation should be recorded. This permits you to rate how the resident is responding to present treatment and physical conditions.

During your period of observation, try to obtain information for the rating—for example, how is the resident's memory and his awareness of time; does he feel happy, depressed, or indifferent? Ask other staff about behaviors during the week that you may not have seen. For example, has the resident been crying or helping or disturbing others when you were not around?

3. RATING

For each of the 42 questions, pick the one alternative that you feel best describes the resident, and circle it. Be sure to answer all of the questions. It may seem that some of the questions are not appropriate for the residents in your institutional setting, but these questions will help distinguish your residents from residents in other settings who are functioning at a higher or lower level. These questions will eventually be very useful in discussing different levels of functioning.

1. DRESSING

On most days in the past week, the resident:

1. Initiated and completed dressing without staff supervision

2. Dressed with only minor supervision (for example, had his clothes laid out or had to be reminded to dress)

3. Partly dressed himself but needed frequent staff assistance

4. Was either totally dressed by staff or remained in bedclothes

2. BATHING (include baths and showers)

When bathing in the past week, the resident:

1. Prepared and completed his own bathing without staff supervision

2. Bathed himself with only minor supervision (for example, had towels and soap set out or water run but needed urging to get started)

3. Partly bathed himself but needed frequent staff assistance (for example, needed physical aid getting in and out of the tub, whirlpool, or shower or needed parts of his body washed or towel-dried)

4. Was totally bathed by staff (include bed baths, unless given only for practice purposes by students)

3. GROOMING (include care of hair, nails, teeth, and shaving; do not include dressing or bathing)

In the past week, the resident:

1. Completed all aspects of grooming without staff supervision

2. Looked after certain aspects of grooming independently but needed staff supervision or assistance with other aspects

3. Helped with parts of his grooming but needed frequent staff assistance with all aspects of his grooming

4. Was totally groomed by staff

4. INCONTINENCE (of either urine or feces)

In the past week, how often was the resident incontinent?

1. Not at all

2. Only during the night

3. Occasionally during the daytime

4. Frequently during the daytime (more than once a day)

5. USING THE TOILET

Most of the times that the resident did use the toilet in the past week, he:

1. Initiated going to and properly used the toilet without staff supervision

2. Used the toilet himself with only minor supervision (for example, had to be reminded to go or reminded to wipe, or occasionally made a mess on the floor)

3. Helped with his toileting but needed frequent staff assistance (for example, needed help in taking down pants, wiping, and getting on and off the toilet)

4. Was totally toileted by staff (had to be lifted on and off the toilet, including use of bed pans and staff-attended catheters or colostomies)

6. PHYSICAL MOBILITY

On most days in the past week, when getting around inside the building, the resident:

1. Walked without any assistance

2. Moved independently with mechanical assistance (for example, walked alone with a cane, walker, or crutches or propelled himself in a wheelchair)

3. Walked with the physical assistance of staff

4. Remained bedbound or chairbound (chair-bound refers to residents who were moved from the bed to a chair during the daytime but were otherwise quite immobile)

7. GETTING IN AND OUT OF BED

On most days in the past week, the resident:

1. Got in and out of bed without any type of physical assistance

2. Got in and out of bed independently of staff but with the help of some equipment (for example, using a trapeze or sliding board by himself)

3. Got in and out of bed with the physical assistance of staff

4. Remained in bed all day

8. USE OF RESTRAINTS (for example, bed rails, soft ties, or geri-chairs)

How often during the daytime in the past week were restraints used with this resident?

1. Not at all

2. Seldom (on 1 to 3 days for only short periods of time)

3. At times (either on more than 3 days for only short periods of time or on 1 to 3 days for most of the day)

4. Often (on more than 3 days for most of the day)

9. UNDERSTANDING COMMUNICATION (speaking, writing, or gesturing)

Most of the times that you communicated with the resident in the past week, he:

1. Understood clearly

2. Understood only brief communications (such as short sentences or gestures)

3. Understood brief communications only if they were repeated

4. Did not understand any communications

10. TALKING

Most of the times that the resident spoke during the past week, his speech:

1. Was coherent and logical

2. Began logically but wandered off topic while talking

3. Sounded coherent, but his conversation was irrelevant (for example, his speech was unrelated to the question being asked or the event taking place)

4. Made very little sense (for example, word jumbles or meaningless phrases or meaningless noises)

5. Question does not apply — the resident did not speak in the past week

11. FINDING WAY AROUND INSIDE (for example, ability to find his room, the washroom, the dining room)

How often during the daytime in the past week did the resident become disoriented (confused) in finding his way around the inside of his residence?

1. Not at all

2. Seldom (only 1 to 3 times during the week)

3. At times (either once or twice a day on more than 3 days or several times a day on 1 to 3 days)

4. Often (several times a day on more than 3 days)

5. Question does not apply (resident never moved around inside the building without assistance from the staff)

12. RECOGNIZING STAFF

On most days in the past week, the resident:

1. Recognized several members of the staff by name or by exact role (for example, doctor, nurse, or physiotherapist)

2. Recognized one or two members of the staff by name or by exact role

3. Could tell members of the staff apart from residents or visitors but did not know the name or exact role of any staff member

4. Could not tell members of the staff apart from residents or visitors

13. AWARENESS OF PLACE

During the past week, the resident:

1. Knew exactly where he was living (knew the institution's name and the city or town where it is located)

2. Knew the type of place he was living in but was confused about its name or location

3. Sometimes seemed to understand the type of place he was living in but at other times was confused about this

4. Was confused about the type of place he was living in (for example, thought he was living at home or somewhere else)

5. This information could not be obtained (the resident did not communicate appropriately)

14. AWARENESS OF TIME

Consider whether on most days in the past week the resident was aware of (a) the year (within 1), (b) the season, and (c) the approximate time of day (for example, whether it was morning or after lunch or after supper)?

1. He was aware of all three (year, season, and time of day)

2. He was aware of two of the three

3. He was aware of one of the three

4. He was confused about all three

5. This information could not be obtained (the resident did not communicate appropriately)

15. MEMORY FOR RECENT EVENTS (day-to-day events, such as recreation, meals, visits occurring within the past week)

During the past week, the resident:

1. Could remember most recent events clearly

2. Could remember most recent events but only in a vague way

3. Could remember some recent events but completely forgot others

4. Seemed to forget most events a few minutes after they occurred

5. This information could not be obtained (the resident did not communicate appropriately)

16. MEMORY FOR IMPORTANT PAST EVENTS (for example, his year of birth, his past occupation, and names of members of his family and whether they are still living)

During the past week, the resident:

1. Could easily remember many past events correctly

2. Could remember many past events correctly but with some effort

3. Could remember some past events but forgot others

4. Was confused about most events in his past life

5. This information could not be obtained (the resident did not communicate appropriately)

17. **LOOKING SAD AND DEPRESSED** (for example, looking gloomy, unhappy, or mournful; do not include looking bored, indifferent, worried, or anxious)

How often during the past week did the resident look sad and depressed?

1. Not at all

2. Seldom (on 1 to 3 days for only short periods of time)

3. At times (either on more than 3 days for only short periods of time or on 1 to 3 days for most of the day)

4. Often (on more than 3 days for most of the day)

5. Could not tell—the resident has some facial paralysis or physical problem (for example, parkinsonism) that gives his face a gloomy look

18. **REPORTING SADNESS AND DEPRESSION** (talking about being sad or depressed or wanting to be somewhere else; do not include complaints about his care; also do not include talking about being worried)

How often during the past week did the resident say (or write) something to indicate that he was sad or depressed?

1. Not at all

2. Seldom (only one to three times during the week)

3. At times (either once or twice a day on more than 3 days or several times a day on 1 to 3 days)

4. Often (several times a day on more than 3 days; also include here any resident who specifically said he wanted to be dead)

5. Question does not apply (the resident did not speak or write in the past week)

19. **SOUNDING SAD AND DEPRESSED** (using a tone of voice when speaking that suggests sadness or depression, or making sad noises like moans or sighs; do not include sounding angry or worried or in acute pain.)

How often during the past week did the resident sound sad and depressed?

1. Not at all

2. Seldom (on 1 to 3 days for only short periods of time)

3. At times (either on more than 3 days for only short periods of time or on 1 to 3 days for most of the day)

4. Often (on more than 3 days for most of the day)

5. Question does not apply (the resident did not speak or make any sounds in the past week)

20. **LOOKING WORRIED AND ANXIOUS** (do not include looking sad or depressed)

How often during the past week did the resident look worried, tense, or anxious?

1. Not at all

2. Seldom (on 1 to 3 days for only short periods)

3. At times (either on more than 3 days for only short periods of time or on 1 to 3 days for most of the day)

4. Often (on more than 3 days for most of the day)

5. Do not know

21. REPORTING WORRY AND ANXIETY (talking about being worried about certain things; do not include talking about being unhappy)

How often during the past week did the resident say (or write) something to indicate that he was worried or anxious about something?

1. Not at all

2. Seldom (only one to three times during the week)

3. At times (either once or twice a day on more than 3 days or several times a day on 1 to 3 days)

4. Often

5. Question does not apply (the resident did not speak or write)

6. Do not know

22. CRYING (do not include moaning or sighing or yelling)

How often during the past week did the resident cry?

1. Not at all

2. Seldom (on one to three days for only short periods of time)

3. At times (either once or twice a day on more than 3 days or several times a day on 1 to 3 days)

4. Often (on more than 3 days for long periods of time)

5. Do not know

23. PESSIMISM ABOUT THE FUTURE (talking about the future being hopeless or unbearable or about how things will not improve)

How often during the past week did the resident say (or write) something to indicate that he felt pessimistic about his future?

1. Not at all

2. Seldom (only one to three times during the week)

3. At times (either once or twice a day on more than 3 days or several times a day on 1 to 3 days)

4. Often (several times a day on more than 3 days)

5. Question does not apply (the resident did not speak or write in the past week)

24. SELF CONCERN

How often during the past week did the resident have trouble concentrating on events happening to him or around him because he was so upset or concerned about his troubles?

1. Not at all

2. Seldom (only one to three times during the week)

3. At times (either once or twice a day on more than 3 days or several times a day on 1 to 3 days)

4. Often (several tines a day on more than 3 days)

25 COOPERATION WITH NURSING CARE (cooperation with feeding, bathing, grooming, and medication)

On most days in the past week, when interacting with nurses and orderlies, the resident:

1. Actively cooperated in his own care (attempted to help and participate when possible)

2. Passively cooperated in his own care (quietly allowed himself to be cared for)

3. Resisted care attempts in a minor way (would give an initial argument or whine or physical resistance but quickly gave in)

4. Resisted care attempts in a major way (getting him to cooperate was a real chore)

26. FOLLOWING STAFF REQUESTS AND INSTRUCTIONS

Most of the requests or instructions made by the staff of the resident in the past week:

1. Were followed without resistance or resentment

2. Were followed without resistance but with quiet resentment (for example, were responded to with quiet muttering or nasty looks)

3. Were responded to with an argument or physical resistance before being complied with

4. Were responded to with resistance and finally had to be physically enforced by the staff

5. Were not understood by the resident (include residents who were so mentally or physically disabled that staff never gave them even simple instructions)

27. IRRITABILITY

How often during the past week was the resident irritable and grouchy?

1. Not at all

2. Seldom (on 1 to 3 days for only short periods of time)

3. At times (on more than 3 days for only short periods of time, or on 1 to 3 days for most of the day)

4. Often (on more than 3 days for most of the day)

28. REACTIONS TO FRUSTRATION (reacting with abuse or whining when requests were denied or when he had to wait for something)

During the past week, when the resident experienced frustrations, how often did he lose his temper?

1. Not at all

2. Seldom (only one to three times during the week)

3. At times (either once or twice a day on more than 3 days, or several times a day on 1 to 3 days)

4. Often (several times a day on more than 3 days)

29. VERBAL ABUSE OF STAFF (include yelling at, swearing at, cursing, threatening)

How often during the past week did the resident verbally abuse staff members?

1. Not at all

2. Sometimes

3. Frequently (at least once a day on more than 3 days) when asked to do something he did not want to do

4. Frequently (at least once a day on more than 3 days) with no apparent provocation or cause

5. Question does not apply (the resident did not speak or make any sounds in the past week)

30. VERBAL ABUSE OF OTHER RESIDENTS (Include yelling at, swearing at, cursing threatening.)

How often during the past week did the resident verbally abuse other residents?

1. Not at all

2. Sometimes

3. Frequently (at least once a day on more than 3 days) when they interfered with him

4. Frequently (at least once a day on more than 3 days) with no apparent provocation or cause

5. Question does not apply (the resident either did not speak or had no access to other residents)

31. PHYSICAL ABUSE OF OTHERS (hitting or shoving other residents or staff)

How often during the past week did the resident physically strike anyone?

1. Not at all

2. On one occasion, after being provoked

3. On one occasion, without apparent cause or provocation

4. More than once (include residents who actually had to be put in restraints to keep them from striking others)

5. Question does not apply (the resident is physically incapable of striking someone)

32. PROVOKING ARGUMENTS WITH OTHER RESIDENTS

How often during the past week did the resident start or provoke an argument with another resident?

1. Not at all

2. Seldom (only one to three times during the week)

3. At times (either once or twice a day on more than 3 days or several times a day on 1 to 3e days)

4. Often (several times a day on more than 3 days)

5. Question does not apply (the resident had no access to other residents)

33. PREFERRING SOLITUDE (keeping to himself)

When not receiving physical care in the past week, did the resident seem to prefer being left alone?

1. No. He always enjoyed company when it was available.

2. He seemed indifferent about whether he had company or was left alone.

3. At least some of the time he actively discouraged company.

4. Most of the time he actively discouraged company.

34. INITIATING SOCIAL CONTACTS (by speaking, gesturing, or smiling first or by approaching)

In the past week, the resident:

1. Frequently (several times a day on more than 3 days) initiated social contacts with both staff members and other residents

2. Frequently (several times a day on more than 3 days) initiated social contacts with either staff or other residents, but not both

3. Sometimes initiated social contacts with either staff or other residents

4. Never initiated social contacts with either staff or other residents

35. RESPONDING TO SOCIAL CONTACTS (do not consider simply following instructions or looking at the person as responding to social contacts)

How often during the past week did the resident respond to social contacts made by other people?

1. Most of the time and tried to keep the contact going (for example, by continuing the conversation or holding on to the person)

2. Most of the time but only briefly (for example, simply answered the question or nodded or smiled but made no effort to keep the contact going)

3. Only some of the time (less than half of the times that others tried to make contact)

4. Not at all

36. FRIENDSHIPS WITH OTHER RESIDENTS

In the past week, the resident:

1. Was close friends with more than one other resident (this implies a real relationship)

2. Was close friends with only one other resident

3. Established a casual friendship with at least one other resident (for example, tagged along with for a while, but no real bond)

4. Did not have any type of friendship with another resident

5. Question does not apply (the resident had no access to other residents)

37. INTEREST IN DAY-TO-DAY EVENTS (for example, watching or listening and reacting to things going on around him)

In the past week, how often did the resident pay active attention to the things happening around him?

1. Often (on more than 3 days for most of the day)

2. At times (either on more than 3 days for only short periods or on 1 to 3 days for most of the day)

3. Seldom (on 1 to 3 days for only short periods of time)

4. Not at all

38. INTEREST IN OUTSIDE EVENTS (for example, taking an interest in the activities of his family and absent friends, news, or sports)

In the past week, how often did the resident seem to take any interest in events happening outside of his residence?

1. Daily

2. Some days

3. Rarely (for example, he might show mild interest in his family, but only to be concerned about future visits)

4. Not at all

39. KEEPING OCCUPIED (on his own, by reading, actively watching the television or listening to radio, engaging in hobbies, chatting with others, going on walks; do not include organized recreational activities)

How often during the past week did the resident keep himself occupied on his own?

1. Often (on more than 3 days for most of the day)

2. At times (either on more than 3 days for only short periods of time or on 1 to 3 days for most of the day)

3. Seldom (on 1 to 3 days for only short periods of time)

4. Not at all

40. HELPING OTHER RESIDENTS (include any kind of help that seems to reflect concern for the other person; for example, physically helping them or comforting or entertaining them)

How often during the past week did the resident volunteer to help other residents?

1. Often (several times a day on more than three days)

2. At times (either once or twice a day on more than 3 days or several times a day on 1 to 3 days)

3. Seldom (only 1 to 3 times during the week)

4. Not at all

5. Question does not apply (the resident was either physically immobile [needed staff assistance to move around inside] or was kept in restraints on most days)

41. AGITATION OR RESTLESSNESS (walking or pacing the halls, rocking, repeatedly banging things with hands or feet, repeatedly picking at real or imagined objects, verbal outburst directed at no one)

How often during the past week was the resident very restless or agitated?

1. Not at all

2. Sometimes

3. Frequently (at least once a day on more than three days)

4. Resident is continuously restrained

5. Do not know

42. UNUSUAL EVENTS

Did anything unusual happen to the resident during the past week (such as, the death of a loved one, physical injury or illness, surgery) that might make his behavior atypical?

☐ No

☐ Yes

☐ Do not know

Please specify:_____

_____

_____

_____

_____

Note. From "Standardization and Validation of the Multidimensional Observation Scale for Elderly Subjects (MOSES)" by E. Helmes, K. Csapo, & J.A. Short, 1987, *Journal of Gerontology, 42*(4), 395-405. Reprinted with permission of E. Helmes.

APPENDIX B

RESOURCES FOR AD PATIENTS AND CAREGIVERS

The purpose of this appendix is to provide the reader with various forms of resources. The resources are grouped based on type of information.

BOOKS FOR CAREGIVERS

Caring for Your Aging Parents: A Planning and Action Guide by D. Cohen & C. Eisdorfer, 1995. New York: Tarcher/Putnam.

Spiritual Care: Nursing Theory, Research, and Practice by E.J. Taylor, 2002. New Jersey: Prentice Hall.

Tangled Minds: Understanding Alzheimer's Disease and Other Dementia's by M.R. Gillick & M. Gallick, 1999. New York: Plume.

Understanding Difficult Behaviors: Some Practical Suggestions for Coping With Alzheimer's Disease and Related Illnesses by A. Robinson, B. Spencer, & L. White (eds.), 1991. Available through Alzheimer's Program, P.O. Box 994, Ann Arbor, MI 48106.

RESEARCH RESOURCES

The following list of web sites may help you gather more information about studies that are presently being conducted to further the research on Alzheimer's disease:

- The www.clinicaltrials.gov web site developed by National Institutes of Health through its National Library of Medicine contains about 5,000 clinical studies sponsored primarily by the National Institutes of Health.

  http://www.clinicaltrials.gov

- ADEAR: Alzheimer's Disease Education & Referral Center. A service of the National Institute of Aging.

  http://www.alzheimers.org/trials

- The Center Watch Clinical Trials Listing Service web site is less detailed but includes trials not listed in the Alzheimer's Disease Clinical Trials Database.

  http://www.centerwatch.com

- Mental Health: A Report of the Surgeon General: Alzheimer's disease. General information on Alzheimer's disease
  http://www.surgeongeneral.gov/library/mental health/chapter5/sec4.html

NUTRITIONAL RESOURCES

- Dietary guidelines for Americans: Food Guide Pyramid
  Modified food guide pyramid for people over age 70.
  http://commentator.tufts.edu/archive/nutrition/pyramid.html
  http://www.fda.gov/opacom/lowlit/eatage.html

- Nutrition Insights: Food insufficiencies and the nutritional status of the elderly population
  http://www.usda.gov/cnpp/Insights/Insight18.pdf

- Florida International University – National Policy and Research Center on Nutrition and Aging
  http://www.fiu.edu/~nutreldr

- Administration on Aging
  http://www.aoa.dhhs.gov

INCONTINENCE RESOURCES

- National Association for Continence
  http://www.nafc.org

- National Institute on Aging
  http://www.nia.publications.org/engagepages/urinary.asp

- Overactive Bladder Relief Center
  http://www.oabrelief.com

- Healthology
  New York-based online health media company founded and managed by physicians. Once at the site click on "Health Topics" and look under Elder Care or Urology.
  http://www.healthology.com

- National Kidney and Urologic Diseases Information Clearinghouse
  Urinary Incontinence in Women
  http://www.niddk.nih.gov/kudiseases/pubs/uiwomen/index.htm

MISCELLANEOUS ONLINE RESOURCES FOR PROFESSIONAL AND FAMILY CAREGIVERS

ALZ Well
Alzheimer's caregivers page
http://www.alzwell.com

Alzheimer Disease Genetics Initiative Data Archive
http://zork.wustl.edu/nimh/ad.html

Alzheimer Disease Overview
Information about the disease including prevalence and heredity
http://www.geneclinics.org/profiles/alzheimer

Alzheimer Europe
Nonprofit organization that aims to improve the care and treatment of patients with Alzheimer's disease (AD)
http://www.alzheimer-europe.org

Alzheimer Research Forum
A nonprofit organization supporting the information needs of researchers and promoting openness and collaboration with colleagues worldwide
http://www.alzforum.org

Alzheimer Society of Canada
Information on the Alzheimer Society, the disease, care, research, news, events, and more
http://www.alzheimer.ca

Alzheimer's Association
Resources on Alzheimer's research, treatment, and news
http://www.alz.org

Alzheimer's Disease Education & Referral Center
Information, news, and publications about AD and related dementias
http://www.alzheimers.org

Alzheimer's: Few Clues on the Mysteries of Memory

http://www.fda.gov/fdac/features/1998/398_alz.html

Cognitive Enhancement Research Institute

Smart Drug News chronicles the latest developments in the field of cognitive drugs and related technologies

http://www.ceri.com

Dementia Research Centre

A resource based in the United Kingdom

http://dementia.ion.ucl.ac.uk

Early Alzheimer's Disease

A patient and family guide

http://www.ahcpr.gov/clinic/alzcons.htm

ElderWeb

A listing of sites with information pertaining to AD

http://www.elderweb.com

National Cell Repository for Alzheimer Disease

http://ncrad.iu.edu

National Institute on Aging

AD Progress Report and latest news

http://www.alzheimers.org

Neuroscience and Neuropsychology of Aging (NNA) Program

http://www.nia.nih.gov/research/extramural/neuroscience/index.htm

Resources for Enhancing Alzheimer's Caregiver Health (REACH)

http://www.edc.gsph.pitt.edu/reach

CAREGIVERS RESOURCES

Alzheimer's Association

http://www.alz.org

Family Caregiver Alliance

Caregiving and long-term care information

http://www.caregiver.org

Caregiver.com

Online magazine for caregivers

http://www.caregiver.com

Centers for Medicare & Medicaid Services

National regulatory information about elder care

http://cms.gov

Gives information on every Medicare/Medicaid certified nursing home in the country

http://www.medicare.gov

DyingWell.org

A reading list on dying well with web links for anyone facing end-of-life illnesses

http://www.dyingwell.org/links.htm

The Elder Care Locator

Finds services in the local community or helps to locate elder services.

1-800-677-1116
http://www.eldercare.gov

The Elderly Place

Highlights caregiving of Alzheimer's patients

http://www.elderlyplace.com

National Family Caregivers Association

Promotes healthier and happier caregivers

http://www.nfcacares.org

Senior Options

Provides a comprehensive guide for older adults and caregivers in almost any region. The following is an example from Washington Association of Housing and Services for the Aging (WAHSA)

http://www.wahsa.com/senior_options.htm

GLOSSARY

acetylcholine: A chemical neurotransmitter found in neurons that carries information across the synaptic cleft (space between two nerve cells) and is deficient in patients with Alzheimer's disease.

acetylcholinesterase inhibitors: A substance such as a drug that prevents an enzyme from breaking down unused acetylcholine in synaptic cleft.

agitation: A state of anxiety accompanied by motor restlessness.

agnosia: Inability to recognize familiar objects, people, sounds, shapes, tastes, or smells. Although agnosia often is present in the early stages of Alzheimer's disease, it may be so subtle and slight that it goes unnoticed.

Aids Dementia Complex (ADC): A subcortical type of dementia with changes noted in attention, apathy, and impaired motor control affecting the ability to function in a social or occupational setting.

akathisia: A condition of motor restlessness in which there is a feeling of muscular quivering, an urge to move about constantly, and an inability to sit still; a common extrapyramidal side effect of psychotropic drugs.

Alzheimer's disease: A progressive, neurodegenerative disease characterized by loss of function and death of nerve cells in several areas of the brain, leading to loss of cognitive function (such as memory and language).

amnesia: Memory impairment.

anorexia: Loss of appetite, especially when prolonged.

anticholinergic effects: Side effects produced by medications that inhibit the parasympathetic branch of the autonomic nervous system (such as dry mouth, blurred vision, and urinary retention). Medications with anticholinergic side effects include antihistamines, psychotropic drugs, cardiovascular drugs, corticosteroids, and antibiotics.

aphasia: Impairment of the speech process. Receptive aphasia is an inability to comprehend what one hears. Expressive aphasia is an inability to express oneself, even though the question has been heard and understood. The two types of aphasia can be differentiated by asking the patient to perform a certain command, such as closing the eyes, sticking out the tongue, or raising the left arm. If the patient hears and understands what is being said, the command will be followed. If the patient cannot hear or cannot comprehend what is heard (receptive aphasia), the patient will be unable to comply.

apolipoprotein E: Type of protein that is attached to a fat molecule and transports cholesterol in the bloodstream.

apraxia: Inability to carry out purposeful movements and actions despite intact motor and sensory systems.

autosomal gene: A chromosome other than a sex chromosome.

best practice: Interventions or tools suggested or used by practitioners or experts in the care of patients.

biochemical: Characterized by, produced by, or involving chemical reactions in living organisms.

burnout: An excessive stress reaction to one's occupational or professional environment that is manifested by feelings of emotional and physical exhaustion coupled with a sense of frustration and failure.

catastrophic reactions: The loss of emotional control, nearly always involving extreme anger, often accompanied by fear, hostility, and anxiety. Behaviors include screaming, hitting, throwing things, and sobbing. Happens most frequently during personal care with patients in the middle stages of dementia, and most often in the late afternoon.

Creutzfeldt-Jakob disease: A very rare form of encephalopathy thought to be caused by a slow virus, termed a prion. The disease occurs primarily in adults, with peak incidence in the late fifties. Infection results in dementia, myoclonus, ataxia, and other neurologic symptoms.

dehydration: An abnormal depletion of body fluids. The lack of adequate fluid levels needed in the body to carry on normal function. Can be caused by fluid loss (vomiting or diarrhea), inadequate intake, or both.

delirium: An acute medical condition manifested by disorientation, confusion, and fluctuating levels of consciousness.

dementia: A nonspecific deterioration of intellectual functioning characterized by failing memory, distractibility, impairment in judgment and abstraction, reduced language capability, alterations in mood and affect, changes in personality, and disturbance of orientation. There are more than 70 causes of dementia, with the most common one being Alzheimer's disease.

depression: A psychoneurotic or psychotic disorder marked especially by sadness, inactivity, difficulty in thinking and concentration, a significant increase or decrease in appetite and time spent sleeping, feelings of dejection and hopelessness, and sometimes suicidal tendencies. Older adults often exhibit atypical symptoms, such as agitation, anxiety, decreased verbalization, decreased physical functioning, and unspecific somatic complaints.

dysphagia: Difficulty swallowing.

environment: The circumstances, objects, or conditions by which one is surrounded. The aggregate of social and cultural conditions that influence the life of an individual or community.

ethnicity: Ethnic quality or affiliation.

folate: Folic acid, one of the B vitamins that is a key factor in the synthesis of nucleic acid (deoxyribonucleic acid and ribonucleic acid).

functional incontinence: The type of incontinence occurring most frequently in Alzheimer's disease. Occurs when urine is lost because the person is unaware of the need to urinate or cannot reach a toilet because of immobility or some other barrier.

hematocrit: The ratio of the volume of packed red blood cells to the volume of whole blood.

hemoglobin: An iron-containing respiratory pigment of vertebrate red blood cells that functions in oxygen transport to the tissues after conversion to oxygenated form in the lungs and assists in carbon dioxide transport back to the lungs after surrender of its oxygen.

holistic: Relating to or concerned with wholes or with complete systems rather than with the analysis of, treatment of, or dissection into parts.

homocysteine: An amino acid produced by the body, usually a by-product of consuming meat. Elevated levels of homocysteine appear to increase the chance of Alzheimer's disease.

Huntington's chorea: Also called Huntington's disease. Genetic neurological disorder, usually appearing in midlife, that is characterized by memory loss, mood swings, and involuntary movements affecting gait and speech.

iatrogenic: Inadvertently induced by medical treatment.

incontinence: Inability of the body to control the evacuative functions.

Korsakoff's psychosis: Also called Korsakoff's syndrome. A memory disorder caused by a deficiency of vitamin B that may occur as a result of chronic alcohol abuse. Features include personality changes, ataxia, confabulation, psychosis, disorientation, polyneuritis, insomnia, and hallucinations.

Lewy bodies: Small, round structures first identified in parts of the brain in the basal ganglia of patients with Parkinson's disease. They are also sometimes seen throughout the brains of patients with Alzheimer's disease, often when the patient has both conditions.

life review: Introduced by Butler in 1963 as a way to review the past in an attempt to examine conflicts and resolve and reconcile them or make order and meaning from them.

mad cow disease (bovine spongiform encephalopathy [BSE]): A new disease of cattle, first reported in 1986 in Great Britain, characterized clinically by apprehensive behavior, hyperesthesia, and ataxia and histopathologically by spongiform changes in the gray-matter of the brain stem. May be a variation of Creutzfeldt-Jakob disease.

malnutrition: Faulty or inadequate nutrition.

Medicaid: A program of medical aid designed for people unable to afford regular medical service and financed by the state and federal governments.

Medicare: A government program of medical care especially for those over age 65, some disabled persons under 65, and renal dialysis or transplant patients.

Mini-Mental Status Exam: The accepted standard for mental status examinations used to estimate the current level of cognitive function.

Montessori methods: Maria Montessori designed an educational program in which children engaged in a series of individualized activities to foster independence and meaningful choices. Founded on rehabilitation concepts by breaking down tasks into simple steps and guiding individuals though one step at a time. Recognizing and maintaining residents' strengths is the goal.

Mozart effect: Discovered in 1993 at the University of California, theorized that for demented individuals, music may form a bridge between the cognitive and creative sides of the brain. Listening to music may improve concentration and enhance remaining abilities.

multi-infarct dementia: Condition in which dementia is caused by repeated small strokes.

Need-Driven Dementia-Compromised Behavior Model: Looks at disruptive behaviors of demented persons as "potentially understandable needs." The interaction of background and proximal issues produce the need-driven behavior. The model provides a framework for understanding and researching behavior.

neuritic plaques: Abnormal clusters of dead and dying nerve cells, other brain cells, and protein.

neurofibrillary tangles (tangles of tau): Aggregations of neurofilaments and neurotubules in neurons, which are noted through microscopy. Neurofibrillary tangles are commonly seen in normal aged brains but usually are few in number. In Alzheimer's disease, however, these tangles are widespread throughout the cortex and are quite dense.

neuroleptic malignant syndrome: This medical emergency is characterized by muscular rigidity, high fever, elevated levels of creatine phosphokinase, unstable blood pressure, and confusion.

neuroleptics: Drugs used to treat psychotic symptoms. They include phenothiazines (such as Thorazine, Mellaril, Stelazine), butyrophenones (such as Haldol), and thioxanthenes (such as Navane).

neurotransmitters: Chemical substances that conduct electrical impulses from one cell to another and thus enable an electrical impulse to proceed. The main neurotransmitters that are deficient in Alzheimer's disease are acetylcholine, somatostatin and, to a lesser extent, serotonin and dopamine.

nootropic: Word coined to describe a new class of drugs that act as cognitive enhancers with no side effects or toxicity. From the Greek words *noos*, meaning mind, and *tropein*, meaning toward.

nutrient dense: More nutrients in a smaller amount of food, such as supercereal or soup.

Omnibus Budget Reconciliation Act (OBRA) of 1987: Federal legislation emphasizing nursing home responsibility for ensuring that residents reach their maximal level of function and well-being in an environment that respects their dignity and autonomy. Mandated a reduction in use of chemical and physical restraints.

organizational environment: The philosophy of the institution, including the policies and procedures, staffing patterns, staff education, and availability of equipment and supplies.

pathophysiology: The physiology of abnormal states; the functional changes that accompany a particular syndrome or disease.

Patient Self-Determination Act of 1991: Mandates that agencies and institutions receiving Medicare and Medicaid reimbursement provide written information to individuals about their rights to participate in medical decision-making (outlined in state laws) and to put together advance directives.

pharmacokinetics: The characteristic interactions of a drug and the body in terms of its absorption, distribution, metabolism, and excretion.

Pick's disease: A form of dementia characterized by slowly progressive deterioration of social skills and changes in personality, leading to impairment of intellect, memory, and language.

progressively lowered stress threshold model: A model for explaining dysfunctional behavior that indicates a progressive lowering of the threshold for stress, which hinders the individual's functioning in the environment.

protein-calorie malnutrition: Also called kwashiorkor. Severe deficiency of protein plus inadequate caloric intake with decrease in serum albumin.

psychotropic drugs: Drugs that affect the mind or behavior, such as antidepressants, anxiolytics, and neuroleptic medications.

reality orientation: The repetition of specific information to confused and disoriented persons.

religion: A system of beliefs and formal practices that are practiced individually or in a community group to provide focus and meaning to life, understand death, and maintain hope for the future.

reminiscence: The process or practice of thinking or telling about past experiences.

respite care: Short-term supervisory, personal, and nursing care to impaired elderly who cannot be left alone.

sarcopenia: Loss of muscle mass due to aging and the combined effects of inactivity, poor nutrition, and illness.

serum albumin level: The protein with the highest concentration in plasma. Maintains oncotic pressure of the blood, which keeps fluid from leaking into the tissues. Decreased serum albumin may result from liver or kidney disease or may indicate malnutrition.

special care units: Segregated units designed to reduce the anxiety and agitation of people with dementia. Several different theoretical frameworks guide the programs and interventions for individuals with dementia.

spirituality: The individuality of each person's beliefs about relationships, love and intimacy, forgiveness, hopes for the future, and methods of making peace with the past.

therapeutic activities: What people do to search for meaning and purpose in life.

urinary tract infection: Also called cystitis. An inflammation of the bladder or urethra usually caused by bacteria. Some people are at higher risk for bladder and other urinary tract infections than others. Common symptoms include a frequent urge to urinate and a painful burning when urinating.

universality: Existence or prevalence everywhere.

validation therapy: An interdisciplinary helping method based on the principle that when emotions are expressed to someone who listens with empathy, the person is relieved. The goal is to improve the quality of life for demented persons. Individuals with Alzheimer's disease may return to the past to survive present-day loses.

vascular: Of or relating to a channel for the conveyance of a body fluid (such as blood of an animal or sap of a plant) or to a system of such channels.

wandering: A purposeful behavior (from the context of the wanderer) that attempts to fulfill a particular need, is initiated by a cognitively impaired and disoriented individual, and is characterized by excessive ambulation that often leads to safety- or nuisance-related problems.

BIBLIOGRAPHY

Abbasi, A.A. & Rudman, D. (1994). Undernutrition in the nursing home: Prevalence, consequences, causes, and prevention. *Nutrition Reviews, 52*(4), 113-22.

Abraham, I., Bottrell, M., Dash, K., Fulmer, T., Mezey, M., O'Donnell, L., et al. (1999). *Nurses Improving Care for Health System Elders: A planning and implementation guide* (3rd ed.). New York: Hartford Foundation Institute for Geriatric Nursing.

Administration on Aging. (2002). Nutrition Screening Initiative (NSI). Older Americans Act Nutrition Program. Retrieved March 2003, from http://www.aoa.dhhs.gov/press/medadv/2002/03_Mar/Tommynutrition030102.pdf

Administration on Aging (AOA). (March 8, 2004). Nutrition. *Announcement from the Assistant Secretary.* Retrieved August 13, 2004 from http://www.aoa.dhhs.gov/eldfam/Nutrition/Nutrition.asp

Aldridge, D. (2000). *Music therapy in dementia care.* London: Jessica Kingsley Publishers.

Alexopoulous, G.S., Abrams, R.C., Young, R.C., Shamoian, C.A. (1988). Cornell Scale for Depression in Dementia. *Biological Psychiatry, 23*(3), 21-84.

Alexopoulous, G. (1995). Mood disorders. In H. Kaplan & B.J. Sadock (Eds.), *Kaplan & Sadock's comprehensive textbook of psychiatry: Vol. 2* (6th ed.). Baltimore: Williams & Wilkins.

Allen, P.N. (2002). Indiana University School of Nursing Course: K492 Multidisciplinary Care of Older Adults.

Allen, P.N. (2003). Indiana University School of Nursing Course: Excerpts from K492 Multidisciplinary Care of Older Adults (Web-based).

Allen, R.S, Thorn, B.E., Fisher, S.E., Gerstle, J., Quarles, K., Bourgeois, M.S., et al. (2003). Prescription and dosage of analgesic medication in relation to resident behaviors in the nursing home. *Journal of the American Geriatrics Society, 51*(4), 534-38.

Alzheimer's Association. (n.d.). *Fact Sheets: Hospitalization* (ED247ZN). Retrieved September 16, 2004, from http://www.alz.org/Resources/FactSheets/FSHospitalization.pdf

Alzheimer's Association. (1990). *Male caregiver's guidebook: Caring for your loved one with Alzheimer's at home.* Des Moines: Author.

Alzheimer's Association. (2004). *Day to Day Care, Communication.* Retrieved August 31, 2004 from http://www.alz.org/Care/DaytoDay/communication.asp

Alzheimer's Association. (2002). Statistics: About Alzheimer's Disease. Retrieved October 12, 2003, from http://www.alz.org

Alzheimer's Organization. (April 5, 2004). *Alzheimer's Disease Statistics.* Fact Sheet. Retrieved August 25, 2004 from http://www.alz.org/Resources/FactSheets/FSAlzheimerStats.pdf

Amella, E.J. (1998). Assessment and management of eating and feeding difficulties for older persons: A NICHE protocol. *Geriatric Nursing, 19*(5), 269-74.

American Psychiatric Association. (1994). *Diagnostic and statistical manual of mental disorders* (4th ed.). Washington, DC: Author.

American Psychiatric Association. (2000). *Practice guidelines for the treatment of patients with Alzheimer's disease & other dementias of late life.* Retrieved October 12, 2003, from http://www.psych.org/psych_pract/treatg/pg/pg_dementia_9.cfm

Andrews, J.C. & Andrews, N.C. (2003). Counseling Alzheimer's patients and their families. *Clinician Reviews, 13*(4), 56-61.

Andrieu, S., Reynish, E., Nourhashemi, F., Shakespeare, A., Moulias, S., Ousset, P.J., et al. (2002). Predictive factors of acute hospitalization in 134 patients with Alzheimer's disease: A one year prospective study. *International Journal of Geriatric Psychiatry, 17*(5), 422-26.

Area Agency on Aging of Pasco-Pinellas, Inc. (n.d.). *Caregiver's Checklist.* Retrieved May 16, 2004, from www.agingcarefl.org/caregiver/alzheimers/checklist

Astra Zeneca. (July 22, 2004). Study Examines SEROQUEL for the Treatment of Agitation in Elderly Patients with Dementia. Retrieved October 4, 2004 from http://www.alzheimersupport.com/articles/pastdrugnews.cfm

Baer, W.M. & Hanson, L.C. (2000). Families' perception of the added value of hospice in the nursing home. *Journal of the American Geriatrics Society, 48*(8), 879-82.

Bailey, J., Gilbert, E., & Herweyer, S. (1992). To find a soul...doll therapy to reach out to Alzheimer's patients. *Nursing, 22*(7), 63-4.

Beers, M.H. (1997). Explicit criteria for determining potentially inappropriate medication use by the elderly. An update. *Archives of Internal Medicine, 157*(14), 1531-36.

Berger, A., Fratiglioni, L., & Forsell, Y. (2000). Depression may be a component of preclinical Alzheimer's disease. *Geriatrics, 55*(2), 102.

Bentue-Ferrer, D., Tribut, O., Polard, E., & Allain, H. (2003). Clinically significant drug interactions with cholinesterase inhibitors: A guide for neurologists. *CNS Drugs, 17*(13), 947-63.

Bethea, L.S., Travis, S.S., & Pecchioni, L. (2000). Family caregivers' use of humor in conveying information about caring for dependent older adults. *Health Communication, 12*(4), 361-76.

Better eldercare: A nurse's guide to caring for older adults. (2002). Springhouse, PA: Springhouse Corp.

Bieber, M.R. (2003). Mild cognitive impairment: Aging to Alzheimer's disease. New York: Oxford University Press.

Black, S.E. (1999). The search for diagnostic and progression markers in AD: So near but still too far? *Neurology, 52*(8), 1533-34.

Blasi, Z.V., Hurley, A.C., & Volicer, L. (2002). End-of-life care in dementia: A review of problems, prospects, and solutions in practice. *Journal of the American Medical Directors Association, 3*(2), 57-65.

Borson, S., Scanlan, J., Brush, M., Vitaliano, P., & Dokmak, A. (2000). The Mini-Cog: A cognitive "vital signs" measure for dementia screening in multi-lingual elderly. *International Journal of Geriatric Psychiatry, 15*(11), 1021-27.

Bosek, M.S., Lowry, E., Lindeman, D.A., Burck, J.R., & Gwyther, L.P. (2003). Promoting a good death for persons with dementia in nursing facilities: Family caregivers' perspectives. *JONA's Healthcare Law, Ethics, and Regulation, 5*(2), 34-41.

Bottrell, M. (2001). Advanced directives. In M. Mezey (Ed.), *Encyclopedia of elder care: The comprehensive resource on geriatric and social care.* New York: Springer Publishing Co.

Boyd, S. (1999). *50 excuses for a closed mind (or how to kill an idea). Fluid Power Journal.* Retrieved May 5, 2004, from http://www.fluidpower journal.com/1999issues/06JulyAugust99/ articles/02/steppingout.htm

Brawley, E.C. (2002). How to improve the bathing experience. *Alzheimer's Care Quarterly, 3*(1), 38.

Breitner, J.C. & Zandi, P.P. (2003). Effects of estrogen plus progestin on risk of dementia. *Journal of the American Medical Association, 290*(13), 1706-07.

Brett, A.S. & Jersild, P. (2003). "Inappropriate" treatment near the end of life: Conflict between religious convictions and clinical judgment. *Archives of Internal Medicine, 163*(14), 1645-49.

Briggs, E. (2003) The nursing management of pain in older people. *Nursing Standard, 17*(18), 47-55.

Brilliant, A. (1981). *I have abandoned my search for truth and am now looking for a good fantasy.* Santa Barbara, CA: Woodbridge Press.

Bruce, A.W. & Kopp, P. (2001). Pain experienced by older people. *Professional Nurse, 16*(11), 1481-85.

Bruek, L. (2001). Montessori comes to dementia care. *Nursing Homes, 50*(8), 33-34.

Brummel-Smith, K., London, M.R., Drew, N., Krulewitch, H., Singer, C., & Hanson, L. (2002). Outcomes of pain in frail older adults with dementia. *Journal of the American Geriatrics Society, 50*(11), 1847-51.

Buckwalter, G.L. (2003). Addressing the spiritual & religious needs of persons with profound memory loss. *Home Healthcare Nurse, 21*(1), 20-24.

Buckwalter, K.C., Davis, L.L., Wakefield, B.J., Kienzle, M.G., & Murray, M.A. (2002). Telehealth for elders and their caregivers in rural communities. *Family & Community Health, 25*(3), 31-40.

Buettner, L. (1999). Simple pleasures: A multilevel sensori-motor intervention for nursing home residents with dementia. *American Journal of Alzheimer's Disease,* Nov-Dec, 10-19.

Burns, A., Howard, R. & Pettit, W. (1995). *Alzheimer's disease: A medical companion.* Cambridge, MA: Blackwell Science.

Butler, R.N. (1963). The life review: An interpretation of reminiscence in the aged. *Psychiatry, 26,* 65-76.

Butts, J.B. (2001). Outcomes of comfort touch in institutionalized elderly female residents. *Geriatric Nursing, 22*(4), 180-84.

Cable News Network. (1999). Test of Alzheimer's vaccine in mice shows promise. Retrieved March 6, 2004, from www.cnn.com/ health/9907/07/alzheimers.vaccine.02/

Cable News Network. (2004). *Study: Vitamins C, E cut Alzheimer's risk.* Retrieved October 11, 2004, from http://www.cnn.com/2004/HEALTH/ conditions/01/20/alzheimers.vitamins.reut/

Calaprice, A. (2000). *The Expanded Quotable Einstein.* Princeton, NJ: Princeton University Press.

Campbell, A.J., Robertson, M.C., Gardner, M.M., Norton, R.N., Tilyard, M.W., Bushner, D.M. (1997). Randomised controlled trial of a general practice programme of home based exercise to prevent falls in elderly women. *BMJ, 315*(7115), 1065-9.

Carbonell, J.G. (2004). Administration on Aging. Retrieved July 30, 2004, from http://www.aoa .dhhs.gov/eldfam/nutrition/nutrition.asp

Carvey, P.M. (1998). *Drug action in the central nervous system.* New York: Oxford University Press.

Cavanaugh, J.C. & Blanchard-Fields, F. (2002). *Adult development and aging* (4th ed.). Belmont, CA: Wadsworth Publishing Co.

Centers for Disease Control and Prevention. (2002). Bovine spongiform encephalopathy and variant Creutzfeldt-Jakob disease. Retrieved October 12, 2003, from http://www.cdc.gov/ncidod/diseases/cjd/bse_cjd.htm

Centers for Disease Control and Prevention. (2003). National Center for Health Statistics. *Nursing homes, beds, occupancy, and residents, according to geographic division and state: United States, 1995-2001.* Retrieved July 30, 2004, from http://www.cdc.gov/nchs/hus.htm

Centers for Medicare and Medicaid Services. (2000). *Choosing Long Term Care – 02223, revised 11/1/2001.* Washington, DC: U.S. Government Printing Office. Retrieved October 6, 2003, from http://www.medicare.gov/publications/

Centers for Medicare and Medicaid Services. (2002a). *Final draft of technical information for the quality measures included in the nursing home quality initiative.* Retrieved October 21, 2004, from http://www.cms.hhs.gov/quality/nhqi/NH20021029More.pdf

Centers for Medicare and Medicaid Services. (2002b). *Long Term Care Resident Assessment Instrument,* Version 2.0. Now called *Long Term Care Resident Assessment Instrument (RAI) User's Manual for the Minimum Data Set (MDS),* Version 2.0. Oral/Nutritional Status, 3-149. Baltimore, MD.

Centers for Medicare and Medicaid Services. (April 1, 2002c). Medicare News. *Statement of Tom Scully, Administrator, Centers for Medicare & Medicaid Services on therapy coverage of Alzheimer's Disease patients.* Retrieved October 30, 2003, from http://hcfa.gov/media/press/release.asp?Counter=435

Centers for Medicare and Medicaid Services. (2002d). *RAI Version 2.0 Manual,* Appendix A, page C7. Retrieved August 31, 2004, from http://cms.hhs.gov/quality/mds20/rai1202app.pdf

Chang, S.O. (2001). The conceptual structure of physical touch in caring. *Journal of Advanced Nursing, 33*(6), 820-27.

Chemerinski, E., Petracca, G., Sabe, L., Kremer, J., & Starkstein, S.E. (2001). The specificity of depressive symptoms in patients with Alzheimer's disease. *American Journal of Psychiatry, 158*(1), 68-72.

Chisholm, M.A. & DiPiro, J.T. (2002). Pharmaceutical manufacturer assistance programs. *Archives of Internal Medicine, 162*(7), 780-84.

CIBA Foundation Symposium, No. 196. (1996). *Growth Factors as drugs for neurological and sensory disorders.* New Jersey: Wiley Publishers.

Clabaugh, J. (July 29, 2004). Celera, Merck to Tackle Alzheimer's, *American City Business Journals, Inc.* Retrieved October 4, 2004 from http://www.alzheimersupport.com/articles/past drugnews.cfm

Clark, C.M. & Karlawish, J.H. (2003). Alzheimer disease: Current concepts and emerging diagnostic and therapeutic strategies. *Annals of Internal Medicine, 138*(5), 400-10.

Clayton, J. (1991). Let there be life: An approach to worship with Alzheimer's patients and their families. *Journal of Pastoral Care, 45*(2), 177-79.

Cohen-Mansfield, J. (2001). Managing agitation in elderly patients with dementia. *Geriatric Times, II,* (3).

Cohen-Mansfield, J. & Lipson, S. (2002). Pain in cognitively impaired nursing home residents: How well are physicians diagnosing it? *Journal of the American Geriatrics Society, 50*(6), 1039-44.

Colling, K.B. & Buettner, L.L. (2002). Simple pleasures: Interventions from the Need-Driven Dementia-Compromised Behavior Model. *Journal of Gerontological Nursing, 28*(10), 16-20.

Colombo, M., Vitali, S., Cairati, M., Perelli-Cippo, R., Bessi, O., Gioia, P., et al. (2001). Wanderers: Features, findings, issues. *Archives of Gerontology & Geriatrics, Suppl 1*, 99-106.

Coltharp, W., Jr., Richie, M.F., & Kaas, M.J. (1996). Wandering. *Journal of Gerontological Nursing, 22*(11), 5-10.

Compton, S.A., Flanagan, P., & Gregg, W. (1997). Elder abuse in people with dementia in Northern Ireland: Prevalence and predictors in cases referred to a psychiatry of old age service. *International Journal of Geriatric Psychiatry, 12*(6), 632-35.

Copstead, L.C. & Banasik, J.L. (2000). *Pathophysiology: Biological and behavioral perspectives* (2nd ed.). Philadelphia: W.B. Saunders.

Cousins, N. (1989). *Head first: The biology of hope.* New York: E.P. Dutton & Co.

Covinsky, K.E., Eng, C., Lui, L.Y., Sands, L.P., Sehgal, A.R., Walter, L.C., et al. (2001). Reduced employment in caregivers of frail elders: Impact of ethnicity, patient clinical characteristics, and caregiver characteristics. *Journal of Gerontology, 56*(11), M707-13.

Crogan, N.L., Shultz, J.A., Adams, C.E., & Massey, L.K. (2001). Barriers to nutrition care for nursing home residents. *Journal of Gerontological Nursing, 27*(12), 25-31.

Croog, S.H., Sudilovsky, A., Burleson, J.A., & Baume, R.M. (2001). Vulnerability of husband and wife caregivers of Alzheimer disease patients to caregiving stressors. *Alzheimer Disease and Associated Disorders, 15*(4), 201-10.

Crystal, H.A. (2001). The differential diagnosis of dementia. *The Clinical Advisor, 4*(11/12), 9-15.

Cuellar, N.G. (2002). A comparison of African-American & Caucasian American female caregivers of rural, post-stroke, bedbound older adults. *Journal of Gerontological Nursing, 28*(1), 36-45.

Cummings, J.L. & Cole, G. (2002). Alzheimer disease. *Journal of the American Medical Association, 287*(18), 2335-38.

Czaja, S.J. & Rubert, M.P. (2002). Telecommunications technology as an aid to family caregivers of persons with dementia. *Psychosomatic Medicine, 64*(3), 469-76.

Czaja, S.J., Schulz, R., Lee, C.C., & Belle, S.H. REACH Investigators. (2003). A methodology for describing and decomposing complex psychosocial and behavioral interventions. *Psychology & Aging, 18*(3), 385-95.

Danner, D.D., Snowdon, D.A., & Friesen, W.V. (2001). Positive emotions in early life and longevity: Findings from the nun study. *Journal of Personality and Social Psychology, 80*(5), 804-13.

Davidhizar, R. & Bowen, M. (1992). The dynamics of laughter. *Archives of Psychiatric Nursing, 6*(2), 132-37.

DeLaine, C., Scammell, J., & Heaslip, V. (2002). Continence care and policy initiatives. *Nursing Standard, 17*(7), 45-51, 53-54.

Delafuente, J. (2000). Principles of practical medication prescribing: Avoiding common complications and pitfalls. Paper presented at Geriatric Health Care Conference in Orlando, FL (Sept. 2000).

Desbiens, N.A. & Mueller-Rizner, N. (2000). How well do surrogates assess the pain of seriously ill patients? *Critical Care Medicine, 28*(5), 1347-52.

DiMaria-Ghalili, R.A. (2002). Changes in nutritional status and postoperative outcomes in elderly CABG patients. *Biological Research for Nursing, 4*(2), 73-84.

Dossey, L. (1996). Now you are fit to live: Humor and health. *Alternative Therapies in Health and Medicine, 2*(5), 8-13 & 98-100.

Dossey, B.M. & Guzzetta, C.E. (2000). Holistic nursing practice (Chapter 1). In B.M. Dossey, L. Keegan, & C.E. Guzzetta (Eds.), *Holistic nursing: A handbook for practice* (3rd ed.) (p. 5-26). Gaithersburg, MD: Aspen Publishers, Inc.

Dougherty, J. & Long, C.O. (2003). Techniques for bathing without a battle. *Home Healthcare Nurse, 21*(1), 38-39.

Ebersole, P. & Hess, P. (2001). *Geriatric Nursing & Healthy Aging.* St. Louis: Mosby.

Eliopoulos, C. (1995). *Manual of gerontologic nursing.* St. Louis: Mosby.

Endo, J. (2001). The greatest gift. *Journal of the American Medical Directors Association, 2*(6), 331-32.

Everett, D. (1996). *Forget me not: The spiritual care of persons with Alzheimer's.* Edmonton, AB: Inkwell Press.

Ewers, M. (1983). *Humor: The tonic you can afford: A handbook on the ways of using humor in long term care.* Los Angeles, CA: Ethel Percy Andrus Gerontology Center, University of Southern CA.

Feil, N. (1982). *Validation: The Feil method.* Cleveland: Edward Feil Productions.

Feil, N. (2001). Validation therapy. In M. Mezey (Ed.), *Encyclopedia of elder care: The comprehensive resource on geriatric and social care.* New York: Springer Publishing Co.

Feldman, H., Gauthier, S., Hecker, J., Vellas, B., Subbiah, P. & Whalen, E. Donepezil MSAD Study Investigators Group (2001). A 24-week, randomized, double-blind study of donepezil in moderate to severe Alzheimer's disease. *Neurology, 57*(4), 481-88.

Feldt, K.S., Warne, M.A., & Ryden, M.B. (1998). Examining pain in aggressive cognitively impaired older adults. *Journal of Gerontological Nursing, 24*(11), 14-22.

Ferrell, B.A. (2000). Pain management. *Clinics in Geriatric Medicine, 16*(4), 853-74.

Fick, D.M., Cooper, J.W., Wade, W.E., Waller, J.L., Maclean, J.R., & Beers, M.H. (2003). Updating the Beers criteria for potentially inappropriate medication use in older adults: Results of a U.S. consensus panel of experts. *Archives of Internal Medicine, 163*(22), 2716-24.

Fillit, H.M. (2002). The role of hormone replacement therapy in the prevention of Alzmeimer disease. *Archives of Internal Medicine, 162*(17), 1934-42.

Finnema, E., de Lange, J., Droes, R.M., Ribbe, M., & van Tilburg, W. (2001). The quality of nursing home care: Do the opinions of family members change after implementation of emotion-oriented care. *Journal of Advanced Nursing, 35*(5), 728-40.

Fisher, S.E., Burgio, L.D., Thorn, B.E., Allen-Burge, R., Gerstle, J., Roth, D.L., et al. (2002). Pain assessment and management in cognitively impaired nursing home residents: Association of certified nursing assistant pain report, Minimum Data Set pain report, and analgesic medication use. *Journal of the American Geriatrics Society, 50*(1), 152-56.

Fisher, S.M., Kutner, J.S., & Maier, D. (2003). Pain assessment in persons with advanced dementia: In search of a gold standard. *Journal of the American Geriatrics Society, 51*(4), 155.

Fitchett, G. (1993). *Assessing spiritual needs: A guide for caregivers.* Minneapolis: Augsberg Fortress Publications.

Folstein, M.F., Folstein, S.E., & McHugh, P.R. (1975). "Mini-mental state:" A practical method for grading the cognitive state of patients for the clinician. *Journal of Psychiatric Research, 12*(3), 189-98.

Foreman, M.D., Fletcher, K., Mion, L.C., & Simon, L. (1996). Assessing cognitive function. *Geriatric Nursing, 17*(5), 228–33.

Fuller, G.F. (2000). Falls in the elderly. *American Family Physician, 61*(7), 2159-68, 2173-4.

Fulmer, T., Mezey, M., Bottrell, M., Abraham, I., Sazant, J., Grossman, S., et al. (2002). Nurses Improving Care for Healthsystem Elders (NICHE): Using outcomes and benchmarks for evidenced-based practice. *Geriatric Nursing, 23*(3), 121-27.

Fulmer, T.T., Mion, L.C., & Bottrell, M.M. (1996). Pain management protocol. NICHE Faculty. *Geriatric Nursing, 17*(5), 222-27.

Gallinagh, R., Nevin R., McIlroy, D., Mitchell, F., Campbell, L., Ludwick, R., et al. (2002). The use of physical restraints as a safety measure in the care of older people in four rehabilitation wards: Findings from an exploratory study. *International Journal of Nursing Studies, 39*(2), 147-56.

Gauthier, S. (2002). Advances in the pharmacotherapy of Alzheimer's disease. *Canadian Medical Association Journal, 166*(5), 616-23.

Geerlings, M.I., Schmand, B., Braam, A.W., Jonker, C., Bouter, L.M., & van Tilburg, W. (2000). Depressive symptoms and risk of Alzheimer's disease in more highly educated older people. *Journal of the American Geriatrics Society, 48*(9), 1092-97.

Geldmacher, D., Heck, E., & O'Toole, E. (2001). Providing care for the caregiver. *Patient Care for the Nurse Practitioner,* February, 36-48.

George, L. (2001). Respite care. In M. Mezey (Ed.), *Encyclopedia of elder care: The comprehensive resource on geriatric and social care.* New York: Springer Publishing Co.

Gerdner, L.A. (2000). Effects of individual versus classical "relaxation" music on the frequency of agitation in elderly persons with Alzheimer's disease and related disorders. *International Psychogeriatrics, 12*(1), 49-65.

Gerdner, L.A. & Beck, C.K. (2001). Statewide survey to compare services provided for residents with dementia in special care units and non-special-care units. *American Journal of Alzheimer's Disorders and Other Dementias, 16*(5), 289-95.

Gerdner, L.A., Buckwalter, K.C., & Reed, D. (2002). Impact of a psychoeducational intervention on caregiver response to behavioral problems. *Nursing Research, 51*(6), 363-74.

Gibb, H., Morris, C., & Gleisberg, J. (1997). A therapeutic programme for people with dementia. *International Journal of Nursing Practice, 3*(3), 191–99.

Glaser, V. (2001). Strategies for early diagnosis of AD. *Patient Care for the Nurse Practitioner, 4*(2), 12-22.

Goodman, J. (2001). Taking humor seriously. Retrieved March 8, 2002, from http://www.humorproject.com

Grady, D. (April 8, 2004). Alzheimer's Drugs Frustrate Doctors. *The New York Times.* Retrieved October 4, 2004 from http://www.alzheimersupport.com/articles/past drugnews.cfm

Griffith, V.T. (2002). Diagnose and treat mild to moderate Alzheimer's disease. *The Nurse Practitioner, 27*(12), 13-25.

Greubel, D.L., Stokesberry, C., & Jelley, M.J. (2002). Preventing costly falls in long-term care. *Nurse Practitioner, 27*(3), 83-85.

Gwyther, L.P. (2001). *Caring for people with Alzheimer's disease: A manual for facility staff* (2nd ed.). Durham, NC: American Health Care Association & Alzheimer's Association.

Haak, N.J. (2002). Maintaining connections: Understanding communication from the perspective of persons with dementia. *Alzheimer's Care Quarterly, 3*(2), 116-131

Hagen, B.F. & Sayers, D. (1995). When caring leaves bruises: The effects of staff education on resident aggression. *Journal of Gerontological Nursing, 21*(11), 7-16.

Hall, G.R. (2003a). *Travel guidelines for people with dementing illness.* University of Iowa Center of Aging. Retrieved July 29, 2004, from http://www.vh.org/adult/patient/neurology/alzheimers/travelinfo.html

Hall, G.R. (2003b). *Understanding and coping with problem behaviors related to memory loss.* University of Iowa College of Nursing, Gerontology Nursing Intervention Center. Retrieved July 29, 2004, from http://www.vh.org/adult/patient/neurology/alzheimers/learningguide.html

Harrington, C., Kovner, C., Mezey, M., Kayser-Jones, J., Burger, S., Mohler, S., et al. (2000). Experts recommend minimum nurse staffing standards for nursing facilities in the United States. *Gerontologist, 40*(1), 5-16.

Harrold, J.K. (1998). Pain, symptoms, and suffering: Possibilities and barriers. *Hospice Journal, 13*(1), 37-40.

Hauer, K., Pfisterer, M, Weber, C., Wezler, N., Kliegel, M., & Oster, P. (2003). Cognitive impairment decreases postural control during dual tasks in geriatric patients with a history of severe falls. *Journal of the American Geriatrics Society, 51*(11), 1638-44.

Head, B. (2003). Palliative care for persons with dementia. *Home Healthcare Nurse, 21*(1), 53-60.

Health Care Financing Administration, (1990). *Survey Procedures and Interpretive Guidelines for Skilled Nursing Facilities and Intermediate Care Facilities.* Baltimore: U.S. Dept. of Health and Human Services.

Helmes, E., Csapo, K.G. & Short, J.A. (1987). Standardization and validation of the Multidimensional Observation Scale for Elderly Subjects (MOSES). *Journal of Gerontology, 42*(4), 395-405.

Hepburn, K.W., Tornatore, J., Center, B., & Ostwald, S.W. (2001). Dementia family caregiver training: Affecting beliefs about caregiving and caregiver outcomes. *Journal of the American Geriatrics Society, 49*(4), 450-57.

Highfield, M.F. (1993). PLAN: A spiritual care model for every nurse. *Quality of Life, 2*(3), 80-84.

Hilton, C., Ghaznavi, F., & Zuberi, T. (2002). Religious beliefs and practices in acute mental health patients. *Nursing Standard, 16*(38), 33-36.

Hines, S. (2001). Alzheimer's Disease: Contemporary drug treatment for AD. *Patient Care, 3*, 54-67. Retrieved August 13, 2004 from http://www.drugtopics.com/be_core/content/journals/p/data/2001/0215/02a01treatad.html

Holtzer, R., Tang, M.X., Devanand, D.P., Albert, S.M., Wegesin, D.J., Marder, K., et al. (2003). Psychopathological features in Alzheimer's disease: Course and relationship with cognitive status. *Journal of the American Geriatrics Society, 51*(7), 953-60.

Hope, T., Keene, J., McShane, R.H., Fairburn, C.G., Gedling, K., & Jacoby, R. (2001). Wandering in dementia: A longitudinal study. *International Psychogeriatrics, 13*(2), 137-47.

Horgas, A.L. (2003). Pain management in elderly adults. *Journal of Infusion Nursing, 26*(3), 161-65.

Humphrey, C.J. (2002). Medicare now covers certain treatments for patients with Alzheimer's disease. *Home Healthcare Nurse, 20*(7), 414.

Hurdle, J. (July 23, 2004). Two Alzheimer's Drugs Show Potential – U.S. Studies. *Yahoo News, Reuters.* (2004) Retrieved October 4, 2004 from http://www.alzheimersupport.com/articles/pastdrugnews.cfm

Hurley, A.C. & Volicer, L. (2002). Alzheimer Disease: "It's okay, Mama, if you want to go, it's okay." *JAMA, 288*(18), 2324-31.

Hurley, A.C., Volicer, B.J., Hanrahan, P.A., Houde, S., & Volicer, L. (1992). Assessment of discomfort in advanced Alzheimer patients. *Research in Nursing & Health, 15*(5), 369-77.

Hussain, R. (1985). Severe behavioral problems. In L. Terri & E. Lewishohon (Eds.), *Geropsychological assessment and treatment* (pp. 121–144). New York: Springer Publishing Co.

Hussain, R.A. & Brown, D.C. (1987). Use of two dimensional grid patterns to limit hazardous ambulation in demented patients. *Journal of Gerontology, 42*, 558-560.

Hutchinson, S., Leger-Krall, S., & Skodol Wilson, H. (1996). Toileting: A behavioral challenge in Alzheimer's dementia care. *Journal of Gerontological Nursing, 22*(10), 18-27.

Janevic, M.R. & Connell, C.M. (2001). Racial, ethnic, and cultural differences in the dementia caregiving experience: Recent findings. *The Gerontologist, 41*(3), 334-47.

Janssen Pharmaceutica Products, L.P. (2003). Titusville, N.J. Retrieved December 12, 2003 from http://www.us.reminyl.com

Jech, A.O. (2002). The healing power of humor. *Nursing Spectrum (South), 3*(5), 38-43.

Jensen, J., Lundin-Olsson, L., Nyberg, L., & Gustafson, Y. (2002). Fall and injury prevention in older people living in residential care facilities: A cluster randomized trial. *Annals of Internal Medicine, 136*(10), 733-41.

Johansson, C. (2003). Geriatric rehabilitation for the Soul Preface. *Topics in Geriatric Rehabilitation, 10*(4), 228-230.

Joint Commission on Accreditation of Healthcare Organizations. (2003). *Pain assessment and management: An organizational approach.* Retrieved December 17, 2003, from http://www.jcaho.org/standards_frm.html

Jones, D. (1995). Seating problems in long-term care. In J. Rader & E. Youngquist (Eds.), *Individualized dementia care: Creative, compassionate approaches* (pp. 169–189). New York: Springer Publishing Co.

Jones, R.W. (2003). Have cholinergic therapies reached their clinical boundary in Alzheimer's disease? *International Journal of Geriatric Psychiatry, 18*(Supp #1), S7-S13.

Jonsson, L. (2003). Pharmacoeconomics of cholinesterase inhibitors in the treatment of Alzheimer's disease. *Pharmacoeconomics, 21*(14), 1025-1037.

Kamel, H.K., Phlavan, M., & Malekgoudarzi, B. (2000). Falls in the nursing home: Frequency and determining factors. *Journal of the American Medical Directors Association, 1,* A5.

Kamel, H.K., Phlavan, M., Malekgoudarzi, B., Gogel, P., & Morley, J.E. (2001). Utilizing pain assessment scales increases the frequency of diagnosing pain among elderly nursing home residents. *Journal of Pain Symptom Management, 21*(6), 450-55.

Kanski, G.W., Janelli, L.M., Jones, H.M., & Kennedy, M.C. (1996). Family reactions to restraints in an acute care setting. *Journal of Gerontological Nursing, 22*(6), 17-22.

Kawas, C.H. (2003). Clinical Practice: Early Alzheimer' disease. *The New England Journal of Medicine, 349*(11), 1056-63.

Kayser-Jones, J. & Pengilly, K. (1999). Dysphagia among nursing home residents. *Geriatric Nursing, 20*(2), 77-84.

Keller, H.H., Gibbs, A.J., Boudreau, L.D., Goy, R.E., Pattillo, M.S., & Brown, H.M. (2003) Prevention of weight loss in dementia with comprehensive nutritional treatment. *Journal of the American Geriatrics Society, 51*(7), 945-52.

Kemper, S., Greiner, L.H., Marquis, J.G., Prenovost, K., & Mitzner, TL. (2001). Language decline across the life span: Findings from the Nun Study. *Psychology & Aging, 16*(2), 227-39.

Kennedy, G.J. (2001). Diagnosis of Alzheimer's disease. *The Clinical Advisor,* November/ December Supplement, 2001, 3-8.

Kepfer, P. & Eisendrath, S.J. (2003). Consultations & comments: Reader reaction and timely answers from experts. Chronic pain and trauma: A psychiatric perspective. *Consultant, 43*(13), 1508.

Kerley, L. & Turnbull, J. (1998). In R.C. Hamdy, J.M. Turnball, J. Edwards, & M.M. Lancaster (Eds.), *Alzheimer's disease: A handbook for caregivers* (3rd ed.). St. Louis: Mosby.

Keyes, K. (1989). *Handbook of higher consciousness: The workbook: A daily practice book to help you increase your heart-to-heart loving and happiness.* Love Line Books.

Kiely, D.K., Simon, S.E., Jones, R.N., & Morris, J.N. (2000). The protective effect of social engagement on mortality in long-term care. *Journal of the American Geriatrics Society, 48*(11), 1367-72.

Killiany, R.J., Gomez-Isla, T., Moss, M., Kikinis, R., Sandor, T., Jolesz, F., et al. (2000). Use of structural magnetic resonance imaging to predict who will get Alzheimer's disease. *Annals of Neurology, 47*(4), 430-39

Kinosian, B.P., Stallard, E., Lee, J.H., Woodbury, M.A., Zbrozek, A.S., & Glick, H.A. (2000). Predicting 10-year care requirements for older people with suspected Alzheimer's disease. *Journal of the American Geriatrics Society, 48*(6), 631-38.

Kolanowski, A.M. (1999). An overview of the Need-Driven Dementia-Compromised Behavior Model. *Journal of Gerontological Nursing, 25*(9), 7-9.

Kolanowski, A.M. & Whall, A.L. (2000). Toward holistic theory-based intervention for dementia behavior. *Holistic Nursing Practice, 14*(2), 67-76.

Koppel, R. (2002). *Alzheimer's disease: The costs to U.S. businesses in 2002.* Washington, DC: Alzheimer's Association.

Kroenke, K. (2002). A 75-year-old man with depression. *Journal of the American Medical Association, 287*(12), 1568-76.

Lai, C.K. & Arthur, D.G. (2003). Wandering behaviour in people with dementia. *Journal of Advanced Nursing, 44*(2), 173-82.

Lancaster, M. (1998). Managing incontinence. In R.C. Hamdy, J.M. Turnball, J. Edwards, & M.M. Lancaster (Eds.), *Alzheimer's disease: A handbook for caregivers* (3rd ed.). St. Louis: Mosby.

Lanctot, K.L., Herrmann, N., Yau, K.K., Khan, L.R., Liu, B.A., LouLou, M.M., et al. (2003). Efficacy and safety of cholinesterase inhibitors in Alzheimer's disease: A meta-analysis. *Canadian Medical Association Journal, 169*(6), 557-64.

Landes, A.M., Sperry, S.D., Strauss, M.E., & Geldmacher, D.S. (2001). Apathy in Alzheimer's disease. *Journal of the American Geriatrics Society, 49*(12), 1700-07.

Lane, P., Kuntupis, M., MacDonald, S., McCarthy, P., Panke, J.A., Warden, V., et al. (2003). A pain assessment tool for people with advanced Alzheimer's and other progressive dementias. *Home Healthcare Nurse, 21*(1), 32-37.

Lantz, M. & Shelkey, M. (2001). Psychotropic medications. In M. Mezey (Ed.), *Encyclopedia of elder care: The comprehensive resource on geriatric and social care.* New York: Springer Publishing Co.

Larrimore, K.L. (2003). Alzmeimer disease support group characteristics: A comparison of caregivers. *Geriatric Nursing, 24*(1), 32-35, 49.

Laurenhue, K. (1996). *Caregiving with humor and creativity.* Seminar presented for the Alzheimer's Association, Fort Myers, FL.

Lehne, R.A. (2004). *Pharmacology for Nursing Care* (5th ed.). St. Louis: Mosby.

Lemere, C.A., Spooner, E.T., Leverone, J.F., Mori, C., Iglesias, M., Bloom, J.K., et al. (2003). Amyloid-beta immunization in Alzheimer's disease transgenic mouse models and wildtype mice. *Neurochemical Research, 28*(7), 1010-27.

Lindgren, C. (1993). The caregiver career. IMAGE: *The Journal of Nursing Scholarship, 25*(3), 214–219.

Lindgren, C., Connelly, C. & Gaspar, H. (1999). Grief in spouse & children caregivers of dementia patients. *Western Journal of Nursing Research, 21*(4), 521–537.

Loefler, I. (2003). Health, science, and religion in contemporary American culture. *Mayo Clinic Proceedings, 78*(7), 893-95.

Lonergan, E.T. (Ed.). (1991). Institute of Medicine (U.S.), Committee on a national research agenda on aging. *Extending life, enhancing life: A national research agenda on aging.* Washington, D.C.: National Academy Press.

Long, C.O. & Dougherty, J. (2003). What's new in Alzheimer's disease? *Home Healthcare Nurse, 21*(1), 8-14.

Luggen, A.S., Miller, J.M., & Jett, K. (2003) General nurse practitioner care guidelines: Dementia with Lewy bodies. *Geriatric Nursing, 24*(1), 56-57.

Lutz, C.A. & Przytulski, K.R. (2001). *Nutrition and Diet Therapy* (3rd ed.). Philadelphia: F.A. Davis.

Maas, M.L., Specht, J.P., Weiler, K., Buckwalter, K.C., & Turner, B. (1998). Special care units for people with Alzheimer's disease. Only for the privileged few? *Journal of Gerontological Nursing, 24*(3), 28-37.

Maas, M.L., Swanson, E., Specht, J., & Buckwalter, K.C. (1994). Alzheimer's special care units. *Nursing Clinics of North America, 29*(1), 39-46.

Mace, N.L. & Rabins, P.V. (2001). *The 36-hour day* (Revised ed.). New York: Warner Books.

Mahi, J. (1999) Herbspotlight. Huperzine A for improved memory, focus and attention span. *totalhealth magazine, 21*(1), 19.

Mahoney, D.F., Jones, R.N., Coon, D.W., Mendelsohn, A.B., Gitlin, L.N., & Ory, M. (2003). The Caregiver Vigilance Scale: Application and validation in the Resources for Enhancing Alzheimer's Caregiver health (REACH). *American Journal of Alzheimer's Disease and Other Dementias, 18*(1), 39-48.

Mahoney, D.F, Tarlow, B., & Sandaire, J. (1998). A computer-mediated intervention for Alzheimer's caregivers. *Computers in Nursing, 16*(4), 208-16.

Mariano, C., Gould, E., Mezey, M., & Fulmer, T. (Eds.) (1999). *Best nursing practices in care for older adults.* New York: The John A. Hartford Foundation Inc.

Marx, V. (August 5, 2004). Merck Signs Deals In Oncology And Alzheimer's Drug major will work with Pierre Fabre and Celera Diagnostics. *Chemical and Engineering News.* Retrieved October 4, 2004 from http://www.alzheimer support.com/articles/pastdrugnews.cfm

Matthiesen, V., Lamb, K.V., McCann, J., Hollinger-Smith, L., & Walton, J.C. (1996). Hospital nurses' views about physical restraints use with older patients. *Journal of Gerontological Nursing, 22*(6), 8-16.

Maugans, T.A. (1996). The SPIRITual history. *Archives of Family Medicine, 5*(1), 11-16.

McCurry, S.M., Gibbons, L.E, Logsdon, R.G., Vitiello, M., & Teri, L. (2003). Training caregivers to change the sleep hygiene practices of patients with dementia: The NITE- AD project. *Journal of the American Geriatrics Society, 51*(10), 1455-60.

Merriam-Webster, Inc. (1989). *The new Merriam Webster dictionary.* Springfield, MA: Author.

Merz, Lundbeck, Neurobiological Technologies Inc (NTI). (2004). *New Study Results Demonstrate Beneficial Effects of Axura (Memantine) on Brain Activity in Patients With Mild to Moderate Alzheimer's Disease.* Retrieved August 12, 2004 from http://www.memantine. com/en/news/releases/2004/

Meuser, T.M. & Marwit, S.J. (2001). A comprehensive, stage-sensitive model of grief in dementia caregiving. *Gerontologist, 41*(5), 658-70.

Micelli, B. (1999). Nursing unit meal management maintenance program. *Journal of Gerontological Nursing, 25*(8), 22-36.

Migliaccio-Walle, K., Getsios, D., Caro, J.J., Ishak, K.J., O'Brien, J.A., & Papadopoulos, G. AHEAD Study Group. (2003). Economic evaluation of galantamine in the treatment of mild to moderate Alzheimer's disease in the United States. *Clinical Therapeutics, 25*(6), 1806-25.

Miller, C.A. (2001). Newest developments in dementia treatment and prevention. *Geriatric Nursing, 22*(4), 216, 218.

Mobius, H.J. (2003). Memantine: update on the current evidence. *International Journal of Geriatric Psychiatry, 18*(Supp #1), S47-S54.

Moffat, N. (1994). Strategies of memory therapy. In B. Wilson & N. Moffat (Eds.), *Clinical management of memory problems* (2nd ed.). San Diego: Singular.

Mohs, R.C., Doody, R.S., Morris, J.C., Ieni, J.R., Rogers, S.L., Perdomo, C.A., et al. (2001). A 1-year, placebo-controlled preservation of function survival study of donepezil in AD patients [corrected]. *Neurology, 57*(3), 481-88.

Mooney, N.E. (2000). The therapeutic use of humor. *Orthopaedic Nursing, 19*(3), 88-92.

Moore, L.A. & Davis, B. (2002). Quilting narrative: Using repetition techniques to help elderly communicators. *Geriatric Nursing, 23*(5), 262-66.

Morley, J. & Omran, M. (2001). In M. Mezey (Ed.), *Encyclopedia of elder care: The comprehensive resource on geriatric and social care.* New York: Springer Publishing Co.

Mosqueda, L., Heath, J., & Burnight, K. (2001). Recognizing physical abuse and neglect in the skilled nursing facility: The physician's responsibilities. *Journal of the American Medical Directors Association, 2*(4),183-86.

Moss, M., Braunschweig, H., & Rubinstein, R. (2002). Terminal care for nursing home residents with dementia. *Alzheimer's Care Quarterly, 3*(3), 233.

Moss, S.E., Polignano, E., White, C.L., Minichiello, M.D., & Sunderland, T. (2002). Reminiscence group activities and discourse interaction in Alzheimer's disease. *Journal of Gerontological Nursing, 28*(8), 36-44.

Mueller, P.S., Plevak, D.J., & Rummans, T.A. (2001). Religious involvement, spirituality, and medicine: Implications for clinical practice. *Mayo Clinic Proceedings, 76*(12), 1225-35.

Murman, D.L, Chen, Q., Powell, M.C., Kuo, S.B., Bradley, C.J. & Colenda, C.C. (2002). The incremental direct costs associated with behavioral symptoms in AD. *Neurology, 59*(11), 1721-29.

National Center for Injury Prevention and Control. (2002). *Preventing falls among seniors.* Retrieved July 2, 2004, from http://www.cdc.gov/ncipc/duip/spotlite/falls.htm

Neal, M. & Briggs, M. (2003). Validation therapy for dementia. *Cochrane Database of Systematic Reviews*, (3), CD001394.

Neumann, P.J., Hermann, R.C., Kuntz, K.M., Araki, S.S., Duff, S.B., Leon, J., et al. (1999). Cost-effectiveness of donepezil in the treatment of mild or moderate Alzheimer's disease. *Neurology, 52*(6), 1138-45. Retrieved August 30, 2004 from http://www.neurology.org/cgi/content/abstract/52/6/1138

Neville, P., Boyle, A., & Baillon S. (1999). A descriptive survey of acute bed usage for dementia care in old age psychiatry. *International Journal of Geriatric Psychiatry, 14*(5), 348-354.

Newsview. (2001). *Geriatric Nursing, 22*(6), 286-87. Author.

Novartis Pharmaceuticals of Canada. (2003). *Prescribing Information Rivastigmine/Exelon.* Retrieved December 12, 2003 from http://www.pharma.ca.novartis.com/downloads/e/exelon_scrip_e.pdf

Optima. (2000). *Non-pharmacological interventions for the Alzheimer's resident.* Adapted from a 1999 Optima Awards entry. Medquest Communications.

Orhon A. (2002). The healing power of humor. *Utah Nurse, 11*(3). 20-21.

Osato, E.E., Stone, J., Phillips, S.L., & Winne, D.M. (1993). Clinical manifestations: Failure to thrive in the elderly. *Journal of Gerontological Nursing, 19*(8), 28-34.

Panda, M. & Desbiens, N.A. (2001). Pain in elderly patients: How to achieve control. *Consultant, 10*(1), 1597-1604.

Parmelee, P.A. (1996). Pain in cognitively impaired older persons. *Clinics in Geriatric Medicine, 12*(3), 473-87

Pepping, J. (2000). Alternative therapies. Huperzine A...a potent and selective acetylcholinesterase inhibitor. *American Journal of Health-System Pharmacy, AJHP, 57*(6), 530, 533-4.

Phillips, V.L. & Diwan, S. (2003). The incremental effect of dementia-related problem behaviors on the time to nursing home placement in poor, frail, demented older people. *Journal of the American Geriatrics Society, 51*(2), 188-93.

Pietrukowicz, M.E. & Johnson, M.M. (1991). Using life histories to individualize nursing home staff attitudes towards residents. *The Gerontologist, 31*(1), 102–06.

Pittiglio, L. (2000). Use of reminiscence therapy in patients with Alzheimer's Disease. *Lippincott's Case Management, 5*(6), 216-220.

Poole, J. & Mott, S. (2003). Agitated older patients: Nurses' perceptions and reality. *International Journal of Nursing Practice, 9*(5), 306-12.

Pollmann, J.W. (1999). *The use of humor by caregivers of spouses with Alzheimer's disease.* [Doctoral Dissertation. Research.] University of Cincinnati (p.125).

Pouncey, M. (n.d.) Understanding Medicare, Medigap and Medicaid. *AARP The Magazine.* Retrieved September 20, 2004 from http://www.aarpmagazine.org/family/Articles/a2003-01-21-understanding med.html

ProHealth (n.d.). Recently Published Alzheimer's Drug News. Retrieved September 23, 2004 from http://www.alzheimersupport.com/articles/pastdrugnews.cfm

Rader, J. (1995). Use of skillful, creative psychosocial interventions. In J. Rader & E.M. Youngquist (Eds.), *Individualized dementia care: Creative, compassionate approaches.* New York: Springer Publishing Co.

Rader, J., Jones, D., & Miller, L. (2000). The importance of individualized wheelchair seating for frail older adults. *Journal of Gerontological Nursing, 26*(11), 24-32.

Reisberg, B., Ferris, S.H., deLeon, M.J., & Crook, T. (1982). The Global Deterioration Scale for assessment of primary degenerative dementia. *American Journal of Psychiatry, 139*(9), 1136-39.

Remington, R. (2002). Calming music and hand massage with agitated elderly. *Nursing Research, 51*(5), 317-23.

Resnick, B. (2001). Promoting health in older adults: A four-year analysis. *Journal of American Academy of Nurse Practitioners, 13*(1), 23-33.

Resnick, S.M. & Henderson, V.W. (2002). Hormone therapy and risk of Alzheimer disease: A critical time. *Journal of the American Medical Association, 288*(17), 2170-72.

Richards, M. (1990). Meeting the spiritual needs of the cognitively impaired. *Generations, 14*, 63-64.

Roach, M. (1996). The laughing clubs of India. *Health,* September, 93-97.

Robinson, K.M., Adkisson, P., & Weinrich, S. (2001). Problem behaviours, caregiver reactions, and impact among caregivers of persons with Alzheimer's disease. *Journal of Advanced Nursing, 36*(4), 573-82.

Rogawski, M.A., & Wenk, G.L. (2003). The neuropharmacological basis for the use of memantine in the treatment of Alzheimer's disease. *CNS Drug Reviews, 9*(3), 275-308.

Rogers, W.A. & Fisk, A.D. (2000). Human factors, applied cognition, and aging. In F.I.M. Craik & T.A. Salthouse (Eds.), *The Handbook of Aging and Cognition* (2nd ed.). (pp. 559-591). Mahwah, NJ: Lawrence Erlbaum Associates, Publishers.

Rogers, S.L., Doody, R.S., Mohs, R.C., & Friedhoff, L.T. Donepezil Study Group. (1998). Donepezil improves cognition and global function in Alzheimer disease: A 15-week, double-blind, placebo-controlled study. *Archives of Internal Medicine, 158*(9), 1021-31.

Rogers, S.L. & Friedhoff, T. Donepezil Study Group. (1996). The efficacy and safety of donepezil in patients with Alzheimer's disease: Results of a US multicentre, randomized, double-blind, placebo-controlled trial. *Dementia, 7*(6), 293-303.

Ronch, J. (1987). Specialized Alzheimer's units in nursing homes: Pros and cons. American *Journal of Alzheimer Care and Research, 2,* 10-19.

Rowe, M. & Alfred, D. (1999). The effectiveness of slow-stroke massage in diffusing agitated behaviors in individuals with Alzheimer's disease. *Journal of Gerontological Nursing, 25*(6), 22-34.

Rowe, M.A. (2003). People with dementia who become lost: Preventing injuries and death. *American Journal of Nursing, 103*(7), 32-39.

Royall, D. (2003). The "Alzheimerization" of dementia research. *Journal of the American Geriatrics Society, 51*(2), 277-78.

Rubenstein, L.Z., Powers, C.M., & MacLean, C.H. (2001). Quality indicators for the management and prevention of falls and mobility problems in vulnerable elders. *Annals of Internal Medicine, 135*(8 Pt 2), 686-93.

Rubin, A. & Rubin, H. (n.d.). A website for senior citizens and those who care about them. Retrieved February 10, 2003 from www.therubins.com

Sandbandham, M. & Sphirm, M. (1995). Music as a nursing intervention for residents with Alzheimer's disease in long term care. Geriatric nursing: *American Journal of Care for the Aging. 16*(2): 79.

Santo Pietro, M.J., (2002). Training nursing assistants to communicate effectively with persons with Alzheimer's disease: A call for action. *Alzheimer's Care Quarterly, 3*(2), 157-64.

Sarkisian, C.A. & Lachs, M.S. (1996). "Failure to thrive" in older adults. *Annals of Internal Medicine, 124*(12), 1072-78.

Savell, K. & Krinsky, A. (1998). *Cognitive behavioral alternatives to pharmacological intervention and physical restraint within long term care.* ATRA Annual Conference, Boston, MA.

Schulz, R., Mendelsohn, A.B., Haley, W.E., Mahoney, D., Allen R.S., Zhang, S., et al. (2003). End-of-life care and the effects of bereavement on family caregivers of persons with dementia. *New England Journal of Medicine, 349*(20), 1936-42.

Schultz, S.K., Ellingrod, V.L., Turvey, C., Moser, D.J., & Arndt, S. (2003). The influence of cognitive impairment and behavioral dysregulation on daily functioning in the nursing home setting. *American Journal of Psychiatry, 160*(3), 582-84.

Scott, L.J. & Goa, K.L. (2000). Galatamine: A review of its use in Alzheimer's disease. *Drugs, 60*(5), 1095-122.

Seiler, W.O. & Stahelin, H.B. (1999). *Malnutrition in the elderly.* New York: Springer/Berlin.

Seiler, W.O. (2001). Clinical pictures of malnutrition in ill elderly subjects. *Nutrition, 17*(6), 496-98.

Serby, M. & Yu, M. (2003). There's good news about depression in the elderly. *The Clinical Advisor, September,* 64-75.

Shaw, C. & Taylor, S. (1992). A survey of wheelchair seating problems of the institutionalized elderly. *Assistive Technology, 3*(1), 5–10.

Shega, J.W., Levin, A., Hougham, G.W., Cox-Hayley, D., Luchins, D., Hanrahan, P., et al. (2003). Palliative Excellence in Alzheimer Care Efforts (PEACE): A program description. *Journal of Palliative Medicine, 6*(2), 315-20.

Sheikh, J.I. & Yesavage, J.A. (1985). A knowledge assessment test for geriatric psychiatry. *Hospital & Community Psychiatry, 36*(11), 1160-66.

Sherder, E.J. (2000). Low use of analgesics in Alzheimer's disease: Possible mechanisms. *Psychiatry, 63,* 1-12.

Sheridan, P.L., Solomont, J., Kowall, N., & Hausdorff, J.M. (2003). Influence of executive function on locomotor function: Divided attention increases gait variability in Alzheimer's disease. *Journal of the American Geriatrics Society, 51*(11), 1633-37.

Shumaker, S.A., Legault, C., Rapp, S.R., Thal, L., Wallace, R.G., Ockene, J.K., et al. (2003). Estrogen plus progestin and the incidence of dementia and mild cognitive impairment in postmenopausal women: The Women's Health Initiative Memory Study: A randomized controlled trial. *Journal of the American Medical Association, 289*(20), 2651-62.

Sloane, P. & Hargett, F. (1997). Institutionalized care. In R. Ham & P. Sloane (Eds.), *Primary care geriatrics: A case-based approach.* St. Louis: Mosby.

Sloane, P.D., Mitchell, C.M., Preisser, J.S., Phillips, C., Commander, C., & Burker, E. (1998) Environmental correlates of resident agitation in Alzheimer's disease special care units. *Journal of the American Geriatrics Society, 46*(7), 862-9.

Small, J.A., Gutman, G., Makela, S., & Hillhouse, B. (April, 2003). Effectiveness of communication strategies used by caregivers of persons with Alzheimer's disease during activities of daily living. *Journal of Speech, Language, and Hearing Research, 46,* 353-367.

Smith, G.B. (2002). Case management guideline: Alzheimer disease and other dementias. *Lippincott's Case Management: Managing the Process of Patient Care, 7*(2), 77-84.

Smith, J.D. & Levin-Allerhand, J.A. (2003). Potential use of estrogen-like drugs for the prevention of Alzheimer's disease. *Journal of Molecular Neuroscience, 20*(3), 277-81.

Smith, M.A., Perry, G., Atwood, C.S., & Bowen, R.L. (2003). Estrogen replacement and risk of Alzmeimer disease. *Journal of the American Medical Association, 289*(9), 1100.

Snow, A.L., Hovanec, L., Passano, J., & Brandt, J. (2001). In A.L. Horgas (2003). *Development of a pain assessment instrument for use with severely demented patients.* Poster presented at: Annual Meeting of the American Psychological Association; August 2001; Washington, D.C.

Snyder, M., Yuen-hsia, T., Brandt, C., Crochan, C., Hanson, S., Constantine, R., et al. (2001). A glider-swing intervention for people with dementia. *Geriatric Nursing, 22*(2), 86–90.

Southam, M. (2003). Therapeutic humor: Attitudes and actions by occupational therapists in adult physical disabilities settings. *Occupational Therapy in Health Care, 17*(1), 23-41.

Spector, A. & Orrell, M. (2001). Reality orientation. In M. Mezey (Ed.), *Encyclopedia of elder care: The comprehensive resource on geriatric & social care.* New York: Springer Publishing Co.

Stewart, J.T. (1995). Management of problems in the demented patient. *American Academy of Family Physicians, 52*(8), 2311-17, 2321-22.

Stewart, J. (2000). *Management of the dementia patient.* Paper presented at Geriatric Health Care Conference in Orlando, FL, September 2000.

Strumpf, N., Evans, L., & Bourbonniere, M. (2001). Restraints. In M. Mezey (Ed.), *Encyclopedia of elder care: The comprehensive resource on geriatric and social care.* New York: Springer Publishing Co.

Stuckey, J.C., Post, S.G., Ollerton, S., FallCreek, S.J., & Whitehouse, P.J. (2002). Alzheimer's disease, religion, and the ethics of respect for spirituality: A community dialogue. *Alzheimer's Care Quarterly, 3*(3), 199-207.

Sullivan, M., Smidt-Jernstrom, K. & Rader, J. (1995). Assessing the resident's needs. In J. Rader & E.M. Youngquist (Eds.), *Individualized dementia care: Creative, compassionate approaches.* New York: Springer Publishing Co.

Szwabo, P. & Tideiksaar, R. (1991) Alzheimer's disease and senile dementia. *Physician Assistant, 15*(9), 19-22, 25-6, 29.

Talerico, K.A., Evans, L.K., & Strumpf, N.E. (2002). Mental health correlates of aggression in nursing home residents with dementia. *Gerontologist, 42*(2), 169-77.

Tappen, R., Williams, C., Barry, C., & DiSesa, D. (2001). Conversation intervention with Alzheimer's patients: Increasing the relevance of communication. *Clinical Gerontologist, 24*(3/4), 63-75.

Tariot, P.N., Cummings, J.L., Katz, I.R., Mintzer, J., Perdomo, C.A., Schwam, E.M., et al. (2001). A randomized, double-blind, placebo-controlled study of the efficacy and safety of donepezil in patients with Alzheimer's disease in the nursing home setting. *Journal of the American Geriatrics Society, 49*(12), 1590-99.

Teno, J.M., Weitzen, S., Wetle, T., & Mor, V. (2001) Persistent pain in nursing home residents. *Journal of the American Medical Association, 285*(16), 2081.

Teresi, J., Abrams, R., Holmes, D., Ramirez, M., & Eimicke, J. (2001). Prevalence of depression and depression recognition in nursing homes. *Social Psychiatry and Psychiatric Epidemiology, 36*(12), 613-20.

Thomas, D.W. (1995). Wandering: A proposed definition. *Journal of Gerontological Nursing, 21*(9), 35-41.

Thome, B., Dykes, A.K., & Hallberg, I.R. (2003). Home care with regard to definition, care recipients, content, and outcome: Systematic literature review. *Journal of Clinical Nursing, 12*(6), 860-72.

Thorogood, M., Hillsdon, M., & Summerbell, C. (2003). Physical activity and falls in elderly people, physical activity. *Clinical Evidence Concise, 10:* 17. London, UK: BMJ Publishing Group, Ltd.

Thompson, T.G. (2004). Administration on Aging. Retrieved July 30, 2004, from http://www.aoa .dhhs.gov/eldfam/nutrition/nutrition.asp

Thyer, B. (1986). Clinical Anxiety Scale. University of Georgia School of Social Work. In K. Corcoran & J. Fischer (Eds.), *Measures for clinical practice: A source book* (4th ed.) (p. 187). New York: Free Press.

Tideiksaar, R. (2003). Best practice approach to fall prevention in community-living elders. *Topics in Geriatric Rehabilitation, 19*(3), 199-205.

Todd, B. (1986). Drugs and the elderly: When the benefits outweigh the risks. *Geriatric Nursing, 7*(4), 212, 222.

Touhy, T.A. (2001). Nurturing hope and spirituality in the nursing home. *Holistic Nursing Practice, 15*(4), 45-56.

Turnbull, J.M. & Turnbull, E.A. (1998). Developing a day's activity. In R. Hamdy, J. Turnbull, J. Edwards, & M. Lancaster (Eds.), *Alzheimer's disease: A handbook for caregivers* (3rd ed.). St. Louis: Mosby.

U.S. Department of Health and Human Services. (1997). *Surveyor's guidebook on dementia* (Publication No. 386-897/33457). Washington, DC: U.S. Government Printing Office.

U.S. Department of Health and Human Services. (March, 1999). Office of the Inspector General. *Quality of care in nursing homes: An overview.* OEI-02-99-00060. Retrieved March 6, 2004, from www.oig.hhs.gov/oei/reports/oei-02-99-00060.pdf

U.S. Department of Health and Human Services. Centers for Medicare and Medicaid Services. (2000). *Medicare state operations manual provider certification.* Retrieved October 21, 2004, from http://www.cms.hhs.gov/manuals/pm_trans/R20SOM.pdf

U.S. Department of Health and Human Services. (January, 2001). Office of the Inspector General. *Nursing Home Resident Assessment Quality of Care.* OEI-02-99-00040. New York. Available online from http://oig.hhs.gov/oei/reports/oei-02-99-00040.pdf

U.S. Department of Health and Human Services. (October, 2002). *Provider Education Article: Psychotropic Drug Use in Skilled Nursing Facilities.* Program Memorandum, CMS Publication 60AB.

U.S. Food and Drug Administration (FDA, www.fda.gov) & National Consumers League (NCL, www.nclnet.org). (1998). Food and Drug Interactions. Retrieved September 21, 2004, from http://vm.cfsan.fda.gov/~lrd/fdinter.html

Verdery, R.B. (1995). Failure to thrive in elderly. *Clinics of Geriatric Medicine, 11*(4), 653-59.

Verghese, J., Lipton, R.B., Hall, C.B., Kuslansky, G., Katz, M.J., & Buschke, H. (2002). Abnormality of gait as a predictor of non-Alzheimer's dementia. *New England Journal of Medicine, 347*(22), 1761-68.

Volicer, L. (2001). Management of severe Alzheimer's disease and end-of-life issues. *Clinics in Geriatric Medicine, 17*(2), 377-91.

Volicer, L. (2002). Commentary on "Terminal care for nursing home residents with dementia". *Alzheimer's Care Quarterly, 3*(3), 247.

Volicer, L. & Ganzini, L. (2003). Health professionals' views on standards for decision-making capacity regarding refusal of medical treatment in mild Alzheimer's disease. *Journal of the American Geriatrics Society, 51*(9), 1270-74.

Volicer, L. & Hurley, A.C. (2003). Management of behavioral symptoms in progressive degenerative dementias. *Journals of Gerontology Series A – Biological Sciences and Medical Sciences, 58*(9), M837-45.

Vollen, K.H. (1996). Coping with difficult resident behaviors takes time. *Journal of Gerontological Nursing, 22*(8), 22-26.

Wachter, A. (1996). Rethinking psychotropics. *Contemporary Long Term Care, 19*(11) 70H.

Wallace, F. & Buckwalter, K. (2003). *Guidelines for Alzheimer's disease management.* Iowa Geriatric Education Center — Department of Neurology. Retrieved August 20, 2003 from http://www.vh.org/adult/provider/neurology/alzheimers/

Waring, S.C., Rocca, W.A., Petersen, R.C., O'Brien, P.C., Tangalos, E.G., & Kokmen, E. (1999). Postmenopausal estrogen replacement therapy and risk of AD: A population-based study. *Neurology, 52*(5), 965-70.

Watson, N., Hauptmann, M., Brink, C., Powers, B., Taillie, E. & Lash, M. (1997, November). *Small group humor therapy to reduce agitation among nursing home residents with dementia.* Paper presented at the Gerontological Society of America 50th Anniversary Scientific Meeting. Cincinnati, Ohio.

Weiner, C., Tabak, N., & Bergman, R. (2003). The use of physical restraints for patients suffering from dementia. *Nursing Ethics, 10*(5), 512-25.

Wengenack, T.M., Whelan, S., Curran, G.L., Duff, K.E., & Poduslo, J.F. (2000). Quantitative histological analysis of amyloid deposition in Alzheimer's double transgenic mouse brain. *Neuroscience, 101*(4), 939-44.

Wesnes, K.A., McKeith, I.G., Ferrara, R., Emre, M., Del Ser, T., Spano, P.F., et al. (2002). Effects of rivastigmine on cognitive function in dementia with lewy bodies: A randomised placebo-controlled international study using the cognitive drug research computerised assessment system. *Dementia and Geriatric Cognitive Disorders, 13*(3), 183-92.

White, M.H. & Dorman, S.M. (2003). Online support for caregivers: Analysis of an Internet Alzheimer mailgroup. *Computers in Nursing, 18*(4), 168-179.

World Health Organization. (n.d.). *WHO definition of palliative care.* Retrieved September 29, 2004, from http://www.who.int/cancer/palliative/definition/en/

Williams, H. (1986). Humor and healing: Therapeutic effects in geriatrics. *Gerontion 1986, 1*(3), 14-17.

Wilson, R.S., Gilley, D.W., Bennett, D.A., Beckett, L.A., & Evans, D.A. (2000). Hallucinations, delusions, and cognitive decline in Alzheimer's disease. *Journal of Neurology, Neurosurgery, and Psychiatry, 69*(2), 172-77.

Wilson, R.S., Barnes, L.L., Mendes de Leon, C.F., Aggarwal, N.T., Schneider, J.S., Bach, J., et al. (2002). Depressive symptoms, cognitive decline, and risk of AD in older persons. *Neurology, 59*(3), 364-70.

Winblad, B. & Jelic, V. (2003). Treating the full spectrum of dementia with memantine. *International Journal of Geriatric Psychiatry, 18*(Supp 1), S1-46.

Wisniewski, S.R., Belle, S.H, Coon, D.W., Marcus, S.M., Ory, M.G., Burgio, L.D., et al. REACH Investigators. (2003). The Resources for Enhancing Alzheimer's Caregiver Health (REACH): Project design and baseline characteristics. *Psychology and Aging, 18*(3), 375-84.

Wooten, P. (1996). Humor: An antidote for stress. *Holistic Nursing Practice, 10*(2), 49-56.

Womack, P. & Breeding, C. (1998). Position of the American Dietetic Association: Liberalized diets for older adults in long-term care. *Journal of the American Dietetic Association, 98*(2), 201-04.

Wynne, C.F., Ling, S.M., & Remsburg, R. (2000). Comparison of pain assessment instruments in cognitively intact and cognitively impaired nursing home residents. *Geriatric Nursing, 21*(1), 20-23.

Yaffe, K., Fox, P., Newcomer, R., Sands, L., Lindquist, K., Dane, K., et al. (2002). Patient and caregiver characteristics and nursing home placement in patients with dementia. *Journal of the American Medical Association, 287*(16), 2090-97.

Yardley, L. & Smith, H. (2002). A prospective study of the relationship between feared consequences of falling and avoidance of activity in community-living older people. *Gerontologist, 42*(1), 17-23.

Young, M.G. (2001). Providing care for the caregiver. *Patient Care for the Nurse Practitioner, 4*(2), 36-48.

Zandi, P.P., Anthony, J.C., Khachaturian, A.S., Stone, S.V., Gustafson, D., Tschanz, J.T., et al. Cache County Study Group. (2004). Reduced risk of Alzheimer disease in users of antioxidant vitamin supplements: the Cache County Study. *Archives of Neurology, 61*(1), 82-88.

Zeisel, J. & Raia, P. (2000). Nonpharmacological treatment for Alzheimer's disease: A mind-brain appraoch. *American Journal of Alzheimer's Disease and Other Dementias, 15*(6), 331-40.

Zeisel, J., Silverstein, N.M., Hyde, J., Levkoff, S., Lawton, M.P., & Holmes, W. (2003). Environmental correlates to behavioral health outcomes in Alzheimer's special care units. *Gerontologist, 43*(5), 697-711.

Zingmark, K., Sandman, P.O., & Norberg, A. (2002). Promoting a good life among people with Alzheimer's disease. *Journal of Advanced Nursing, 38*(1), 50-58.

INDEX

vascular dementia, 21
Vioxx, 158
visual religious triggers, 101*t*
Vitamin C, 158
Vitamin E, 158

W
wandering behavior
  described, 141
  doll therapy for, 144, 146
  managing, 143-144, 145*t,* 146
  research on, 141-143
  triggers of, 143
  types of, 143
Web sites
  Alzheimer's Association, 163
  on drug development, 163
wheelchair assessment, 81, 82*t*
WHI (Women's Health Initiative), 160
WHO (World Health Organization), 110, 186
Wooten, Patty, 43

Z
zolpidem (Ambien), 135

PRETEST KEY

Alzheimer's Disease:
A Complete Guide for Nurses

1.	d	Chapter 1
2.	b	Chapter 1
3.	a	Chapter 2
4.	c	Chapter 2
5.	d	Chapter 3
6.	d	Chapter 4
7.	c	Chapter 4
8.	b	Chapter 4
9.	d	Chapter 4
10.	a	Chapter 5
11.	c	Chapter 5
12.	c	Chapter 6
13.	d	Chapter 7
14.	b	Chapter 8
15.	d	Chapter 8
16.	a	Chapter 8
17.	a	Chapter 8
18.	c	Chapter 8
19.	a	Chapter 9
20.	c	Chapter 10

Notes

Notes

Notes